Psoriasis: Advances in Knowledge and Care

Editors

M. ALAN MENTER
CHRISTOPHER E. M. GRIFFITHS

DERMATOLOGIC CLINICS

www.derm.theclinics.com

Consulting Editor
BRUCE H. THIERS

January 2015 • Volume 33 • Number 1

ELSEVIER

1600 John F. Kennedy Boulevard • Suite 1800 • Philadelphia, Pennsylvania, 19103-2899

http://www.theclinics.com

DERMATOLOGIC CLINICS Volume 33, Number 1
January 2015 ISSN 0733-8635, ISBN-13: 978-0-323-34174-5

Editor: Joanne Husovski
Developmental Editor: Susan Showalter

Dermatologic Clinics (ISSN 0733-8635) is published quarterly by Elsevier Inc., 360 Park Avenue South, New York, NY 10010-1710. Months of publication are January, April, July, and October. Business and editorial offices: 1600 John F. Kennedy Blvd., Suite 1800, Philadelphia, PA 19103-2899. Customer service office: 11830 Westline Drive, St. Louis, MO 63146. Periodicals postage paid at New York, NY, and additional mailing offices. Subscription prices are USD 365.00 per year for US individuals, USD 559.00 per year for US institutions, USD 425.00 per year for Canadian individuals, USD 681.00 per year for Canadian institutions, USD 495.00 per year for international individuals, USD 681.00 per year for international institutions, USD 165.00 per year for US students/residents, and USD 240.00 per year for Canadian and international students/residents. International air speed delivery is included in all *Clinics* subscription prices. All prices are subject to change without notice. **POSTMASTER:** Send address changes to *Dermatologic Clinics*, Elsevier Health Sciences Division, Subscription Customer Service, 3251 Riverport Lane, Maryland Heights, MO 63043. **Customer Service: 1-800-654-2452 (U.S. and Canada); 314-447-8871 (outside U.S. and Canada). Fax: 314-447-8029. E-mail: journalscustomerservice-usa@elsevier.com (for print support); journalsonlinesupport-usa@elsevier.com (for online support).**

Reprints. For copies of 100 or more, of articles in this publication, please contact the Commercial Reprints Department, Elsevier Inc., 360 Park Avenue South, New York, New York 10010-1710. Tel.: 212-633-3874; Fax: 212-633-3820; Email: repritns@elsevier.com.

The *Dermatologic Clinics* is covered in *MEDLINE/PubMed (Index Medicus), Current Contents/Clinical Medicine, Excerpta Medica, Chemical Abstracts,* and *ISI/BIOMED.*

Contributors

CONSULTING EDITOR

BRUCE H. THIERS, MD
Professor and Chairman, Department of
Dermatology and Dermatologic Surgery,
Medical University of South Carolina,
Charleston, South Carolina

EDITORS

M. ALAN MENTER, MD
Division of Dermatology, Baylor University
Medical Center at Dallas, Dallas, Texas

**CHRISTOPHER E. M. GRIFFITHS, MD,
FMedSci**
Dermatology Centre, Salford Royal Hospital,
The University of Manchester, Manchester
Academic Health Science Centre, Manchester,
United Kingdom

AUTHORS

**JONATHAN N. BARKER, MD, FRCP,
FRCPath**
Division of Genetics and Molecular Medicine,
St John's Institute of Dermatology, Guy's and
St Thomas' NHS Foundation Trust, King's
College London, London, United Kingdom

FRANCESCA CAPON, PhD
Division of Genetics and Molecular Medicine,
King's College London, London, United
Kingdom

ROBERT J.G. CHALMERS, MB, FRCP
Honorary Consultant Dermatologist,
Department of Dermatology, Manchester
Royal Infirmary, Dermatology Centre, Salford
Royal NHS Foundation Trust, University of
Manchester, Manchester, United Kingdom

PETER FOLEY, MD
St Vincent's Hospital Melbourne, The
University of Melbourne, Victoria, Australia

AMY C. FOULKES, MD
The Dermatology Centre, Manchester
Academic Health Science Centre, Salford
Royal NHS Foundation Trust, The University of
Manchester, Salford, Manchester, United
Kingdom

MARISA KARDOS GARSHICK, MD
Department of Dermatology, Massachusetts
General Hospital, Boston, Massachusetts

ALICE B. GOTTLIEB, MD, PhD
Department of Dermatology, Tufts Medical
Center, Boston, Massachusetts

**CHRISTOPHER E. M. GRIFFITHS, MD,
FMedSci**
Dermatology Centre, Salford Royal Hospital,
The University of Manchester, Manchester
Academic Health Science Centre, Manchester,
United Kingdom

JOHN B. KELLY III, MD, PhD
Department of Dermatology, University of
Connecticut Health Center, Farmington,
Connecticut

JAEHWAN KIM, MD, PhD
Laboratory for Investigative Dermatology,
The Rockefeller University, New York,
New York

ALEXA BOER KIMBALL, MD, MPH
Department of Dermatology, Massachusetts
General Hospital, Boston, Massachusetts

BRIAN KIRBY, MD
Consultant Dermatologist, St Vincent's
University Hospital; Associate Clinical
Professor, University College Dublin, Dublin,
Ireland

JAMES G. KRUEGER, MD, PhD
Laboratory for Investigative Dermatology,
The Rockefeller University, New York,
New York

CRAIG L. LEONARDI, MD
Clinical Professor of Dermatology, Saint Louis
University School of Medicine, St Louis,
Missouri

SATVEER K. MAHIL, MA, MRCP
Division of Genetics and Molecular Medicine,
St John's Institute of Dermatology, Guy's
and St Thomas' NHS Foundation Trust,
King's College London, London, United
Kingdom

M. ALAN MENTER, MD
Division of Dermatology, Baylor University
Medical Center at Dallas, Dallas, Texas

Prof. ERROL P. PRENS, MD, PhD
Dermatologist-Immunologist, Department of
Dermatology, Erasmus University Medical
Center Rotterdam, Rotterdam, The
Netherlands

EMOKE RACZ, MD, PhD
Dermatologist, Department of Dermatology,
Erasmus University Medical Center Rotterdam,
Rotterdam, The Netherlands

RICARDO ROMITI, MD
Professor of Dermatology, University of São
Paulo, São Paulo, Brazil

CAITRIONA RYAN, MD
Vice Chair, Department of Dermatology, Baylor
University Medical Center Dallas, Dallas, Texas

BRUCE E. STROBER, MD, PhD
Associate Professor and Vice Chair,
Department of Dermatology, University of
Connecticut Health Center, Farmington,
Connecticut; Probity Medical Research,
Waterloo, Ontario, Canada

PAUL W. TEBBEY, PhD
Director of Medical and Scientific Affairs
International Psoriasis Council, St Louis,
Missouri

SUZANNE J. TINTLE, MD, MPH
Department of Dermatology, Tufts Medical
Center, Boston, Massachusetts

PETER C.M. VAN DE KERKHOF, MD, PhD
Department of Dermatology, Radboud
University Nijmegen Medical Centre,
Nijmegen, The Netherlands

RICHARD B. WARREN, MD, PhD
The Dermatology Centre, Manchester
Academic Health Science Centre, Salford
Royal NHS Foundation Trust, The University
of Manchester, Salford, Manchester,
United Kingdom

Contents

Psoriasis is a common and debilitating immune-mediated skin disease with a complex genetic basis. Genetic studies have provided critical insights into the pathogenesis of disease. This article focuses on the results of genetic association studies, which provide evidence that psoriasis susceptibility genes are involved in innate and adaptive immunity and skin barrier functions. The potential for disease stratification and the development of more effective treatments with fewer side effects using genetic data are highlighted.

Psoriasis vulgaris is a chronic inflammatory skin disease that results from the complex interplay between keratinocytes, dendritic cells, and T cells. Keratinocytes trigger innate and adaptive immune responses. Dermal myeloid dendritic cells regulate T cell activation and production of cytokines and chemokines that amplify inflammation. Most of the psoriatic T cells discretely produce interferon-γ, interleukin (IL)-17, and IL-22. The initiation phase of psoriasis involves Toll-like receptors, antimicrobial peptide LL37, and plasmacytoid dendritic cells. Keratinocytes are the main cutaneous cell type expressing IL-17 receptors and hence the immune circuit is amplified by keratinocytes upregulating mRNAs for a range of inflammatory products.

Psoriasis is associated with significant physical, social, and behavioral comorbidities that create a substantial burden. We outline herein that these comorbidities start early in life and persist for decades, ultimately impacting the entire life course of patients with psoriasis. By highlighting the ages that psoriasis patients are affected with physical, social, behavioral and emotional comorbidities, we demonstrate the age-appropriate considerations for psoriasis patients.

There is evidence that patients with moderate to severe psoriasis have an increased risk of conditions such as cardiovascular disease, obesity, diabetes mellitus, and metabolic syndrome. The precise mechanisms underlying the observed increase in cardiovascular disease in psoriasis remain to be defined but inflammatory pathways mutual to both conditions are probably involved. Suppression of systemic inflammation in psoriasis could help reduce cardiovascular inflammation but robust evidence is still lacking evidence is lacking. This article summarizes the current literature on cardiovascular and metabolic comorbidities in psoriasis, identifies research gaps, and suggests management strategies to reduce cardiovascular risk in patients with moderate to severe psoriasis.

Psoriasis is a complex disease. Dermatologists have not documented psoriasis severity, except in clinical trials; doing so requires tools for assessing psoriasis and an understanding of what changes in those assessments mean in terms of outcome. Two psoriasis assessment tools have dominated: The Psoriasis Area and Severity Index and the Dermatology Life Quality Index. There are advantages and disadvantages to each. Newer instruments may not be more suitable for documenting psoriasis. There may be benefits in terms of patient ownership of disease management from using self-assessment tools for documenting severity, for example, the Self-assessment version of the Simplified Psoriasis Index.

Topical therapies are the mainstream treatment of psoriasis because most patients have mild disease. First-line treatments are vitamin D derivatives and corticosteroids. These treatments are usually given in combination schedules. For topical treatments the selection of the most appropriate vehicle is of major importance, thus improving adherence to the treatment, which frequently is impaired by the complexities of topical therapeutic choices. Evidence for efficacy and safety of topical treatments is readily available for vitamin D treatments and short-term treatment with corticosteroids. However, the scientific evidence for longer-term treatments is limited. Multiple new small molecules are in various stages of development and are reviewed.

Phototherapy is a first-line option for the treatment of moderate to severe psoriasis. Systematic reviews indicate near comparable efficacy of the different forms of phototherapy. Localized phototherapy can be an adjunctive treatment of recalcitrant plaques during systemic treatment of psoriasis. More than 200 psoralen–UV-A therapy treatment sessions is associated with an increased risk of keratinocytic cancers, whereas no increased risk has been demonstrated for narrow-band UV-B therapy. The mechanism of action of phototherapy in psoriasis is via inhibition of keratinocyte proliferation; induction of apoptosis in keratinocytes, dendritic, and T cells; and inhibition of Th1 and Th17 pathways, but activation of Th2.

For patients with moderate to severe psoriasis, there is a large range of variably effective and safe oral, systemic medications. With appropriate monitoring, these therapies may be used as either monotherapy or in combination with other therapies. Newer drugs in the research pipeline hold significant promise.

DERMATOLOGIC CLINICS

RELATED INTEREST

Diagnosis and Management of Psoriasis in Children
Megha M. Tollefson
Pediatric Clinics of North America, April 2014,
Volume 61, Issue 2, pages 261–277

Preface
The International Psoriasis Council: Advancing Knowledge, Enhancing Care

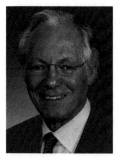

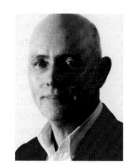

M. Alan Menter, MD   Christopher E. M. Griffiths, MD, FMedSci

Editors

Founded in 2004, the International Psoriasis Council (IPC) is a dermatology-led, voluntary, global nonprofit organization dedicated to innovation across the full spectrum of psoriasis through research, education, and patient care. The IPC's mission is to empower our network of global key opinion leaders to advance knowledge about psoriasis and its associated comorbidities, thereby enhancing the care of patients worldwide. The IPC provides a forum for education, collaboration, and innovation among physicians, researchers, and other professionals working on the physical, economic, and social aspects of psoriasis and its associated comorbidities (www.psoriasiscouncil.org).

The IPC is governed by an eleven-member board of directors and has close to 100 councilors representing 24 countries worldwide. Its councilors specialize primarily in dermatology, but also represent other clinical disciplines, including rheumatology, pediatrics, cardiology, psychology, and experimental, translational, and implementation research. Together, these thought leaders identify and prioritize the key issues germane to global psoriasis research, education, and patient care and set short-term and long-term strategic imperatives to address these issues.

Research into the many facets of psoriasis has yielded important insights resulting in a progression of understanding of the disease. Over the past 30 years, this knowledge progression has been translated into clinical benefit with the advent of immune-targeted systemic and biological therapies and now new oral small molecules that selectively target the extracellular or intracellular proteins involved in the development of psoriasis. Despite this progress, there are still major gaps in our understanding of psoriasis, which continues to attract basic and clinical investigation.

Traditional medical research is organized along geopolitical and departmental divisions, a structure that tends to impede multidisciplinary, national, and international collaboration. To overcome this, one of the IPC's primary objectives is to use its global reach to leverage available expertise and resources across multiple disciplines and geographies, thereby maximizing the opportunity to translate these into improved patient care.

One of the IPC's initial goals was to verify and define the association of psoriasis with comorbid conditions. An initial consensus conference, "Obesity in Psoriasis: Metabolic, Clinical, and Therapeutic Implications," was held in Rhodes, Greece in October 2006 to discuss this emergent field.[1] This was one of the first such conferences to draw attention to the link between psoriasis and metabolic syndrome. Subsequently, the IPC convened a second consensus conference in Dallas, Texas in September 2008, "Psoriasis Interdisciplinary Conference on Co-Morbidities and Lifestyle Modification," which included the participation of Nobel-Prize Winner for Medicine, Professor Michael Brown of University of Texas Southwestern. Professor Brown received the prize for elucidation of the cholesterol synthesis

Dermatol Clin 33 (2015) ix–xii
http://dx.doi.org/10.1016/j.det.2014.10.001

derm.theclinics.com

pathways, leading to the development of statins. Program speakers also included experts from the fields of dermatology, rheumatology, pediatrics, diabetology, cardiology, and metabolic medicine.[2] Collectively, these interactions and evaluations spawned an IPC-sponsored global clinical trial to investigate the relationship of adiposity with pediatric psoriasis. The results of the study indicated that children with psoriasis have excess adiposity and increased central adiposity regardless of psoriasis severity. These findings posed the question whether the increased metabolic risks associated with such adiposity can be ameliorated by early monitoring and lifestyle modification.[3] The IPC continues its focus on the association of psoriasis with comorbidities and in November 2013 held a Think Tank in Boston, Massachusetts, which explored the interrelationship between genetics, inflammation, stress, and psychology, and psoriasis and various comorbid conditions.

Beyond comorbidities, the IPC has advanced knowledge toward a better understanding of the genetic susceptibility to psoriasis. An inaugural genetics workshop was organized in association with the 61st meeting of the American Society of Human Genetics in October 2011, in Montreal, Canada. The objective was to map the current understanding of the genetic architecture of psoriasis to allow greater insight into the disease-specific biological pathways that determine the condition as well as to inform better categorization of the disease and potentially aid in the prediction of response to therapy. As a consequence of this interaction, the IPC initiated a project to exome-sequence the genomes of over 20,000 individuals with psoriasis with a view to systematically evaluate the contribution of rare protein coding variants to psoriasis susceptibility.[4] This project is currently underway and involves an international collaboration of geneticists and dermatologists in the United States, Germany, and the United Kingdom, leading to a bioinformatics phase with the potential to deliver important data on inherited susceptibility to psoriasis.

To better understand the pathogenic mechanisms that underlie psoriasis, IPC hosted a workshop at the 42nd Annual European Society for Dermatological Research in Venice, Italy in September 2012. A panel of global dermatology and immunology experts participated in the workshop with the objective of evaluating our current understanding of the immunology of psoriasis, including dysregulation of the skin immune system and perturbations of epidermal homeostasis. Collectively, the workshop participants demonstrated the significant advances in our understanding of the immune regulation that have occurred over the past decade by virtue of the study of psoriasis phenotypes and genotypes.[5]

In addition, the IPC is one of the leaders in developing the first Global Psoriasis Atlas and is a collaborator in the Psoriasis Stratification to Optimize Relevant Therapy (PSORT) consortium. The Global Psoriasis Atlas is a long-term project jointly led by the International League of Dermatological Societies, the International Federation of Psoriasis Associations and the IPC that will develop standardized methodology to help fill the gaps in our understanding of the prevalence, incidence, and burden of psoriasis worldwide. This is an important parallel project to the genetics project. The vision of the PSORT consortium is to better understand the determinants of response of psoriasis to biological therapies and thereby rationalize and optimize patient care in a cost-effective manner.

Continued progress toward elucidating the pathogenic and genetic basis of psoriasis holds the promise of a complete understanding of disease mechanisms, predictors of treatment response, novel drug development strategies, and customized therapeutic regimens for the individual patient. The IPC plans to be leading that charge toward a world where psoriasis has no meaningful impact.

As the IPC continues to advance the knowledge and understanding of psoriasis from a research perspective, it also focuses on translating this knowledge into practical information for physicians and health care providers who are currently managing patients with the spectrum of psoriasis with the goal of improving patient care. As the landscape of disease management in psoriasis continues to evolve, it is critical to equip health care providers with the latest and most cutting-edge information available to inform and to evoke change.

There are clear and substantial deficits in physician understanding and management of psoriasis. In a survey of dermatology trainees, participants correctly answered only 47% of questions about psoriasis.[6] Yet another study found that evidence-based training is underdeveloped in dermatology programs.[7] Dermatologists are often uncomfortable when prescribing systemic agents. In a National Psoriasis Foundation survey of patients with severe psoriasis, 26% were treated with systemic therapy, phototherapy, or both; 39% were not in treatment, and 35% were treated with topical therapy alone.[8]

Guidelines are available for the diagnosis and management of psoriasis and the identification of comorbidities. Immunomodulatory and biologic drugs are currently recommended in these guidelines for patients with moderate to severe psoriasis and/or psoriatic arthritis.[9,10] However, not all clinicians are clear as to when and how to incorporate these agents into the treatment algorithms for their patients.

To address these issues, the IPC conducts a variety of educational programs and activities that reaches nearly 10,000 health care providers annually. The *IPC Psoriasis Review*, published biannually, is designed to provide practicing physicians with an authoritative review of the most important publications in psoriasis, along with a concise editorial commentary on the value of these publications. The *Review* also provides overviews of important scientific meetings and information on the IPC's education, research, and treatment activities. The publication is translated into Spanish and Portuguese and is distributed throughout South America and Europe. In addition, the English language version is distributed to over 8000 dermatologists worldwide.

The *IPC Meet the Experts* (MTE) case-based educational program is a cornerstone of the IPC's educational initiatives. Initiated in 2008, the MTE events are run as a panel discussion led by local psoriasis experts and chaired by an IPC Board member or councilor to educate dermatologists on various approaches to managing difficult-to-treat psoriasis patients. These difficult-to-treat cases cover topics such as obesity, comorbid conditions, subclassifications, pregnancy, transitioning patients between therapies, combination therapies, and new treatment methods. The interactive program provides attendees with the opportunity to ask questions of the panel and also to provide their own perspective on the cases. Cases for each program are specifically selected for the geographic region in which the program is being held. For instance, our Latin America programs feature cases from local dermatologists. MTE programs draw audiences of up to 150 people. The program has been held in twenty different countries reaching nearly 1000 health care providers annually. In addition to the above programs, the IPC conducts intensive preceptorship programs at leading universities, hosts a variety of Web-based programs, and educates health care providers through accredited continuing medical education programs across the globe.

This collection of *Dermatologic Clinics* articles on psoriasis, written by IPC board members and councilors, covers cutting-edge topics on our understanding of the pathogenesis and treatment of the disease and how these may inform future research and management. The treatise provides a comprehensive, yet manageable, primer of advances in psoriasis.

M. Alan Menter, MD
Division of Dermatology
Baylor University Medical Center at Dallas
Dallas, TX, USA

Christopher E. M. Griffiths, MD, FMedSci
Dermatology Centre
Salford Royal Hospital
The University of Manchester
Manchester Academic Health Science Centre
Manchester M6 8HD, UK

E-mail addresses:
amderm@gmail.com (M. Alan Menter)
Christopher.Griffiths@manchester.ac.uk
(C.E. M. Griffiths)

REFERENCES

1. Sterry W, Strober BE, Menter A. Obesity in psoriasis: the metabolic, clinical and therapeutic implications. Report of an interdisciplinary conference and review. Br J Dermatol 2007;157:649–55.
2. Menter A, Griffiths CEM, Tebbey PW, et al, on behalf of the International Psoriasis Council. Exploring the association between cardiovascular and other disease-related risk factors in the psoriasis population: the need for increased understanding across the medical community. J Eur Acad Dermatol Venereol 2010;24:1371–7.
3. Paller AS, Mercy K, Kwasny MJ, et al. Association of pediatric psoriasis severity with excess and central adiposity: an international cross-sectional study. JAMA Dermatol 2013;149(2):166–76.
4. Capon F, Barker JN. The quest for psoriasis susceptibility genes in the post-GWAS era: charting the road ahead. Br J Dermatol 2012;166:1173–5.
5. Bachelez H, Viguier M, Tebbey PW, et al. The mechanistic basis for psoriasis immunopathogenesis: translating genotype to phenotype. Br J Dermatol 2013;169:283–6.
6. Greist HM, Pearce DJ, Blauvelt M, et al. Resident education: effect of the sixth national psoriasis foundation chief residents' meeting. J Cutan Med Surg 2006;10:16–20.
7. Dellavalle RP, Stegner DL, Deas AM, et al. Assessing evidence-based dermatology and evidence-based internal medicine curricula in US residency training programs: a national survey. Arch Dermatol 2003;139:369–72 [discussion: 372].
8. Horn EJ, Fox KM, Patel V, et al. Are patients with psoriasis undertreated? Results of National Psoriasis

Foundation survey. J Am Acad Dermatol 2007;57: 957–62.

9. American Academy of Dermatology Work Group, Menter A, Korman NJ, Elmets CA, et al. Guidelines of care for the management of psoriasis and psoriatic arthritis: section 6. Guidelines of care for the treatment of psoriasis and psoriatic arthritis: case-based presentations and evidence-based conclusions. J Am Acad Dermatol 2011;65:137–74.

10. Menter A, Gottlieb A, Feldman SR, et al. Guidelines of care for the management of psoriasis and psoriatic arthritis: section 1. Overview of psoriasis and guidelines of care for the treatment of psoriasis with biologics. J Am Acad Dermatol 2008;58:826–50.

Genetics of Psoriasis

Satveer K. Mahil, MA, MRCP[a], Francesca Capon, PhD[b],
Jonathan N. Barker, MD, FRCP, FRCPath[a],*

KEYWORDS

- Psoriasis • Genetics • Genome-wide association studies • Stratification

KEY POINTS

- Psoriasis is a common and clinically heterogeneous group of immune-mediated skin diseases that includes psoriasis vulgaris and pustular variants, amongst others. Although most research has involved psoriasis vulgaris, emerging data suggest that the different clinical phenotypes may have unique immunogenetic profiles.
- Greater than 40 regions of the genome (susceptibility loci) have been found to be associated with psoriasis using genome-wide and further targeted association studies.
- Each psoriasis susceptibility locus contains many genes; the candidate causal genes within the loci suggest a key role for adaptive and innate immunity and skin barrier functions in disease pathogenesis.
- Less than 25% of psoriasis heritability has been accounted for by genetic studies and the remaining missing heritability may in part be attributable to genetic variants of low/modest effect and epigenetic mechanisms.
- Future integration of detailed phenotype information with genetic data will enable disease stratification, with potential advances in the development of diagnostic and prognostic markers, predictors of drug responsiveness, and more efficacious, less toxic targeted therapies.

INTRODUCTION

Substantial progress has been made into identifying the genetic determinants of common immune-mediated diseases. This has highlighted biologic pathways involved in disease pathogenesis and also potential novel drug targets. Nevertheless, further advancements are required before this research is translated into the development of diagnostic and prognostic biomarkers and efficacious, targeted treatments without serious side effects. The major health and economic burden associated with these diseases may then start to decline. Psoriasis is a common, chronic, immune-mediated skin disease that affects approximately 2% of the population worldwide.[1] It is associated with considerable psychosocial morbidity and systemic diseases, such as metabolic syndrome, cardiovascular disease, and inflammatory arthritis. There are two peak ages of onset: between 15 and 30 years, and 50 and 60 years. The most common clinical phenotype of psoriasis is psoriasis vulgaris (affecting 85%–90% of patients), characterized by erythematous, scaling plaques. Most research to date (as described in this article) has explored the early onset (before age 40) form of this disease called type 1 psoriasis. Other subtypes include type 2 psoriasis (onset after age 40), guttate psoriasis, nail psoriasis and pustular variants.

Psoriasis is a complex, multifactorial disease, with genetic and environmental factors having an important role in its etiology. A strong genetic

Disclosures: None.
[a] Division of Genetics and Molecular Medicine, St John's Institute of Dermatology, Guy's and St Thomas' NHS Foundation Trust, King's College London, 9th Floor, Tower Wing, London SE1 9RT, UK; [b] Division of Genetics and Molecular Medicine, King's College London, Guy's Hospital, 9th Floor, Tower Wing, London, SE1 9RT, UK
* Corresponding author. Division of Genetics and Molecular Medicine, King's College London, Guy's Hospital, 9th Floor, Tower Wing, London SE1 9RT, UK.
E-mail address: jonathan.barker@kcl.ac.uk

basis for psoriasis is now well established through epidemiologic studies and heritability is estimated at 60% to 90%, which is among the highest for complex genetic diseases.[2] Initial epidemiologic studies revealed a higher incidence of psoriasis in the relatives of patients compared with the general population.[3] Approximately 70% of individuals with childhood psoriasis report a positive family history.[4] Twins studies showed higher concordance rates in monozygotic twins (35%–73%) than dizygotic twins (12%–20%).[5–7] Segregation analyses in large, multigenerational families show that psoriasis is likely to be a polygenic disease.[8]

TOOLS FOR INVESTIGATING THE GENETIC BASIS FOR PSORIASIS; A COMMON, COMPLEX DISEASE

In contrast to mendelian conditions, in which mutations are rare in the population and of large effect, the multiple alleles contributing to susceptibility to complex genetic diseases, such as psoriasis, are common and individually confer modest risk.[9–11] Based on this "common disease–common variant" hypothesis, numerous genome-wide linkage scans and association studies have been performed in the search for the multiple genes that predispose to psoriasis.

Linkage studies identify areas of the genome that confer disease susceptibility by tracing the cosegregation of clinical phenotypes with specific genomic regions. These identified at least nine chromosomal segments (genetic loci) that cosegregate with psoriasis (PSORS1-9); however, except for PSORS1, PSORS2, and PSORS4, the evidence for susceptibility loci found by linkage studies could not be replicated. PSORS1, a 220-kb region found on chromosome 6p21.3, was shown to confer the most risk for psoriasis. It has the largest effect size, is estimated to account for between 35% and 50% of heritability, and is the most replicated locus for psoriasis.[12–14] The presence of strong linkage disequilibrium (LD) across the region has made identification of the underlying disease susceptibility allele difficult. LD is the phenomenon whereby single-nucleotide polymorphisms (SNPs) that are located in close proximity in the genome are inherited together. Distinguishing the disease/causal SNP from other statistically associated ones within the same LD block is thus challenging.

The PSORS1 region contains the candidate genes human leukocyte antigen C (HLA-C), coiled-coil-α-helical rod protein (CCHCR1), and corneodesmosin (CDSN). The HLA-Cw6 allele is associated with psoriasis in many different populations, suggesting that it may be the causal psoriasis susceptibility allele within PSORS1.[15,16] HLA-C encodes a class I major histocompatibility complex molecule that is expressed on antigen-presenting cells and involved in CD8[+] T-cell activation (via antigen presentation), thus highlighting the importance of immune dysregulation in psoriasis pathogenesis. SNPs affecting HLA-Cw6 expression have also recently been found that are likely to contribute to psoriasis susceptibility.[17,18]

The statistical power of linkage studies to discover the causative genes contributing to complex diseases is, however, limited because the risk conferred by each susceptibility locus is only small. Genome-wide association studies (GWAS) soon proved to be more powerful in the analysis of common, complex diseases, such as psoriasis. In GWAS, statistical differences in allele frequencies are found between unrelated cases and control subjects (ethnically matched) within a population, hence alleles that are associated with disease are identified. It is reliant on the careful phenotyping of sufficient numbers of cases and control subjects and the accurate typing of genetic markers (SNPs) that span the genome in each individual. The completion of human genome sequencing and the development of high-throughput genotyping platforms have enabled GWAS to be a powerful and accessible tool. No prior hypotheses regarding candidate causal genes/variants are required before completing a GWAS and the candidate genes that are subsequently identified within disease-associated intervals provide critical insights into the pathogenesis of disease. Increased power to detect associations from GWAS is gained from investigating larger sample numbers, hence promoting collaborations between large centers and meta-analyses.

GWAS provides the stimulus for further work because the lead SNP within the susceptibility interval is not necessarily the causal variant. Each locus can be refined by denser SNP arrays, such as the Immunochip. The Immunochip (Illumina Infinium) contains more than 200,000 SNPs implicated in 12 immune-mediated conditions including psoriasis.[19] In the following section, the findings from psoriasis GWAS and the Immunochip study are reviewed.

FINDINGS FROM GENETIC STUDIES: INSIGHTS INTO PSORIASIS PATHOGENESIS

Greater than 40 regions of the genome have now been found to be associated with psoriasis; 26 were discovered using GWAS and a further 15 psoriasis susceptibility loci were identified in the Immunochip study (Table 1).[20–28] Each region spans many genes; however, specific genes have been highlighted within each locus that are the most biologically plausible candidates given the function of the encoded proteins. Using the results of these investigations, a model for psoriasis pathogenesis is now emerging that combines skin barrier function, innate immunity, and adaptive immunity.

Adaptive Immunity

Antigen presentation to the immune system seems to be critical to the pathogenesis of psoriasis because SNPs that are in strong LD with HLA-Cw6 alleles yield the strongest association signal in all GWAS. Early onset disease (type 1 psoriasis) and a severe clinical course are highly associated with HLA-Cw6. Furthermore, genetic variants within endoplasmic reticulum aminopeptidase 1 (ERAP1) gene are associated with psoriasis. ERAP1 codes for an enzyme that trims peptide antigens into short chains consisting of nine amino acids, which can then be loaded onto major histocompatibility complex class I molecules for presentation to immune cells at the cell surface. ERAP1 alleles have been shown to interact with HLA-Cw6 (genetic epistasis) such that ERAP1 genetic variants only confer susceptibility to psoriasis in individuals also harboring the HLA-C risk allele.[23] This provides further support for the HLA-Cw6 allele as the causal psoriasis susceptibility allele within PSORS1.

The importance of the interleukin (IL)-23/Th17 pathway in psoriasis pathogenesis has been shown in genetic and immunologic studies. Variants in or near the genes IL12B, IL23R, and IL23A are associated with psoriasis susceptibility.[22,29–33] IL-23 is a heterodimer that signals through the IL-23R complex and is composed of IL-23p19 and IL-12p40 subunits. The IL-12p40 subunit is shared with IL-12 and encoded by the gene IL12B. The IL23A gene codes for the IL-23p19 subunit. IL-23 promotes the survival and expansion of Th17 cells and subsequent release of cytokines, such as IL-17, IL-22, and tumor necrosis factor (TNF)-α.

GWAS have shown an association between a nonsynonymous SNP in IL23R (guanine to adenine substitution; R381Q) and protection against developing psoriasis. It is also associated with protection against ankylosing spondylitis and Crohn disease.[34,35] Functional characterization of this SNP has shown that the protective variant causes impaired IL-23–induced Th17 effector cell function, with reduced IL-17A production and reduced STAT3 activation (downstream of IL23R).[36,37] Hence in psoriasis, there may be aberrant IL-23 signaling and Th17 cell activity, which contribute to chronic inflammation. In support, IL12B and IL23A are overexpressed in lesional skin of psoriasis patients.[38] TYK2 encodes a kinase that promotes IL-17 transcription via STAT3 phosphorylation and also regulates type I and II interferon (IFN) signaling. Coding variants in TYK2 have also been shown to be associated with psoriasis in GWAS and the Immunochip study.[23,28]

TRAF3IP2 encodes ACT1, which is an essential signaling adaptor molecule in IL-17 signaling. ACT1 can activate nuclear factor (NF)-κB through phosphorylation of the inhibitor of kappa B kinase complex. A coding variant in TRAF3IP2 (Asp10Asn) is associated with psoriasis and psoriatic arthritis, and leads to almost complete loss of binding of ACT1 to its binding partner TRAF6.[20,39] The functional consequences of this susceptibility allele have been well characterized in Act1-deficient mice, who demonstrate upregulated Th17 responses and spontaneous IL-22–dependent skin inflammation.[40]

Finally, the role of Th2 pathway modulation in psoriasis pathogenesis has been underscored by the strong associations found in GWAS between psoriasis and genes encoding the cytokines IL-4 and IL-13.[22]

Skin Barrier Function

Linkage studies first suggested an association between psoriasis and genes expressed during epidermal differentiation that are contained within the epidermal differentiation complex. PSORS4 is on chromosome 1q21 and contains the epidermal differentiation complex.[41–43] The epidermal differentiation complex encompasses the late cornified envelope (LCE) genes, which encode stratum corneum proteins involved in epidermal terminal differentiation. A GWAS of a large Chinese cohort revealed an association between SNPs in the LCE cluster and psoriasis.[26] Furthermore, a deletion involving LCE3B and LCE3C genes was found to be associated with psoriasis in a European cohort.[27] The expression of LCE3 genes was almost undetectable in normal and nonlesional psoriatic skin; however, it was upregulated in lesional skin and normal skin following skin injury (eg, tape stripping).[44]

Based on the previously mentioned studies, it has been hypothesized that minor skin injury (ie, a compromised barrier) and incomplete barrier repair caused by insufficient LCE3B/3C expression promotes antigen and proinflammatory stimuli penetration, which leads to chronic inflammation.[45]

Innate Immunity

The role of innate immunity in psoriasis pathogenesis is being increasingly recognized.[46] The skin is

Table 1
Genes associated with psoriasis

Gene[a]	Chromosome	Biologic Pathway	Protein Function
TNFRSF9	1	Adaptive immunity	Costimulatory molecule involved in generation of memory T cells
IL-28RA	1	Innate immunity; IFN signaling	IL-29 receptor subunit
RUNX3	1	Adaptive immunity; T-cell activation	Transcription factor involved in promoting Th1 and memory T-cell differentiation
IL23R	1	Adaptive immunity; IL-23/Th17 axis	IL-23 receptor subunit
LCE3B/LCE3C	1	Skin barrier function	Keratinocyte structural protein
REL	2	Innate immunity; NF-κB signaling	Transcription factor (subunit) of the NF-κB family
B3GNT2	2	Adaptive immunity	Enzyme involved in lymphocyte function
IFIH1	2	Innate immunity; innate antiviral signaling	RIG-like helicase; antiviral receptor
ERAP1	5	Adaptive immunity; antigen presentation	Peptidase to trim peptides for binding to MHC I
IL-4, IL-13	5	Adaptive immunity; Th2 signaling	Modulation of Th2 cell response
TNIP1	5	Innate immunity; NF-κB signaling	Regulation of NF-κB signaling
IL12B	5	Adaptive immunity, IL-23/Th17 axis	p40 subunit shared by IL-12 and IL-23
EXOC2	6	Innate immunity; innate antiviral signaling	Promotes the production of type I IFNs in response to intracellular DNA
HLA-C	6	Adaptive immunity; antigen presentation	MHC class I
TRAF3IP2	6	Innate immunity; NF-κB signaling	Signaling adaptor protein
TNFAIP3	6	Innate immunity; NF-κB signaling	TNF-α inducible zinc finger protein that inhibits NF-κB signaling
TAGAP	6	Adaptive immunity	Involved in T-cell activation
ELMO1	7	Innate immunity	Promotes toll-like receptor mediated IFN-α production
DDX58	9	Innate immunity; innate antiviral signaling	RIG-I antiviral receptor
KLF4	9	Innate immunity	Transcription factor that regulates macrophage activation
ZCH12C	11	Innate immunity	Zinc finger protein that regulates macrophage activation
ETS1	11	Adaptive immunity	Transcription factor involved in regulating CD8+ T-cell and Th17 cell differentiation
IL23A	12	Adaptive immunity; IL-23/Th17 axis	p19 subunit of IL-23
NFKBIA	14	Innate immunity; NF-κB signaling	Inhibitor of NF-κB signaling
SOCS1	16	Adaptive immunity	Regulation of Th17 cell differentiation
FBXL19	16	Innate immunity; NF-κB signaling	Putative inhibitor of NF-κB signaling
NOS2	17	Innate immunity	Catalyzes the production of nitric oxide for immune defense against pathogens

(continued on next page)

Table 1
(continued)

Gene[a]	Chromosome	Biologic Pathway	Protein Function
STAT3, STAT5A, STAT5B	17	Adaptive immunity	Participates in signaling downstream of multiple cytokines (eg, IL-6, IL-10, and IL-2)
CARD14	17	Innate immunity; NF-κB signaling	Recruitment and activation of NF-κB pathway
MBD2	18	Adaptive immunity	Transcriptional repressor involved in generation of memory T cells
TYK2	19	Innate immunity; IFN signaling	Tyrosine kinase associated with cytoplasmic domain of cytokine receptors
CARM1	19	Innate immunity; NF-κB signaling	Transcriptional coactivator of NF-κB
RNF114	20	Innate immunity; innate antiviral signaling	E3 ubiquitin ligase
UBE2L3	22	Innate immunity; NF-κB signaling	E2-ubiquitin-conjugating enzyme involved in regulating NF-κB signaling

Abbreviations: IFN, interferon; IL, interleukin; MHC, major histocompatibility complex; NF, nuclear factor; RIG-I, retinoic acid-inducible gene I; TNF, tumor necrosis factor.
[a] For each disease-associated genetic locus, the most likely candidate gene (based on protein function) has been specified.
Data from Refs.[12,20,22–28,30,39,50]

the first line of defense against pathogens because it provides a physical, biochemical (eg, antimicrobial peptides), and immunologic barrier. GWAS and the Immunochip study have identified several psoriasis susceptibility loci that contain genes involved in innate immunity.

NF-κB is a family of dimeric transcription factors involved in apoptosis and innate immune regulation. NF-κB is activated via signaling cascades triggered by toll-like receptors (TLR) and cytokines including TNF, IL-17, and IL-1. Inactive NF-κB associates with cytoplasmic inhibitor proteins of the IκB family and active dimmers translocate to the nucleus. All NF-κB proteins have a Rel homology domain that mediates DNA binding and dimerization. Previous GWAS have revealed that several components of the NF-κB signaling pathway are associated with psoriasis.[20,22,23]

Genetic variants in or near TNIP1[22,25] and NFKBIA[20,23,24] encoding the NF-κB regulatory proteins ABIN-1 and IκBα, respectively, have been shown to be associated with psoriasis. TNFAIP3 encodes the ubiquitin-editing enzyme A20, which regulates NF-κB activation in response to TNF and microbial products that signal through TLRs.[47] The association between TNFAIP3 and psoriasis further underscores the potential relevance of NF-κB in the pathogenesis of psoriasis.[22] Recently the Immunochip study and candidate gene studies have confirmed an association between CARD14 and psoriasis. CARD14 is expressed in keratinocytes and regulates NF-κB.

Linkage studies using large pedigrees originally identified mutations in CARD14 as being responsible for PSORS2.[48] Common and rare coding variants have subsequently been identified, with evidence of altered NF-κB activity.[28,49]

Genetic and immunologic studies are converging to highlight the potential importance of innate antiviral immune pathways in psoriasis pathogenesis. RNF114 was identified as a psoriasis susceptibility gene[50] and found to have a regulatory role in the signaling cascade driven by the RIG-I and MDA5 innate antiviral receptors, which are encoded by DDX58 and IFIH1, respectively.[51] Indeed, RIG-I and MDA5 are significantly upregulated in psoriatic lesions.[52] RIG-I and MDA5 bind viral dsRNA and promote the release of proinflammatory and antiviral cytokines, such as IL-1, IL-6, TNF, type I IFN, and IL-29. The latter cytokine is a type III IFN that signals through the receptor encoded by IL28RA. Finally, the protein encoded by EXOC2 is thought to promote the production of type I IFN in response to intracellular DNA.[53] RNF114, DDX58, IFIH1, IL28RA, and EXOC2 are all contained within psoriasis susceptibility loci identified in GWAS and the Immunochip study.[20,23,28] Thus, altered expression of innate antiviral genes may contribute to disease susceptibility by causing the overproduction of proinflammatory cytokines. Given that the skin provides the first line of defense against pathogens, dysregulation of this antimicrobial function may have a critical role in the pathogenesis of psoriasis.

β-Defensins are antimicrobial peptides that are also proinflammatory because they act as chemokines for immune cells, such as dendritic cells and T cells. High genomic copy number of the β-defensin gene cluster was shown to be associated with risk of psoriasis in a Dutch and German cohort.[54] This finding was replicated in a large, independent cohort (although it showed a weaker association).[55] The β-defensin hBD-2 is highly upregulated in lesional psoriasis skin.[56] This may provide increased protection against infection when the skin barrier is disrupted; however, it may also contribute to an overexaggerated immune response to minor stimuli and thus an increased risk of psoriasis.

Taken together, genetic studies have provided vital mechanistic insights into psoriasis pathogenesis. The psoriasis susceptibility loci have highlighted many genes involved in skin barrier function and innate and adaptive immune responses. It has also been shown that different autoimmune diseases, such as Crohn disease and celiac disease (which are more prevalent in individuals with psoriasis), share susceptibility loci with psoriasis. In support, individuals with psoriasis have an increased risk of developing a second (odds ratio 1.6) or third (odds ratio 1.9) autoimmune disease.[57] There may be shared pathogenic mechanisms among different autoimmune diseases, and further research into these biologic pathways may highlight common, novel drug targets.

OTHER SUBTYPES OF PSORIASIS

Although most research to date has involved patients with type 1 psoriasis, recent genetic studies on pustular psoriasis have revealed the importance of a novel cytokine pathway in its pathogenesis, which has direct translational potential.

Generalized pustular psoriasis, characterized by an acute pustular eruption and systemic upset, was found to segregate as an autosomal-recessive trait in several Tunisian families, so linkage studies followed by direct sequencing were performed.[58] A homozygous missense mutation in IL36RN was found. IL36RN codes for the IL36 receptor antagonist protein (IL36Ra). The mutated IL36RN protein was expressed at lower levels and led to increased production of proinflammatory cytokines, such as IL-8, from keratinocytes. IL36RN missense mutations were also discovered in unrelated individuals with generalized pustular psoriasis by exome sequencing.[59,60] IL-1 production was found to be upregulated in response to IL-36 stimulation in these patients. In contrast, no IL36RN mutations were detected through sequencing studies of a large cohort of patients

with psoriasis vulgaris.[61] Taken together, these data highlight a potential distinct pathogenesis for specific disease subtypes, which has therapeutic implications. There are increasing reports of IL-1 blockade using IL-1Ra as an effective treatment of generalized pustular psoriasis.[62,63]

Recently, whole exome sequencing was used to identify two heterozygous mutations in AP1S3, encoding a small subunit of AP-1 complex, which are associated with pustular psoriasis.[64] Silencing of AP1S3 was demonstrated to disrupt the endosomal translocation of TLR-3, which resulted in inhibition of TLR-3–mediated IFN-β induction. Given that IFN-β downregulates the production of IL-1[65] this study further supports a potential role for IL-1 blockade for treatment of pustular variants of psoriasis.

Type 2 psoriasis (onset after age 40) is also emerging as having a unique genetic profile and hence potential distinct immunopathogenesis to type 1 psoriasis. A recent study revealed that variation in the IL1B gene is associated with type 2 psoriasis rather than type 1 disease.[66] Type 2 disease is also not associated with HLA-Cw6, unlike type 1 psoriasis and guttate psoriasis, which highlights the genetic heterogeneity of different clinical subtypes of psoriasis.

TRANSLATION OF GENETIC STUDIES INTO THE CLINIC

Currently treatments for psoriasis are limited by their side effect profiles and interindividual variation in efficacy. Candidate gene pharmacogenetic studies, investigating whether variants in specific genes are associated with clinical response to treatments, have been undertaken to improve patient care and reduce drug-related costs. Methotrexate is often the first systemic agent used to treat moderate or severe psoriasis. Improved response to methotrexate is associated with SNPs in ABCC1 and ABCG2, which were investigated because they are genes that regulate the intracellular uptake of methotrexate.[67] SNPs in ABCC1 were found to be significantly associated with toxicity to methotrexate. GWAS have also identified candidate genes for further investigation in pharmacogenetic studies. Two SNPs in TNFAIP3 have been found to be associated with clinical response to TNF inhibitors[68] and there is a more rapid response to ustekinumab in patients who are HLA-Cw6 positive.[69] Although this research is promising, the pharmacogenetic studies undertaken to date are limited by low sample sizes and lack of replication studies. There are also multiple potential confounding factors that can affect drug response (eg, body mass index and alcohol intake).

Through advances in genetic research, stratified medicine is now a realistic goal, whereby groups of patients likely to have good or poor responses to specific treatments are identified. Distinct clinical phenotypes of psoriasis may be correlated with genetic data to determine if different subtypes of psoriasis are associated with different mutations. This will provide mechanistic insights into disease, prognostic information (eg, which patients may develop psoriatic arthritis), and help to guide the development of pathogenesis-based treatments. This is a more powerful and less biased approach than previous studies in which single candidate genes were selected based on prior knowledge of pathways involved in drug metabolism or signaling.

The Psoriasis Stratification to Optimize Relevant Therapy (PSORT) consortium was formed to improve understanding of the determinants of responses to biologic therapies for psoriasis (www. psort.org.uk).[70] It uses the large-scale UK-based clinical data resource called British Association of Dermatologists' Biologic Interventions Registry and integrates this with genetic, immune, and transcriptomic data for patients treated with biologics. The study is ongoing and expected outcomes include the development of diagnostic and prognostic markers; predictors of drug responsiveness; and targeted treatments that have improved efficacy, lower cost, and fewer side effects.

The proof of concept of the translational potential of genetic studies is ustekinumab (now approved by the Food and Drug Administration for psoriasis), a fully humanized monoclonal antibody that targets the shared p40 subunit of IL-12/IL-23. GWAS highlighted the importance of the IL-23/Th17 axis, thus informing the development of this highly effective treatment. In clinical trials, PASI-75 was achieved in more than 60% of ustekinumab-treated psoriasis patients at 12 weeks compared with 3% of the placebo group.[71,72] Several other promising drugs targeting different components of the IL-23/Th17 axis are also currently under investigation.[73–75]

Direct-to-consumer genetic testing has also been the focus of recent interest, because it may enable more personalized interventions to take place. However, the use of these publically available tests has raised concerns regarding lack of formal regulation, clinical utility of the results, potential false-positives and -negatives, and problems with genetic counseling and interpretation of the results.[76,77] Nevertheless, when used in the correct context, these tests may stimulate early screening for specific diseases and beneficial preventative interventions. Given that this is a rapidly developing field, it is important to provide education and guidelines to physicians to enable appropriate counseling of patients considering such testing and interpretation of results from patients who have undergone testing.

FUTURE CHALLENGES

Although genetic studies have identified more than 40 susceptibility loci for psoriasis and provided mechanistic insights into its pathogenesis, considerable work remains to be completed to fully elucidate the complex genetic basis of this common and debilitating disease. Most of the identified loci contain multiple genes. Fine mapping using dense SNP arrays, such as the Immunochip, will enable refinement of the association signals (susceptibility loci). A key challenge is then identifying the causal alleles within the refined association signals, which will help to guide the development of targeted treatments. The functional effects of the causal variants need to be investigated, eg, causal variants may alter gene expression regulation if in noncoding promoter/enhancer/repressor elements, or protein function if in coding regions. It is also possible that the disease-associated variant within the susceptibility locus may affect expression of genes megabases away (long range enhancer), as recently demonstrated for type 2 diabetes and obesity, hence assumptions regarding candidate genes within susceptibility loci should be made with caution.[78] The Encyclopedia of DNA Elements consortium have published a map of the functional elements that comprise the human genome.[79] This has transformed the understanding of noncoding regions, indicating that most are likely to be functional and disruption of regulatory elements will have pathogenic consequences.[80] These data will facilitate the identification of regulatory variants associated with complex traits.

Less than 25% of psoriasis heritability has been accounted for by the genetic studies described previously, hence a substantial proportion of the genetic risk for psoriasis is yet to be identified, similar to other common, complex diseases.[81] There are several possible reasons for this missing heritability. The statistical power of GWAS to detect variants of modest effect may be limited. Thus collaborative efforts and meta-analyses will be critical in ensuring large sample sizes such that future studies are adequately powered to detect more disease-associated variants of smaller effect.

GWAS use arrays that feature SNPs that are present commonly in the population (ie, in at least

5% of the population). Rarer variants are not represented on the arrays. Although rare variants (of possibly larger effect) may theoretically contribute to the missing heritability, at present the evidence for this is limited.[82,83] To further investigate, a large multicentre collaborative study based on the analysis of the HumanExome BeadChip (Illumina) is ongoing. This project is funded by the International Psoriasis Council and the first round of its data will be reported in late 2014 (http://www.psoriasis-council.org).[84] There may be contributions from epigenetic effects to the genetic risk for psoriasis that have not yet been accounted for. Epigenetic phenomena are heritable changes in gene expression that are not attributed to changes in the sequence of the underlying DNA (eg, histone modifications, DNA methylation). Preliminary data reveal a potential role for epigenetic factors in the pathogenesis of psoriasis.[85–87] Finally, the lead SNP found in association studies may not be the causal SNP, and it may be an imperfect proxy for the causal SNP. By virtue of next-generation sequencing, SNP arrays have become denser, hence the lead SNP found in future association studies may be a more accurate proxy for the causal SNP and the effect size estimated will be more accurate.

Personalized medicine is a key goal for the future, whereby individual genetic profiles will be used to define the specific subtype of psoriasis, clinical course, whether the patient will respond to specific medications, and whether adverse drugs reactions will be experienced. Before this goal is realized, larger studies into the genetic variants contributing to psoriasis susceptibility are required and their possible association with drugs. With emerging next-generation technologies and larger accessible patient cohorts, it is an exciting time for genetic research into psoriasis. For example, PSORT is one of the new major projects that seek to integrate multidimensional data with direct translational potential. As more is understood about the genetic basis of psoriasis, mechanisms of disease pathogenesis will also become clearer. This wealth of information will help to inform the development of more effective, safer, targeted therapies for this common disease that is currently incurable and associated with high morbidity.

REFERENCES

1. Nestle FO, Kaplan DH, Barker J. Psoriasis. N Engl J Med 2009;361(5):496–509.
2. Elder JT, Nair RP, Guo SW, et al. The genetics of psoriasis. Arch Dermatol 1994;130(2):216–24.
3. Lomholt G. Psoriasis: prevalence, spontaneous course and genetics: a census study on the prevalence of skin disease on the Faroe Islands. Denmark: G. E. C Gad, Copenhagen; 1963.
4. Morris A, Rogers M, Fischer G, et al. Childhood psoriasis: a clinical review of 1262 cases. Pediatr Dermatol 2001;18(3):188–98.
5. Brandrup F, Hauge M, Henningsen K, et al. Psoriasis in an unselected series of twins. Arch Dermatol 1978;114(6):874–8.
6. Duffy DL, Spelman LS, Martin NG. Psoriasis in Australian twins. J Am Acad Dermatol 1993;29(3): 428–34.
7. Farber EM, Nall ML, Watson W. Natural history of psoriasis in 61 twin pairs. Arch Dermatol 1974; 109(2):207–11.
8. Gudjonsson JE, Elder JT. Psoriasis: epidemiology. Clin Dermatol 2007;25(6):535–46.
9. Witte JS, Elston RC, Schork NJ. Genetic dissection of complex traits. Nat Genet 1996;12(4):355–6 [author reply: 357–8].
10. Lander ES. The new genomics: global views of biology. Science 1996;274(5287):536–9.
11. Reich DE, Lander ES. On the allelic spectrum of human disease. Trends Genet 2001;17(9):502–10.
12. Trembath RC, Clough RL, Rosbotham JL, et al. Identification of a major susceptibility locus on chromosome 6p and evidence for further disease loci revealed by a two stage genome-wide search in psoriasis. Hum Mol Genet 1997;6(5):813–20.
13. Nair RP, Henseler T, Jenisch S, et al. Evidence for two psoriasis susceptibility loci (HLA and 17q) and two novel candidate regions (16q and 20p) by genome-wide scan. Hum Mol Genet 1997;6(8):1349–56.
14. Veal CD, Capon F, Allen MH, et al. Family-based analysis using a dense single-nucleotide polymorphism-based map defines genetic variation at PSORS1, the major psoriasis-susceptibility locus. Am J Hum Genet 2002;71(3):554–64.
15. Capon F, Munro M, Barker J, et al. Searching for the major histocompatibility complex psoriasis susceptibility gene. J Invest Dermatol 2002;118(5):745–51.
16. Nair RP, Stuart PE, Nistor I, et al. Sequence and haplotype analysis supports HLA-C as the psoriasis susceptibility 1 gene. Am J Hum Genet 2006;78(5): 827–51.
17. Hundhausen C, Bertoni A, Mak RK, et al. Allele-specific cytokine responses at the HLA-C locus: implications for psoriasis. J Invest Dermatol 2012;132(3 Pt 1):635–41.
18. Clop A, Bertoni A, Spain SL, et al. An in-depth characterization of the major psoriasis susceptibility locus identifies candidate susceptibility alleles within an HLA-C enhancer element. PLoS One 2013;8(8): e71690.
19. Cortes A, Brown MA. Promise and pitfalls of the Immunochip. Arthritis Res Ther 2011;13(1):101.
20. Ellinghaus E, Ellinghaus D, Stuart PE, et al. Genome-wide association study identifies a psoriasis

susceptibility locus at TRAF3IP2. Nat Genet 2010; 42(11):991–5.

21. Ellinghaus D, Ellinghaus E, Nair RP, et al. Combined analysis of genome-wide association studies for Crohn disease and psoriasis identifies seven shared susceptibility loci. Am J Hum Genet 2012;90(4): 636–47.

22. Nair RP, Duffin KC, Helms C, et al. Genome-wide scan reveals association of psoriasis with IL-23 and NF-kappaB pathways. Nat Genet 2009;41(2):199–204.

23. Genetic Analysis of Psoriasis Consortium & the Wellcome Trust Case Control Consortium 2, Strange A, Capon F, et al. A genome-wide association study identifies new psoriasis susceptibility loci and an interaction between HLA-C and ERAP1. Nat Genet 2010;42(11):985–90.

24. Stuart PE, Nair RP, Ellinghaus E, et al. Genome-wide association analysis identifies three psoriasis susceptibility loci. Nat Genet 2010;42(11):1000–4.

25. Sun LD, Cheng H, Wang ZX, et al. Association analyses identify six new psoriasis susceptibility loci in the Chinese population. Nat Genet 2010;42(11): 1005–9.

26. Zhang XJ, Huang W, Yang S, et al. Psoriasis genome-wide association study identifies susceptibility variants within LCE gene cluster at 1q21. Nat Genet 2009;41(2):205–10.

27. De Cid R, Riveira-Munoz E, Zeeuwen PL, et al. Deletion of the late cornified envelope LCE3B and LCE3C genes as a susceptibility factor for psoriasis. Nat Genet 2009;41(2):211–5.

28. Tsoi LC, Spain SL, Knight J, et al. Identification of 15 new psoriasis susceptibility loci highlights the role of innate immunity. Nat Genet 2012;44(12):1341–8.

29. Nair RP, Ruether A, Stuart PE, et al. Polymorphisms of the IL12B and IL23R genes are associated with psoriasis. J Invest Dermatol 2008;128(7):1653–61.

30. Cargill M, Schrodi SJ, Chang M, et al. A large-scale genetic association study confirms IL12B and leads to the identification of IL23R as psoriasis-risk genes. Am J Hum Genet 2007;80(2):273–90.

31. Nair RP, Stuart PE, Kullavanijaya P, et al. Genetic evidence for involvement of the IL23 pathway in Thai psoriatics. Arch Dermatol Res 2010;302(2):139–43.

32. Wu Y, Lu Z, Chen Y, et al. Replication of association between interleukin-23 receptor (IL-23R) and its ligand (IL-12B) polymorphisms and psoriasis in the Chinese Han population. Hum Immunol 2010; 71(12):1255–8.

33. Capon F, Di Meglio P, Szaub J, et al. Sequence variants in the genes for the interleukin-23 receptor (IL23R) and its ligand (IL12B) confer protection against psoriasis. Hum Genet 2007;122(2):201–6.

34. Duerr RH, Taylor KD, Brant SR, et al. A genome-wide association study identifies IL23R as an inflammatory bowel disease gene. Science 2006;314(5804): 1461–3.

35. Rueda B, Orozco G, Raya E, et al. The IL23R Arg381Gln non-synonymous polymorphism confers susceptibility to ankylosing spondylitis. Ann Rheum Dis 2008;67(10):1451–4.

36. Di Meglio P, Di Cesare A, Laggner U, et al. The IL23R R381Q gene variant protects against immune-mediated diseases by impairing IL-23-induced Th17 effector response in humans. PLoS One 2011;6(2):e17160.

37. Di Meglio P, Villanova F, Napolitano L, et al. The IL23R A/Gln381 allele promotes IL-23 unresponsiveness in human memory T-helper 17 cells and impairs Th17 responses in psoriasis patients. J Invest Dermatol 2013;133(10):2381–9.

38. Lee E, Trepicchio WL, Oestreicher JL, et al. Increased expression of interleukin 23 p19 and p40 in lesional skin of patients with psoriasis vulgaris. J Exp Med 2004;199(1):125–30.

39. Hüffmeier U, Uebe S, Ekici AB, et al. Common variants at TRAF3IP2 are associated with susceptibility to psoriatic arthritis and psoriasis. Nat Genet 2010; 42(11):996–9.

40. Wang C, Wu L, Bulek K, et al. The psoriasis-associated D10N variant of the adaptor Act1 with impaired regulation by the molecular chaperone hsp90. Nat Immunol 2013;14(1):72–81.

41. Mischke D, Korge BP, Marenholz I, et al. Genes encoding structural proteins of epidermal cornification and S100 calcium-binding proteins form a gene complex ("epidermal differentiation complex") on human chromosome 1q21. J Invest Dermatol 1996; 106(5):989–92.

42. Capon F, Semprini S, Dallapiccola B, et al. Evidence for interaction between psoriasis-susceptibility loci on chromosomes 6p21 and 1q21. Am J Hum Genet 1999;65(6):1798–800.

43. Capon F, Novelli G, Semprini S, et al. Searching for psoriasis susceptibility genes in Italy: genome scan and evidence for a new locus on chromosome 1. J Invest Dermatol 1999;112(1):32–5.

44. Bergboer JG, Tjabringa GS, Kamsteeg M, et al. Psoriasis risk genes of the late cornified envelope-3 group are distinctly expressed compared with genes of other LCE groups. Am J Pathol 2011;178(4):1470–7.

45. Bergboer JG, Zeeuwen PL, Schalkwijk J. Genetics of psoriasis: evidence for epistatic interaction between skin barrier abnormalities and immune deviation. J Invest Dermatol 2012;132(10):2320–1.

46. Garber K. Genetics: deep exploration. Nature 2012; 492(7429):S56–7.

47. Vereecke L, Beyaert R, van Loo G. The ubiquitin-editing enzyme A20 (TNFAIP3) is a central regulator of immunopathology. Trends Immunol 2009;30(8): 383–91.

48. Jordan CT, Cao L, Roberson ED, et al. PSORS2 is due to mutations in CARD14. Am J Hum Genet 2012;90(5):784–95.

49. Jordan CT, Cao L, Roberson ED, et al. Rare and common variants in CARD14, encoding an epidermal regulator of NF-kappaB, in psoriasis. Am J Hum Genet 2012;90(5):796–808.

50. Capon F, Bijlmakers MJ, Wolf N, et al. Identification of ZNF313/RNF114 as a novel psoriasis susceptibility gene. Hum Mol Genet 2008;17(13):1938–45.

51. Bijlmakers MJ, Kanneganti SK, Barker JN, et al. Functional analysis of the RNF114 psoriasis susceptibility gene implicates innate immune responses to double-stranded RNA in disease pathogenesis. Hum Mol Genet 2011;20(16):3129–37.

52. Prens EP, Kant M, van Dijk G, et al. IFN-alpha enhances poly-IC responses in human keratinocytes by inducing expression of cytosolic innate RNA receptors: relevance for psoriasis. J Invest Dermatol 2008;128(4):932–8.

53. Ishikawa H, Ma Z, Barber GN. STING regulates intracellular DNA-mediated, type I interferon-dependent innate immunity. Nature 2009;461(7265):788–92.

54. Hollox EJ, Huffmeier U, Zeeuwen PL, et al. Psoriasis is associated with increased beta-defensin genomic copy number. Nat Genet 2008;40(1):23–5.

55. Stuart PE, Hüffmeier U, Nair RP, et al. Association of β-defensin copy number and psoriasis in three cohorts of European origin. J Invest Dermatol 2012;132(10):2407–13.

56. Jansen PA, Rodijk-Olthuis D, Hollox EJ, et al. Beta-defensin-2 protein is a serum biomarker for disease activity in psoriasis and reaches biologically relevant concentrations in lesional skin. PLoS One 2009;4(3):e4725.

57. Hsu LN, Armstrong AW. Psoriasis and autoimmune disorders: a review of the literature. J Am Acad Dermatol 2012;67(5):1076–9.

58. Marrakchi S, Guigue P, Renshaw BR, et al. Interleukin-36-receptor antagonist deficiency and generalized pustular psoriasis. N Engl J Med 2011;365(7):620–8.

59. Onoufriadis A, Simpson MA, Pink AE, et al. Mutations in IL36RN/IL1F5 are associated with the severe episodic inflammatory skin disease known as generalized pustular psoriasis. Am J Hum Genet 2011;89(3):432–7.

60. Setta-Kaffetzi N, Navarini AA, Patel VM, et al. Rare pathogenic variants in IL36RN underlie a spectrum of psoriasis-associated pustular phenotypes. J Invest Dermatol 2013;133(5):1366–9.

61. Berki DM, Mahil SK, Burden AD, et al. Loss of IL36RN function does not confer susceptibility to psoriasis vulgaris. J Invest Dermatol 2014;134(1):271–3.

62. Viguier M, Guigue P, Pagès C, et al. Successful treatment of generalized pustular psoriasis with the interleukin-1-receptor antagonist Anakinra: lack of correlation with IL1RN mutations. Ann Intern Med 2010;153(1):66–7.

63. Hüffmeier U, Wätzold M, Mohr J, et al. Successful therapy with anakinra in a patient with generalized pustular psoriasis carrying IL36RN mutations. Br J Dermatol 2014;170(1):202–4.

64. Setta-Kaffetzi N, Simpson MA, Navarini AA, et al. AP1S3 mutations are associated with pustular psoriasis and impaired toll-like receptor 3 trafficking. Am J Hum Genet 2014;94(5):790–7.

65. González-Navajas JM, Lee J, David M, et al. Immunomodulatory functions of type I interferons. Nat Rev Immunol 2012;12(2):125–35.

66. Hébert HL, Bowes J, Smith RL, et al. Polymorphisms in IL-1B distinguish between psoriasis of early and late onset. J Invest Dermatol 2014;134:1459–62.

67. Warren RB, Smith RL, Campalani E, et al. Genetic variation in efflux transporters influences outcome to methotrexate therapy in patients with psoriasis. J Invest Dermatol 2008;128(8):1925–9.

68. Tejasvi T, Stuart PE, Chandran V, et al. TNFAIP3 gene polymorphisms are associated with response to TNF blockade in psoriasis. J Invest Dermatol 2012;132(3 Pt 1):593–600.

69. Talamonti M, Botti E, Galluzzo M, et al. Pharmacogenetics of psoriasis: HLA-Cw6 but not LCE3B/3C deletion nor TNFAIP3 polymorphism predisposes to clinical response to interleukin 12/23 blocker ustekinumab. Br J Dermatol 2013;169(2):458–63.

70. Homepage [Internet]. PSORT. Available at: http://www.psort.org.uk/. Accessed October 10, 2014.

71. Leonardi CL, Kimball AB, Papp KA, et al. Efficacy and safety of ustekinumab, a human interleukin-12/23 monoclonal antibody, in patients with psoriasis: 76-week results from a randomised, double-blind, placebo-controlled trial (PHOENIX 1). Lancet 2008;371(9625):1665–74.

72. Papp KA, Langley RG, Lebwohl M, et al. Efficacy and safety of ustekinumab, a human interleukin-12/23 monoclonal antibody, in patients with psoriasis: 52-week results from a randomised, double-blind, placebo-controlled trial (PHOENIX 2). Lancet 2008;371(9625):1675–84.

73. Crow JM. Therapeutics: silencing psoriasis. Nature 2012;492(7429):S58–9.

74. Papp KA, Leonardi C, Menter A, et al. Brodalumab, an anti-interleukin-17-receptor antibody for psoriasis. N Engl J Med 2012;366(13):1181–9.

75. Leonardi C, Matheson R, Zachariae C, et al. Anti-interleukin-17 monoclonal antibody ixekizumab in chronic plaque psoriasis. N Engl J Med 2012;366(13):1190–9.

76. Goldsmith L, Jackson L, O'Connor A, et al. Direct-to-consumer genomic testing from the perspective of the health professional: a systematic review of the literature. J Community Genet 2013;4(2):169–80.

77. Lancet Oncology. Black-box warning: direct-to-consumer marketing. Lancet Oncol 2014;15(1):1.

78. Smemo S, Tena JJ, Kim KH, et al. Obesity-associated variants within FTO form long-range

functional connections with IRX3. Nature 2014; 507(7492):371–5.

79. ENCODE Project Consortium, Bernstein BE, Birney E, et al. An integrated encyclopedia of DNA elements in the human genome. Nature 2012; 489(7414):57–74.

80. Schaub MA, Boyle AP, Kundaje A, et al. Linking disease associations with regulatory information in the human genome. Genome Res 2012;22(9): 1748–59.

81. Manolio TA, Collins FS, Cox NJ, et al. Finding the missing heritability of complex diseases. Nature 2009;461(7265):747–53.

82. Hunt KA, Mistry V, Bockett NA, et al. Negligible impact of rare autoimmune-locus coding-region variants on missing heritability. Nature 2013; 498(7453):232–5.

83. Tang H, Jin X, Li Y, et al. A large-scale screen for coding variants predisposing to psoriasis. Nat Genet 2014;46(1):45–50.

84. Available at: http://www.psoriasiscouncil.org/. Accessed October 10, 2014.

85. Zhang P, Su Y, Lu Q. Epigenetics and psoriasis. J Eur Acad Dermatol Venereol 2012;26(4):399–403.

86. Zhang P, Zhao M, Liang G, et al. Whole-genome DNA methylation in skin lesions from patients with psoriasis vulgaris. J Autoimmun 2013;41:17–24.

87. Roberson ED, Liu Y, Ryan C, et al. A subset of methylated CpG sites differentiate psoriatic from normal skin. J Invest Dermatol 2012;132(3 Pt 1):583–92.

The Immunopathogenesis of Psoriasis

Jaehwan Kim, MD, PhD, James G. Krueger, MD, PhD*

KEYWORDS

• Psoriasis • Immunology • Immunopathogenesis • Keratinocyte • T cells • Dendritic cells

KEY POINTS

- Keratinocytes recruit inflammatory dendritic cells and IL-17–producing T cells through chemokine CCL20.
- Myeloid dendritic cells drive T-cell activation and psoriatic cytokine production through IL-23 and IL-12.
- IL-23 is required for T cells to produce IL-17. IL-23 is composed of two chains, the unique p19 chain and the p40 chain shared with IL-12.
- Distinct subsets of T cells produce interferon-γ, IL-17, and IL-22 in psoriatic lesions.
- Both αβ T cells and γδ T cells are increased in numbers and able to produce IL-17 in psoriatic skin.
- IL-17 is a key cytokine in psoriatic pathogenesis. Keratinocytes respond strongly to IL-17 but other cell types may also respond to IL-17 by activating inflammation-related genes.
- IL-17 can synergize with other cytokines, such as TNF and IL-22, for induction of key gene products related to the psoriasis phenotype.

INTRODUCTION

Psoriasis vulgaris is the best-understood autoimmune skin disease mediated by the cells and molecules of the innate and adaptive immune systems. In many ways, the immune pathways that become activated in psoriasis represent amplifications of background immune circuits that exist as constitutive or inducible pathways in normal human skin.[1] Keratinocytes are key participants in innate immunity recruiting T cells to the skin, and T cells are important in sustaining disease activity. Inflammatory myeloid dendritic cells (DCs) release interleukin (IL)-23 and IL-12 to activate IL-17–producing T cells, T helper (Th) 1 cells, and Th22 cells to produce abundant psoriatic cytokines IL-17, interferon (IFN)-γ, tumor necrosis factor (TNF)-α, and IL-22.[1,2] These cytokines mediate effects on keratinocytes to amplify psoriatic inflammation.

ROLE OF THE IMMUNE SYSTEM IN PSORIASIS

For many years, there was a debate about whether the dominant process in psoriasis involved primary immune activation with secondary hyperplastic keratinocytes or vice versa.[1] The evidence that the immune system plays a more integral role in

Disclosures: The authors are not aware of any affiliations, memberships, funding, or financial holdings that might be perceived as affecting the objectivity of this review. J.G. Krueger has been a consultant to and receives research support from companies developing therapeutics for psoriasis, including Amgen, Boehringer, Centocor/Janssen, Merck, Pfizer, Idera, Astellas, and Japan Tobacco. J. Kim is cosponsored by the Vilcek Foundation and the Rockefeller University Center for Clinical and Translational Science grant # UL1 TR000043 from the National Center for Advancing Translational Sciences, National Institutes of Health Clinical and Translational Science Award program. J. Kim is also supported by National Psoriasis Foundation Discovery Grant Program.
Laboratory for Investigative Dermatology, The Rockefeller University, 1230 York Ave, New York, NY 10065, USA
* Corresponding author.
E-mail address: kruegej@rockefeller.edu

Dermatol Clin 33 (2015) 13–23
http://dx.doi.org/10.1016/j.det.2014.09.002
0733-8635/15/$ – see front matter © 2015 Elsevier Inc. All rights reserved.

derm.theclinics.com

psoriasis has come with clinical and translational research involving human subjects.

First, DAB$_{389}$IL-2 agent (denileukin diftitox [Ontak]), which causes apoptosis in activated T cells expressing functional IL-2 receptors, resulted in clinical and histologic resolution of psoriasis.[3] This was the first study proposing the general hypothesis that psoriasis is a disease mediated by activated T cells and this view has been solidified by the availability of a series of immune-targeted drugs tested in patients with psoriasis.[1,4]

Second, CTLA-4-Ig (abatacept), which blocks B7-mediated costimulation to T cells, resulted in consistent improvements of psoriasis at high doses (>10 mg/kg).[5] Improvements in psoriasis correlated with a decrease of DCs and T-cell subsets from diseased skin regions. Hence, this study indicated that disease activity could be restrained by a specific T-cell antagonist that did not deplete T cells as its primary mechanism of action. Subsequently, multiple biologics primarily targeting the T-cell activation pathway became Food and Drug Administration approved therapeutics for psoriasis.[6] The roles of different T-cell subsets in psoriasis, including Th1 (IFN-γ), Th17 (IL-17), and Th22 (IL-22), have been dissected through the testing of a range of cytokine antagonists.

CELLULAR PLAYERS IN PSORIASIS
Keratinocytes Triggering Innate and Adaptive Immune Responses

Keratinocytes respond to different danger signals, and orchestrate innate and adaptive immune responses.[1] Also, they produce antimicrobial peptides, such as cathelicidin LL-37, defensins, and S100 proteins. Keratinocytes participate in innate immune responses by increased synthesis of innate effector molecules, and also in adaptive immune responses by directing migration of new T-cell subsets into the skin through production of cytokines.[1,7]

Epidermal injury may trigger keratinocytes to activate immune responses. Injured keratinocytes produce high levels of chemokine CCL20, which functions to recruit myeloid DCs and Th17 cells into active psoriasis skin (**Fig. 1**).[1,8,9] Skin infection may also activate immune pathways leading to production of TNF or IFN-α in the skin.[1] TNF induces CCL20 and mediates recruitment of neutrophils by stimulating keratinocyte-derived CXCL chemokines, such as CXCL8. IFN-γ can induce CXCL10 and CXCL11 in keratinocytes, leading to recruitment of Th1 cells, while also increasing synthesis of Mx-1 and other antiviral gene products in keratinocytes.[10] Thymic stromal lymphopoietin,

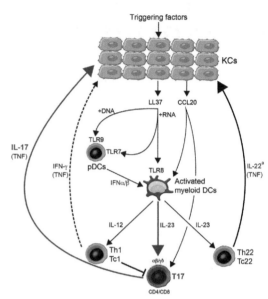

Fig. 1. Immunogenic pathway model of psoriasis. When triggering factors cause skin injury, keratinocytes (KCs) activate myeloid dendritic cells (DCs) with Toll-like receptors (TLRs), antimicrobial peptide LL37, and plasmacytoid DCs (pDCs). KCs also produce CCL20, which attracts myeloid DCs and T17. Activated myeloid DCs stimulate psoriatic T cells producing IL-17 (T17), IFN-γ (Th1, Tc1), and IL-22 (Th22, Tc22). The cytokines released by these cells further stimulate KCs, and the immune circuit is amplified by the feedback cytokines production from KCs. IL-23/T17 axis is the dominant pathogenic pathway in psoriasis (red). It is notable that IL-12/IFN-γ axis potentially suppresses IL-23/T17 axis (blue). [a] IL-19, IL-20 and IL-24 are also upregulated in psoriatic lesions and have biologic effects similar to IL-22.

which is an initiator of Th2-centered immune responses in the skin, can be synthesized by activated keratinocytes.[11]

IL-17 and IL-22 modulate distinct keratinocyte-response pathways. IL-17 is a strong inducer for synthesis of antimicrobial peptides in keratinocytes, and activation of Th22 cells results in increased production of IL-22, which can induce keratinocyte hyperplasia.[10,12]

Resident T Cells and Recruitment of Recirculating T Cells

Skin-homing T cells bind to dermal venules of the skin by interactions between cutaneous lymphocyte antigen (CLA) and E-selectin on the endothelial cells.[13] Approximately 10% of T cells in the peripheral circulation of adults have become differentiated for skin homing immunity through expression of CLA.[1] Beside those CLA$^+$ recirculating T cells, normal human skin also contains CLA$^+$

nonrecirculating resident memory T cells that mediate protective immunity in the skin.[1,14–16] Therefore, healthy skin contains abundant resident T cells and the capacity to recruit additional recirculating T cells.

Psoriatic T Cells Producing Interferon-γ, Interleukin-17, and Interleukin-22

Psoriasis lesions contain increased numbers of T cells that are CD3[+] CD2[+] CD45RO[+] CLA[+] with a subset having activation markers CD25, HLA-DR, and CD27.[17,18] Several CD4[+] T cells discretely produce IFN-γ, IL-17, and IL-22, with initial labeling of these cells as Th1, Th17, and Th22, respectively (see **Fig. 1**).[1,19] There are also CD8[+] T-cell populations that make the same range of cytokines, so these have been termed Tc1, Tc17, and Tc22, respectively. Additionally, not only αβ T cells but also γδ T cells have been found to be IL-17–producing cells in psoriasis.[20] Innate lymphoid cells, which are immune cells that lack a specific antigen receptor yet can produce an array of effector cytokines,[21] may be present and are another potential source of IL-17 in psoriasis.[22] To encompass all the IL-17–producing lymphocyte subsets in the skin, the general term T17 is used in recent papers.[23]

Psoriatic γδ T Cells

Previously, it was assumed that lesional IL-17–producing T cells expressed the αβ T-cell receptor, but recent studies characterized many IL-17–producing T cells in human and murine psoriasis skin as γδ T cells.[20] Psoriasis dermal suspensions and lesions showed significantly more CD3[+] T cells expressing γδ T-cell receptor than is the case in healthy control skin.[24] Also, γδ T cells in peripheral blood have been characterized as Vγ9Vδ2, CLA[+], and CCR6[+], and were able to produce IL-17A and activate keratinocytes via TNF and IFN-γ.[25] Thus, αβ and γδ T cells may be T17 effectors in psoriasis. In psoriasis, these cells accumulated in lesions but apparently were reduced in circulation.[1]

Regulatory T Cells in Psoriasis

Regulatory T cells (Tregs) are a heterogeneous group of cells that maintain antigen-specific self-tolerance and are one immune mechanism to prevent tissue damage caused by inflammation.[1] Tregs use diverse pathways to maintain immune tolerance, including release of inhibitory cytokines, induction of apoptosis, and inhibition of IL-2 secretion.[26] Some naturally occurring circulating Tregs can be identified as CD4[+], CD25 (IL-2R)hi,

Foxp3 (forkhead/winged helix transcription factor 3)[+], and CD127 (IL-7R)[−].[27]

When effector T cells are not being held in check by Tregs, unstrained effector T-cell effects lead to autoimmunity.[28] Some studies have shown Tregs to be dysfunctional in psoriasis, with decreased suppressive capacity, suggesting that psoriasis may result from the inability to suppress autoinflammation.[29] However, the function of skin-derived Tregs has not yet been examined, and further studies are needed to evaluate their contribution to psoriasis.[1]

Dermal Myeloid Dendritic Cells Interplaying with T Cells

DCs may be very central pathogenic players in psoriasis, both by activating T cells and by producing amplifying cytokines and chemokines during inflammation.[30] In the skin, the main DC populations include epidermal DCs (Langerhans cells) and dermal DCs (myeloid DCs and plasmacytoid DCs [pDCs]).

Dermal dendrocytes (considered to be dendritic antigen-presenting cells) were first identified using a marker to the clotting factor XIIIa,[31,32] but in recent years the α_x integrin CD11c has been found as the correct marker of myeloid DCs.[33] In fact, factor XIIIa marks CD163[+] dermal macrophages, which can have dendritic morphology.[33]

A panel of blood DC antigen (BDCA) antibodies was developed to identify human DCs. BDCA-3 (CD141) and BDCA-1 (CD1c) identify distinct circulating myeloid DC subsets.[33,34] BDCA-3[+] DCs, the minor CD11c[+] DC subset in healthy skin, were suggested to have a role in acute response to injury because they were increased two-fold after acute narrow-band UV radiation.[35] However, the major subpopulation of myeloid DCs consists of BDCA-1[+] cells in healthy skin and BDCA-1 expression is used to distinguish two distinct populations of dermal myeloid DCs: BDCA-1[+] "resident" DCs and BDCA-1[−] "inflammatory" DCs.[36] Psoriatic BDCA-1[+] DCs express markers of DC maturity, such as DC-lysosomal–associated membrane protein (DC-LAMP/CD208) and CD205 (DEC-205), in contrast to BDCA-1[−] DCs, which show increased CD209 (DC-SIGN).[1] BDCA-1[+] "resident" DCs and BDCA-1[−] "inflammatory" DCs could both stimulate T cells robustly in an allogeneic mixed lymphocyte reaction and similarly induce allogeneic T cells to produce IFN-γ and IL-17.[1] However, although there is a 30-fold increase in CD11c[+] myeloid DCs in the dermis of psoriatic skin lesions compared with uninvolved psoriatic or normal skin,[2] this increase is in the BDCA-1[−] "inflammatory" DCs, not the BDCA-1[+]

"resident" DCs.[37] Also, effective treatment of psoriasis was correlated with decreased numbers of BDCA-1⁻ "inflammatory" myeloid DCs in psoriasis lesions.[38] Myeloid cells expressing 6-sulfo-LacNAc have been proposed to be BDCA-1⁻ "inflammatory" DC precursors in psoriasis, driving strong Th17 and Th1 responses.[39]

Uncertain Role of Langerhans Cells in Psoriasis

Langerhans cells are a type of immature conventional DC that reside in the epidermis.[13] They are actively phagocytic and contain large granules known as Birbeck granules. CD1a and langerin (CD207) are used as specific markers to distinguish Langerhans cells from other DC subsets. The main role of Langerhans cells is to take up and process antigens and migrate to local skin-draining lymph nodes where they present to antigen-specific T cells.[1] However, the role of Langerhans cells in psoriasis immunopathogenesis is still unclear.[2] Recently, attention has focused on the potential importance of Langerhans cells in uninvolved skin sites of patients with psoriasis and it has been demonstrated that Langerhans cell migration is impaired in early onset psoriasis (onset before 40 years of age).[40,41] Treatment with TNF-α inhibitors (adalimumab, etanercept) and anti-p40 antibody (ustekinumab) significantly restored epidermal Langerhans cell migration in uninvolved skin.[42] Although the influence of impaired Langerhans cell mobilization on the pathogenesis of psoriasis is uncertain, the loss of Langerhans cell motility may have an impact on the ability of these cells to sense the local antigenic microenvironment and regulate cutaneous immune responses.

Macrophages Contributing to Psoriatic Inflammation

Macrophages are phagocytic cells that participate in tissue homeostasis, and in the clearance of erythrocytes and removal of cellular debris generated during tissue remodeling.[43] In normal skin, CD163 is the most useful marker of macrophages.[33] CD163 is a myeloid cell hemoglobin/haptoglobin scavenger receptor that is expressed on most mature tissue macrophages.[44] Although many investigators have used CD68 as a macrophage marker, it is not as specific as CD163 for identifying cutaneous macrophages.[45,46]

Macrophages have long been recognized as antigen-presenting cells, capable of activating memory T cells during stimulation of the adaptive arm of the immune response. However, they were unable to polarize allogeneic T cells to produce IL-17 in psoriasis.[30] Macrophages show a three-fold increase in psoriatic lesional skin and return to nonlesional skin levels after effective treatment.[47] Even though the function of macrophages in psoriasis is not yet fully understood, they likely contribute to the pathogenic inflammation in psoriasis by releasing key inflammatory products.[45]

Neutrophils in Psoriasis

Neutrophils are a first line of defense against an immune attack, possessing many intracellular antimicrobial peptides.[1] Neutrophil extracellular traps, which are weblike extracellular structures primarily composed of DNA from neutrophils, provide for a high local concentration of antimicrobial peptides. Neutrophil extracellular traps have been implicated in disease-associated autoimmune organ damage.[48] In psoriatic skin, neutrophils are predominantly located in the epidermis, and there are abundant neutrophil chemokines, such as CXCL1, CXCL2, and CXCL8/IL-8. However, neutrophils are inconsistently found in chronic psoriasis lesions and are absent from some mouse models of psoriasis.[1] Neutrophil extracellular traps have been identified in psoriasis by staining for nucleic acid with DAPI and neutrophil elastase.[49,50] In addition, neutrophils are positive for IL-17, suggesting another potential role in psoriasis.[50]

Natural Killer and NKT Cells in Psoriasis

Natural killer (NK) cells are a specialized subset of CD56⁺CD16⁺ cells with the ability to kill cancer and virally infected cells in a non–major histocompatibility complex–dependent manner.[51] It has been suggested that NK cells may play a role in psoriasis by releasing cytokines, such as IFN-γ, TNF, and IL-22.[1] NKT cells are a heterogeneous group of innate cells that share some features of NK cells and T cells.[52] There are three subsets in NKT cells, and they may also play a role in psoriasis by releasing cytokines, such as IFN-γ. CD1d, an invariant stimulator of NKT cells, is abundantly expressed in psoriatic epidermis.[53] However, the function of NK and NKT cells has not yet been fully understood, and further studies are required to evaluate their contribution to psoriasis.

IMMUNOGENIC PATHWAY MODELS OF PSORIASIS
A Model of Initiation Phase

Psoriasis can be triggered by many factors including trauma, infection, and medications, but it can be difficult to pinpoint specific triggering factors in individual patients with psoriasis. In mice, a topical biologic response modifier imiquimod (Toll-like receptor [TLR] 7 agonist) induces psoriasiform skin inflammation mediated by the IL-23/T17 axis and activated DCs.[54] Therefore, TLRs may trigger signal-transduction pathways that turn on expression of genes with important functions in psoriasis.

Gilliet and Lande[55–57] have suggested a model of psoriasis initiation involving TLRs, antimicrobial peptide LL37, and pDCs (see **Fig. 1**). When triggering factors cause skin injury, keratinocytes produce LL37 in response. Then, LL37/DNA complexes activate pDCs by binding to intracellular TLR9, and LL37/RNA complexes activate pDCs through TLR7. Activated pDCs produce type I IFN-α and -β, which activate myeloid DCs. In addition, LL37/RNA complexes can directly activate myeloid DCs through TLR8. Extracellular DNA has recently been shown in the epidermis in association with neutrophil extracellular traps, supporting this model of psoriasis initiation.[49,58]

A Model of Immune Circuits

A proximal axis of the next psoriatic immune pathway is through activated myeloid DCs (see **Fig. 1**). These cells can drive T-cell activation and cytokine production through IL-23 and IL-12.[1] Also, they produce IL-20 in psoriasis lesions, and this could be a driver of epidermal hyperplasia.[46] The importance of myeloid DCs in psoriasis was first emphasized by early experiments that demonstrated that psoriasis lesion–derived dermal DCs stimulate a T-cell response with production of IL-2 and IFN-γ.[59] This role of myeloid DCs is now confirmed by recent clinical trials, which have shown that CD11c$^+$ DC cell counts were increased in psoriasis lesions and reduced with all successful treatments studied (alefacept, efalizumab, etanercept, infliximab, narrow-band UV radiation).[1]

In the next steps in the central pathogenic psoriatic pathway, IL-23 is required for expansion and survival of T17 that produces IL-17 (see **Fig. 1**). IL-23 is composed of two chains, the unique p19 chain and the p40 chain shared with IL-12. In psoriasis lesions, abundant IL-23 is available from BDCA-1$^-$ "inflammatory" DCs, BDCA-1$^+$ "resident" DCs, and macrophages.[45,60]

The immune circuit described previously is amplified by the reaction of keratinocytes and myeloid DCs. In response to cytokines from each of T-cell subsets, keratinocytes upregulate mRNAs for a range of inflammatory products, which feedback on immune cells in the skin so that chronic T-cell activation persists.[1] For example, there is a skewed Th1 cell polarization profile in psoriasis, and these Th1 cells migrate into psoriatic lesions by T-cell chemokines, such as CXCL9, CXCL10, and CXCL11, which are produced by myeloid cells and keratinocytes.[61]

Interleukin-17, a Key Cytokine in Psoriasis

The importance of IL-17 has been supported by ex vivo experiments, psoriatic transcriptome studies, and clinical trials with evolving IL-17 antagonists.[1] Ex vivo studies have shown that psoriatic lesional T cells produce abundant IL-17 when activated by anti-CD3/CD28 or PMA/ionomycin, whereas T cells from healthy skin did not produce IL-17 after the same stimuli.[62] Gene set enrichment analysis revealed the enrichment of the keratinocyte IL-17 gene set in the psoriasis transcriptome.[63] Finally, clinical studies have shown that blockade of IL-17A or the IL-17 receptor A subunit can reverse clinical, histologic, and molecular features of psoriasis in approximately 80% of patients with psoriasis given higher levels of the antagonists.[64–67] The strong effect of IL-17 antagonists even raises a question about the pathogenic functions of Th1 and Th22 cell subsets in chronic disease, although there are clear molecular pathways in psoriasis that can be traced to individual cytokines of each T-cell class.[1]

Keratinocytes are the main cell type expressing the receptors for IL-17 (IL-17R) in psoriasis. In previous experiments of human keratinocytes with monolayer culture, IL-17 regulated only a small list of 35 to 40 genes.[10] However, Chiricozzi and colleagues[68] have recently found that IL-17 is able to upregulate 419 gene probes and downregulate 216 gene probes using reconstructed human epidermis model, a three-dimensional epidermal skin model composed of multilayer keratinocytes supported by connective tissue. Furthermore, IL-17 stabilizes chemokine mRNA, such as CXCL1, and synergistic effects exist between IL-17 and TNF, because a combination of the two cytokines induces greater changes in gene expression than either alone.[69,70] TNF-α regulates gene expression through NF-κB, whereas major signaling pathway of IL-17 is through CCAAT/enhancer binding protein transcription.[71,72] IL-17 also induces IL-19 and IL-36γ in psoriasis lesions, which may then lead to proliferative responses in keratinocytes.[1] Therefore, IL-17 is the most important pathogenic stimulant of keratinocytes in psoriasis.

Tumor Necrosis Factor-α

TNF-α can be produced by many cell types including keratinocytes, T cells, and psoriatic BDCA-1$^-$ "inflammatory" DCs.[30,73,74] The multifaceted role of TNF-α in psoriasis has been evaluated in clinical trials of TNF-α inhibitors. When patients with psoriasis received etanercept (TNF-α inhibitor), psoriatic lesional DCs had lower levels of costimulatory molecules.[47] In vitro experiments also revealed that DCs generated in the presence of etanercept downregulated maturation markers and costimulatory molecules (CD86, HLA-DR, and CD11c), and DCs were less able to stimulate allogeneic T-cell proliferation. Therefore, a key effect of TNF-α is regulation of antigen-presenting cells, and TNF-α inhibitors can impair DC–T-cell interactions, resulting in decreased epidermal stimulation by T-cell cytokines.[23,75] More specifically, TNF-α is an activator of IL-23 synthesis in DCs, and the clinical benefit seen with TNF-α blockade is linked to suppression of the IL-23/T17 axis.[47]

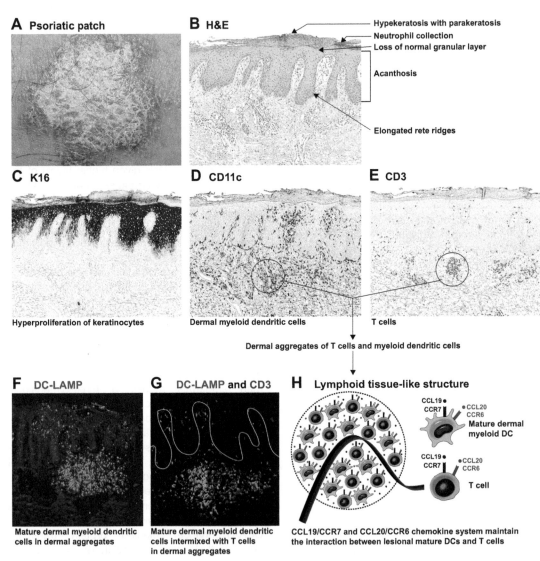

Fig. 2. Clinical and histologic features of psoriasis. (*A*) Erythematous scaly patch of psoriatic lesion. (*B*) Histology of psoriatic skin biopsy with hematoxylin and eosin (H&E) stain. The outermost layer of the epidermis (stratum corneum) is greatly thickened (hyperkeratosis) with the retention of nuclei (parakeratosis). Neutrophils collect in the stratum corneum and epidermis. There is a loss of the normal granular layer. Epidermis is thickened (acanthosis) with elongation into the dermis (rete ridges). (*C*) Keratin 16 (K16) overexpression in the epidermis indicating hyperproliferation of keratinocytes. (*D*) Increased number of CD11c+ dermal myeloid dendritic cells. (*E*) Increased number of CD3+ T cells. (*F*) Immunofluorescence of DC-LAMP+ mature dermal myeloid dendritic cells in dermal aggregates. (*G*) Double-label immunofluorescence of DC-LAMP+ mature dermal myeloid dendritic cells and CD3+ T cells. (*H*) Schematic review of lymphoid tissue–like structure in dermal aggregates. All images original magnification ×10.

Interferon-γ

In the past, Th1 pathway was considered to be the dominant pathogenic model for psoriasis.[76] Th1 cells, producing IFN-γ, are abundant in psoriasis lesions and blood, and they are reduced with successful therapy. Furthermore, approximately 400 of the genes upregulated in psoriasis lesions can be traced to signal transducer and activator of transcription 1 activation, a key IFN-γ transcription factor.[77] However, the dominant role of IFN-γ in psoriasis is now less clear after the discovery of IL-17.[23] Most likely the IL-12/IFN-γ axis does not participate directly in maintaining chronic skin disease in psoriasis, because selective blockade of IL-23 leads to full resolution of psoriasis based on clinical, histologic, and molecular disease markers.[78] In the clinical trial of IL-23–specific monoclonal antibody,[78] high levels of IL-12 and IFN-γ mRNA were maintained, whereas IL-17 levels were dramatically reduced in patients with psoriasis. Direct blockade of IFN-γ with a neutralizing antibody in patients with psoriasis was shown to have little or no therapeutic benefit, suggesting this cytokine does not directly drive the psoriasis phenotype in chronic lesions.[79]

Instead of direct impact on psoriasis pathogenesis, it is likely that the main effect of IFN-γ is activating antigen-presenting cells early in the psoriatic cascade.[80] It has been shown that the IL-12/IFN-γ axis potentially acts to suppress IL-17–modulated tissue injury.[81–83] Hence, theoretically, continued expression of the IL-12/IFN-γ axis in psoriasis while Th17 responses are inhibited via IL-23 or IL-17 blockade might lead to better treatment and suppression of disease, compared with combined blockade of IL-12 and IL-23.

IMMUNOLOGIC CONTRIBUTIONS TO HISTOPATHOLOGIC CHANGES

Psoriatic immune pathways result in the production of psoriatic cytokines, and these contribute to histopathologic changes of skin. Collectively, the cytokines IL-17, IFN-γ, IL-22, and TNF can cause keratinocyte proliferation and cytokine, chemokine, and antimicrobial peptide production (see **Fig. 1**).[10,63,70,84–87] This becomes a self-amplifying loop, where these products act back on the DCs, T cells, and neutrophils to perpetuate the cutaneous inflammatory process.[1]

The result is a well-demarcated, heavily scaled plaque of psoriasis (**Fig. 2**A). Keratinocytes move through the epidermis over 4 to 5 days, a 10-fold acceleration over normal and the epidermis is greatly thickened (acanthosis) (see **Fig. 2**B).[88]

Keratin 16 is overexpressed indicating hyperproliferation of keratinocytes (see **Fig. 2**C). Because the normal process of differentiation cannot occur, there is a loss of the normal granular layer, thickened stratum corneum (hyperkeratosis), and retention of nuclei in the upper layers and stratum corneum (parakeratosis) (see **Fig. 2**B). Scaling and the consequential break in the protective barrier are caused by failure of keratinocytes to stack normally, secrete extracellular lipids, and adhere to one another.[88] There are neutrophils collected in the epidermis and stratum corneum (spongiform pustule of Kogoj and Munro microabscess).

In the dermis, there are abundant mononuclear cells, predominantly myeloid cells and T cells (see **Fig. 2**D, E). Dermal aggregates, manly composed of DC-LAMP+ mature myeloid DCs (see **Fig. 2**F) and T cells (see **Fig. 2**F, G), constitute lymphoid tissuelike structures mimicking the T-cell areas of secondary lymphoid organs.[47,89,90] CCL19, a lymphoid-organizing chemokine, is selectively produced within dermal aggregates and recruits CCR7+ (self-antigen–specific) T cells and DCs into this focus (see **Fig. 2**H).[90] CCR6, a receptor for CCL20 attracting myeloid DCs and T cells, is also coexpressed in T cells and almost all the mature dermal myeloid DCs in the dermal aggregates.[89] These CCL19/CCR7 and CCL20/CCR6 chemokine systems may be crucial in self-maintaining the interaction between lesional mature DCs and T cells where T cells are effectively activated in situ.[89,90]

SUMMARY

Clinical and translational research in human subjects has enabled a better understanding of the immunology of psoriasis, and subsequently the development of novel immune-targeted therapeutics. IL-23/T17 is now recognized as the major axis of the psoriatic immune pathway, and antagonists to IL-23 or IL-17 result in the ability to control most of the signs and symptoms of clinical disease in approximately 80% of patients with psoriasis. However, phase 2 and 3 studies with a range of IL-23 and IL-17 antagonists are just being completed. Further studies must determine whether stable clinical benefits can be obtained by long-term administration of antagonists. Also, the safety of long-term cytokine antagonism must be confirmed. Furthermore, many basic questions about psoriasis remain to be answered. Antigens that drive T-cell response have to be elucidated. Tolerance mechanisms may be defective in psoriasis skin lesions and more work is needed to better understand these mechanisms. These hurdles can be overcome through clinical and translational studies, thus taking many steps forward to the ultimate cure of psoriasis.

REFERENCES

1. Lowes MA, Suárez-Fariñas M, Krueger JG. Immunology of psoriasis. Annu Rev Immunol 2014;32:227–55.

2. Perera GK, Di Meglio P, Nestle FO. Psoriasis. Annu Rev Pathol 2012;7:385–422.

3. Gottlieb SL, Gilleaudeau P, Johnson R, et al. Response of psoriasis to a lymphocyte-selective toxin (DAB389IL-2) suggests a primary immune, but not keratinocyte, pathogenic basis. Nat Med 1995;1:442–7.

4. Valdimarsson H, Bake BS, Jónsdótdr I, et al. Psoriasis: a disease of abnormal keratinocyte proliferation induced by T lymphocytes. Immunol Today 1986;7:256–9.

5. Abrams JR, Lebwohl MG, Guzzo CA, et al. CTLA4Ig-mediated blockade of T-cell costimulation in patients with psoriasis vulgaris. J Clin Invest 1999;103:1243–52.

6. Nograles KE, Krueger JG. Anti-cytokine therapies for psoriasis. Exp Cell Res 2011;317:1293–300.

7. Nestle FO, Di Meglio P, Qin JZ, et al. Skin immune sentinels in health and disease. Nat Rev Immunol 2009;9:679–91.

8. Martin DA, Towne JE, Kricorian G, et al. The emerging role of IL-17 in the pathogenesis of psoriasis: preclinical and clinical findings. J Invest Dermatol 2013;133(1):17–26.

9. Kennedy-Crispin M, Billick E, Mitsui H, et al. Human keratinocytes' response to injury upregulates CCL20 and other genes linking innate and adaptive immunity. J Invest Dermatol 2012;132:105–13.

10. Nograles KE, Zaba LC, Guttman-Yassky E, et al. Th17 cytokines interleukin (IL)-17 and IL-22 modulate distinct inflammatory and keratinocyte-response pathways. Br J Dermatol 2008;159:1092–102.

11. Takai T. TSLP expression: cellular sources, triggers, and regulatory mechanisms. Allergol Int 2012;61:3–17.

12. Eyerich S, Eyerich K, Pennino D, et al. Th22 cells represent a distinct human T cell subset involved in epidermal immunity and remodeling. J Clin Invest 2009;119:3573–85.

13. Murphy K. Janeway's immunobiology. New York: Garland Science; 2011.

14. Streilein JW. Skin-associated lymphoid tissues (SALT): origins and functions. J Invest Dermatol 1983;80(Suppl):12s–6s.

15. Egawa G, Kabashima K. Skin as a peripheral lymphoid organ: revisiting the concept of skin-associated lymphoid tissues. J Invest Dermatol 2011;131:2178–85.

16. Di Meglio P, Perera GK, Nestle FO. The multitasking organ: recent insights into skin immune function. Immunity 2011;35:857–69.

17. Bos JD, De Rie MA. The pathogenesis of psoriasis: immunological facts and speculations. Immunol Today 1999;20:40–6.

18. Ferenczi K, Burack L, Pope M, et al. CD69, HLA-DR and the IL-2R identify persistently activated T cells in psoriasis vulgaris lesional skin: blood and skin comparisons by flow cytometry. J Autoimmun 2000;14:63–78.

19. Bos JD, Hulsebosch HJ, Krieg SR, et al. Immunocompetent cells in psoriasis. In situ immunophenotyping by monoclonal antibodies. Arch Dermatol Res 1983;275:181–9.

20. Cai Y, Fleming C, Yan J. New insights of T cells in the pathogenesis of psoriasis. Cell Mol Immunol 2012;9:302–9.

21. Spits H, Cupedo T. Innate lymphoid cells: emerging insights in development, lineage relationships, and function. Annu Rev Immunol 2012;30:647–75.

22. Villanova F, Flutter B, Tosi I, et al. Characterization of innate lymphoid cells in human skin and blood demonstrates increase of NKp44+ ILC3 in psoriasis. J Invest Dermatol 2014;134:984–91.

23. Lowes MA, Russell CB, Martin DA, et al. The IL-23/T17 pathogenic axis in psoriasis is amplified by keratinocyte responses. Trends Immunol 2013;34:174–81.

24. Cai Y, Shen X, Ding C, et al. Pivotal role of dermal IL-17-producing gammadelta T cells in skin inflammation. Immunity 2011;35:596–610.

25. Laggner U, Di Meglio P, Perera GK, et al. Identification of a novel proinflammatory human skin-homing Vgamma9Vdelta2 T cell subset with a potential role in psoriasis. J Immunol 2011;187:2783–93.

26. Goodman WA, Cooper KD, McCormick TS. Regulation generation: the suppressive functions of human regulatory T cells. Crit Rev Immunol 2012;32:65–79.

27. Palmer MT, Weaver CT. Autoimmunity: increasing suspects in the CD4+ T cell lineup. Nat Immunol 2010;11:36–40.

28. Buckner JH. Mechanisms of impaired regulation by CD4(+)CD25(+)FOXP3(+) regulatory T cells in human autoimmune diseases. Nat Rev Immunol 2010;10:849–59.

29. Sugiyama H, Gyulai R, Toichi E, et al. Dysfunctional blood and target tissue CD4+CD25high regulatory T cells in psoriasis: mechanism underlying unrestrained pathogenic effector T cell proliferation. J Immunol 2005;174:164–73.

30. Zaba LC, Fuentes-Duculan J, Eungdamrong NJ, et al. Psoriasis is characterized by accumulation of immunostimulatory and Th1/Th17 cell-polarizing myeloid dendritic cells. J Invest Dermatol 2009;129:79–88.

31. Nestle FO, Zheng XG, Thompson CB, et al. Characterization of dermal dendritic cells obtained from

normal human skin reveals phenotypic and functionally distinctive subsets. J Immunol 1993;151: 6535–45.

32. Cerio R, Griffiths CE, Cooper KD, et al. Characterization of factor XIIIa positive dermal dendritic cells in normal and inflamed skin. Br J Dermatol 1989;121: 421–31.

33. Zaba LC, Fuentes-Duculan J, Steinman RM, et al. Normal human dermis contains distinct populations of CD11c+BDCA-1+ dendritic cells and CD163+FXIIIA+ macrophages. J Clin Invest 2007;117:2517–25.

34. Dzionek A, Fuchs A, Schmidt P, et al. BDCA-2, BDCA-3, and BDCA-4: three markers for distinct subsets of dendritic cells in human peripheral blood. J Immunol 2000;165:6037–46.

35. Kennedy Crispin M, Fuentes-Duculan J, Gulati N, et al. Gene profiling of narrowband UVB-induced skin injury defines cellular and molecular innate immune responses. J Invest Dermatol 2013;133: 692–701.

36. Hyder LA, Gonzalez J, Harden JL, et al. TREM-1 as a potential therapeutic target in psoriasis. J Invest Dermatol 2013;133:1742–51.

37. Johnson-Huang LM, McNutt NS, Krueger JG, et al. Cytokine-producing dendritic cells in the pathogenesis of inflammatory skin diseases. J Clin Immunol 2009;29:247–56.

38. Johnson-Huang LM, Lowes MA, Krueger JG. Putting together the psoriasis puzzle: an update on developing targeted therapies. Dis Model Mech 2012;5: 423–33.

39. Hansel A, Gunther C, Ingwersen J, et al. Human slan (6-sulfo LacNAc) dendritic cells are inflammatory dermal dendritic cells in psoriasis and drive strong TH17/TH1 T-cell responses. J Allergy Clin Immunol 2011;127:787–94.e1-9.

40. Cumberbatch M, Singh M, Dearman RJ, et al. Impaired Langerhans cell migration in psoriasis. J Exp Med 2006;203:953–60.

41. Shaw FL, Cumberbatch M, Kleyn CE, et al. Langerhans cell mobilization distinguishes between early-onset and late-onset psoriasis. J Invest Dermatol 2010;130:1940–2.

42. Shaw FL, Mellody KT, Ogden S, et al. Treatment-related restoration of Langerhans cell migration in psoriasis. J Invest Dermatol 2014;134:268–71.

43. Mosser DM, Edwards JP. Exploring the full spectrum of macrophage activation. Nat Rev Immunol 2008;8: 958–69.

44. Fabriek BO, Dijkstra CD, van den Berg TK. The macrophage scavenger receptor CD163. Immunobiology 2005;210:153–60.

45. Fuentes-Duculan J, Suarez-Farinas M, Zaba LC, et al. A subpopulation of CD163-positive macrophages is classically activated in psoriasis. J Invest Dermatol 2010;130:2412–22.

46. Wang F, Lee E, Lowes MA, et al. Prominent production of IL-20 by CD68+/CD11c+ myeloid-derived cells in psoriasis: gene regulation and cellular effects. J Invest Dermatol 2006;126:1590–9.

47. Zaba LC, Cardinale I, Gilleaudeau P, et al. Amelioration of epidermal hyperplasia by TNF inhibition is associated with reduced Th17 responses. J Exp Med 2007;204:3183–94.

48. Knight JS, Carmona-Rivera C, Kaplan MJ. Proteins derived from neutrophil extracellular traps may serve as self-antigens and mediate organ damage in autoimmune diseases. Front Immunol 2012;3:380.

49. Aubert P, Suarez-Farinas M, Mitsui H, et al. Homeostatic tissue responses in skin biopsies from NOMID patients with constitutive overproduction of IL-1beta. PLoS One 2012;7:e49408.

50. Lin AM, Rubin CJ, Khandpur R, et al. Mast cells and neutrophils release IL-17 through extracellular trap formation in psoriasis. J Immunol 2011;187:490–500.

51. Dunphy S, Gardiner CM. NK cells and psoriasis. J Biomed Biotechnol 2011;2011:248317.

52. Simoni Y, Diana J, Ghazarian L, et al. Therapeutic manipulation of natural killer (NK) T cells in autoimmunity: are we close to reality? Clin Exp Immunol 2013;171:8–19.

53. Bonish B, Jullien D, Dutronc Y, et al. Overexpression of CD1d by keratinocytes in psoriasis and CD1d-dependent IFN-gamma production by NK-T cells. J Immunol 2000;165:4076–85.

54. van der Fits L, Mourits S, Voerman JS, et al. Imiquimod-induced psoriasis-like skin inflammation in mice is mediated via the IL-23/IL-17 axis. J Immunol 2009;182:5836–45.

55. Ganguly D, Chamilos G, Lande R, et al. Self-RNA-antimicrobial peptide complexes activate human dendritic cells through TLR7 and TLR8. J Exp Med 2009;206:1983–94.

56. Gilliet M, Lande R. Antimicrobial peptides and self-DNA in autoimmune skin inflammation. Curr Opin Immunol 2008;20:401–7.

57. Lande R, Gregorio J, Facchinetti V, et al. Plasmacytoid dendritic cells sense self-DNA coupled with antimicrobial peptide. Nature 2007;449:564–9.

58. Kumar V, Sharma A. Neutrophils: Cinderella of innate immune system. Int Immunopharmacol 2010;10: 1325–34.

59. Nestle FO, Turka LA, Nickoloff BJ. Characterization of dermal dendritic cells in psoriasis. Autostimulation of T lymphocytes and induction of Th1 type cytokines. J Clin Invest 1994;94:202–9.

60. Zaba LC, Fuentes-Duculan J, Eungdamrong NJ, et al. Identification of TNF-related apoptosis-inducing ligand and other molecules that distinguish inflammatory from resident dendritic cells in patients with psoriasis. J Allergy Clin Immunol 2010;125:1261–8.e9.

61. Austin LM, Ozawa M, Kikuchi T, et al. The majority of epidermal T cells in psoriasis vulgaris lesions

can produce type 1 cytokines, interferon-gamma, interleukin-2, and tumor necrosis factor-alpha, defining TC1 (cytotoxic T lymphocyte) and TH1 effector populations: a type 1 differentiation bias is also measured in circulating blood T cells in psoriatic patients. J Invest Dermatol 1999;113: 752–9.

62. Lowes MA, Kikuchi T, Fuentes-Duculan J, et al. Psoriasis vulgaris lesions contain discrete populations of Th1 and Th17 T cells. J Invest Dermatol 2008;128:1207–11.

63. Suárez-Fariñas M, Lowes MA, Zaba LC, et al. Evaluation of the psoriasis transcriptome across different studies by gene set enrichment analysis (GSEA). PLoS One 2010;5:e10247.

64. Krueger JG, Fretzin S, Suarez-Farinas M, et al. IL-17A is essential for cell activation and inflammatory gene circuits in subjects with psoriasis. J Allergy Clin Immunol 2012;130:145–54.e9.

65. Papp KA, Leonardi C, Menter A, et al. Brodalumab, an anti-interleukin-17-receptor antibody for psoriasis. N Engl J Med 2012;366:1181–9.

66. Papp KA, Reid C, Foley P, et al. Anti-IL-17 receptor antibody AMG 827 leads to rapid clinical response in subjects with moderate to severe psoriasis: results from a phase I, randomized, placebo-controlled trial. J Invest Dermatol 2012; 132:2466–9.

67. Leonardi C, Matheson R, Zachariae C, et al. Anti-interleukin-17 monoclonal antibody ixekizumab in chronic plaque psoriasis. N Engl J Med 2012;366: 1190–9.

68. Chiricozzi A, Nograles KE, Johnson-Huang LM, et al. IL-17 induces an expanded range of downstream genes in reconstituted human epidermis model. PLoS One 2014;9:e90284.

69. Datta S, Novotny M, Pavicic PG Jr, et al. IL-17 regulates CXCL1 mRNA stability via an AUUUA/tristetraprolin-independent sequence. J Immunol 2010;184:1484–91.

70. Chiricozzi A, Guttman-Yassky E, Suarez-Farinas M, et al. Integrative responses to IL-17 and TNF-alpha in human keratinocytes account for key inflammatory pathogenic circuits in psoriasis. J Invest Dermatol 2011;131:677–87.

71. Ruddy MJ, Wong GC, Liu XK, et al. Functional cooperation between interleukin-17 and tumor necrosis factor-alpha is mediated by CCAAT/enhancer-binding protein family members. J Biol Chem 2004;279:2559–67.

72. Shen F, Hu Z, Goswami J, et al. Identification of common transcriptional regulatory elements in interleukin-17 target genes. J Biol Chem 2006;281: 24138–48.

73. Lowes MA, Chamian F, Abello MV, et al. Increase in TNF-alpha and inducible nitric oxide synthase-expressing dendritic cells in psoriasis and reduction with efalizumab (anti-CD11a). Proc Natl Acad Sci U S A 2005;102:19057–62.

74. Zaba LC, Krueger JG, Lowes MA. Resident and "inflammatory" dendritic cells in human skin. J Invest Dermatol 2009;129:302–8.

75. Summers deLuca L, Gommerman JL. Fine-tuning of dendritic cell biology by the TNF superfamily. Nat Rev Immunol 2012;12:339–51.

76. Lew W, Bowcock AM, Krueger JG. Psoriasis vulgaris: cutaneous lymphoid tissue supports T-cell activation and "type 1" inflammatory gene expression. Trends Immunol 2004;25:295–305.

77. Johnson-Huang LM, Suarez-Farinas M, Pierson KC, et al. A single intradermal injection of IFN-gamma induces an inflammatory state in both non-lesional psoriatic and healthy skin. J Invest Dermatol 2012; 132:1177–87.

78. Sofen H, Smith S, Matheson RT, et al. Guselkumab (an IL-23–specific mAb) demonstrates clinical and molecular response in patients with moderate-to-severe psoriasis. J Allergy Clin Immunol 2014;133: 1032–40.

79. Harden J, Johnson-Huang LM, Chamian MF, et al. Humanized anti-IFN-gamma (HuZAF) in the treatment of psoriasis. J Allergy Clin Immunol 2014. [Epub ahead of print].

80. Kryczek I, Bruce AT, Gudjonsson JE, et al. Induction of IL-17+ T cell trafficking and development by IFN-gamma: mechanism and pathological relevance in psoriasis. J Immunol 2008;181:4733–41.

81. Zhang J. Yin and yang interplay of IFN-gamma in inflammation and autoimmune disease. J Clin Invest 2007;117:871–3.

82. Cua DJ, Sherlock J, Chen Y, et al. Interleukin-23 rather than interleukin-12 is the critical cytokine for autoimmune inflammation of the brain. Nature 2003;421:744–8.

83. Becher B, Durell BG, Noelle RJ. Experimental autoimmune encephalitis and inflammation in the absence of interleukin-12. J Clin Invest 2002;110: 493–7.

84. Banno T, Gazel A, Blumenberg M. Effects of tumor necrosis factor-alpha (TNF alpha) in epidermal keratinocytes revealed using global transcriptional profiling. J Biol Chem 2004;279:32633–42.

85. Wolk K, Kunz S, Witte E, et al. IL-22 increases the innate immunity of tissues. Immunity 2004; 21:241–54.

86. Harper EG, Guo C, Rizzo H, et al. Th17 cytokines stimulate CCL20 expression in keratinocytes in vitro and in vivo: implications for psoriasis pathogenesis. J Invest Dermatol 2009;129:2175–83.

87. Blumenberg M. SKINOMICS: transcriptional profiling in dermatology and skin biology. Curr Genomics 2012;13:363–8.

88. Lowes MA, Bowcock AM, Krueger JG. Pathogenesis and therapy of psoriasis. Nature 2007;445:866–73.

89. Kim TG, Jee H, Fuentes-Duculan J, et al. Dermal clusters of mature dendritic cells and T cells are associated with the CCL20/CCR6 chemokine system in chronic psoriasis. J Invest Dermatol 2014;134:1462–5.

90. Mitsui H, Suarez-Farinas M, Belkin DA, et al. Combined use of laser capture microdissection and cDNA microarray analysis identifies locally expressed disease-related genes in focal regions of psoriasis vulgaris skin lesions. J Invest Dermatol 2012;132:1615–26.

Psoriasis and the Life Cycle of Persistent Life Effects

Marisa Kardos Garshick, MD[a], Alexa Boer Kimball, MD, MPH[b],*

KEYWORDS

- Psoriasis • Physical comorbidities • Psychological comorbidities • Stigma • Life effects

KEY POINTS

- People with psoriasis suffer from multiple medical and psychological comorbidities.
- Many of the comorbidities affect patients with psoriasis at a younger age than they do the general population and can persist throughout the lives of these individuals.
- Dermatologists should be able to identify these comorbidities and facilitate intervention when appropriate.

INTRODUCTION

Psoriasis is a chronic, systemic, inflammatory disease affecting about 1% to 3% of the population worldwide.[1] Although psoriasis may occur at any age, the peak periods of onset are 16 to 22 and 50 to 60 years of age, with majority of patients developing the disease before age 40.[1,2] Psoriasis primarily affects the elbows, knees, scalp, genitals, and trunk, but can involve any body location.[3]

In addition to cutaneous manifestations, psoriasis is associated with significant physical and behavioral comorbidities.[4,5] Moreover, the visibility of the skin lesions creates a strong psychological burden involving relationships, work, social activities and overall well-being (**Table 1**).[6] It is known that psoriasis has a serious impact on health-related quality of life (HRQL)[7] and it has been proposed that the various physical, social, and psychological impairments may have a cumulative impact on a patient's life course.[5] Persons with psoriasis have a greater prevalence of

comorbidities across all age groups when compared with those without.[8] We emphasize here that some comorbidities start early in life and have implications throughout the following stages of life (**Figs. 1** and **2**). Ultimately, some comorbidities are difficult to reverse and may have serious health consequences, even if the skin disease is well-controlled. Herein, we highlight the relevant age groups most affected or affected differently than the general population.

CHILDHOOD (BIRTH TO 21 YEARS OLD)

The prevalence of psoriasis in children up to 18 years of age is approximately 0.71%, with rates increasing with age.[9] Among children, the mean age at onset of psoriasis is between 6 and 10 years old.[10,11] The rate of associated medical conditions in psoriasis patients under 20 years old is twice as high as those without psoriasis.[9] Childhood psoriasis has been associated with an increased prevalence rate of hyperlipidemia (2.15), obesity

Funding Sources: None.

Conflict of Interest: Dr M.K. Garshick has no conflicts of interest to declare. Dr A.B. Kimball is an Investigator and Consultant and receives grants and honoraria from Abbott, Centocor, and Amgen.

[a] Department of Dermatology, Massachusetts General Hospital, Boston, MA 02114, USA; [b] Department of Dermatology, Massachusetts General Hospital, 50 Staniford Street, Suite 240, Boston, MA 02114, USA

* Corresponding author.

E-mail address: akimball@mgh.harvard.edu

Dermatol Clin 33 (2015) 25–39

http://dx.doi.org/10.1016/j.det.2014.09.003

Table 1
Social periods and physical and behavioral comorbidities affecting psoriasis patients at different life stages

Childhood	Young Adulthood	Mid Adulthood	Late Adulthood
Birth to 21 y old	21 to 35 y old	35 to 65 y old	65 to death
Hyperlipidemia	Stigma	Career	Atherosclerosis
Obesity	Relationships	Psoriatic arthritis	Chronic kidney disease
Hypertension	Pregnancy	Metabolic syndrome	Stroke
Diabetes mellitus	Tobacco use	Diabetes mellitus	Parkinsonism
Rheumatoid arthritis	Alcohol	Dyslipidemia	Malignancy
Crohn's disease	Depression	Hypertension	Mortality
Depression	Obesity	Chronic obstructive pulmonary disease	
Anxiety	Inflammatory bowel disease	Hepatic disease	
	Celiac disease		
	Nonmelanoma skin cancer		
	Myocardial infarction		

(1.70), hypertension (1.89), diabetes mellitus (DM; 2.01), rheumatoid arthritis (5.21), and Crohn's disease (3.69).[9]

Teasing, taunting, and bullying have been identified against patients with psoriasis, particularly during adolescence, but even as early as kindergarten.[12] Prior studies have shown that being bullied and teased as a school-aged child is associated with loneliness, ostracism, and development of social phobia.[13,14] Moreover, pediatric

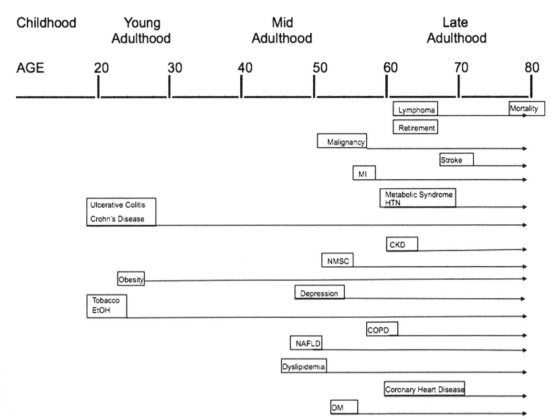

Fig. 1. Age of onset and duration of comorbidities in the general population.

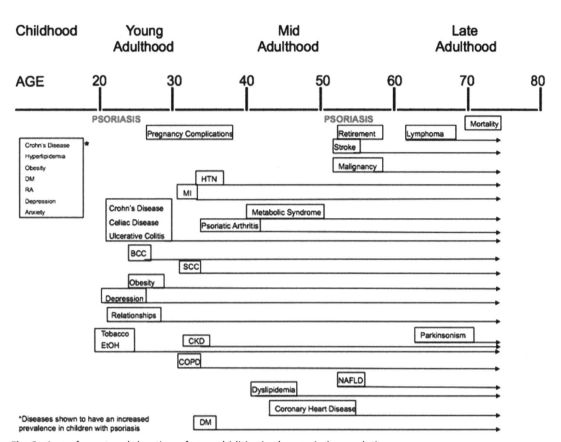

Fig. 2. Age of onset and duration of comorbidities in the psoriasis population.

patients with psoriasis are at increased risk of psychiatric disorders, including depression and anxiety, compared with those without psoriasis.[15] Depression at a young age strongly increases the risk of more depressive episodes and anxiety disorders later in life,[16] suggesting the long-term impact of childhood psoriasis on psychiatric outcomes and psychosocial growth.

YOUNG ADULTHOOD (21 TO 35 YEARS OLD)
Stigma

Stigmatization has long been reported in patients with psoriasis.[17,18] As a result of the visibility of psoriatic lesions, patients experience rejection from common places, including gyms, pools, hairdressers, and jobs,[17] and describe being subject to ridicule by some health professionals.[12] Even when compared with a group of patients with other skin conditions, patients with psoriasis reported significantly more experiences of stigmatization.[18]

Feelings of stigmatization affect self-confidence and cause embarrassment that results in avoidance of relationships, and social and employment opportunities,[6] leading to feelings of restriction in everyday life.[19] Perceptions of stigmatization are significantly related to the psychological distress and the degree of disability that psoriasis patients experience.[20] Psychological factors were stronger determinants of disability than disease location, duration, or severity.[20] Even after improvement in the skin condition, feelings of stigmatization do not always decrease.[21]

Relationships

During a stage in life when there is an emphasis on creating and maintaining relationships, it is crucial to recognize that psoriasis can also affect partners and relatives.[22] In a survey given to relatives and partners of patients, only 8% described that psoriasis had no effect on their quality of life. Of the respondents, 44% described limitations with holiday plans, sport and leisure activities, and evenings out, and 70% reported that treatment of their relative or partner resulted in them having to spend extra time on housework. Additionally, the quality of life of psoriasis patients was more closely related to the number of aspects of their relatives' lives that were affected than objective disease severity.[22] The negative impact of psoriasis on relationships is reflected by the higher divorce rates in psoriasis patients, compared with that in patients with other chronic conditions.[23]

More than 50% of patients, males and females, have genital involvement of their psoriasis at some stage of their lives and more than one third of psoriasis patients report often or always feeling inhibited in their sexual relationships owing to their psoriasis.[6] About 35.5% to 71.3% of patients with psoriasis report sexual problems related to their psoriasis. A reduction of greater than 75% in disease severity was associated with a twofold probability of improvement in sexual life.[24] In patients with psoriasis, 44% report feeling physically unattractive or sexually undesirable or both,[25] demonstrating the impact of psoriasis on an individual's self-image and relationships with others.

Pregnancy

Because the first peak of psoriasis onset is between ages 16 and 22, affected females are commonly of reproductive age, raising concern for the impact of psoriasis on pregnancy. Some data suggest that women with psoriasis are significantly more likely to experience pregnancy complications, including recurrent abortions, chronic hypertension, and cesarean delivery.[26] In a retrospective cohort study, psoriasis patients had a greater odds of a poor outcome composite (preterm birth and low birth weight), but not associated cesarean delivery, preeclampsia/eclampsia, or spontaneous abortion.[27] When comparing more than 3000 pregnancies in women with inflammatory skin disease to those without, there was no difference in incidence or outcome of pregnancy.[28] In 1 study, pregnant women with psoriasis (mean age, 32) were more likely to smoke, have a diagnosis of depression, and be overweight or obese before pregnancy, and were less likely to take preconceptional vitamin supplements, suggesting that the increased risk for adverse outcomes may be related to comorbidities and health behaviors in women with psoriasis.[29] Given the limited data on pregnancy outcomes in women with psoriasis, it has been recommended that pregnant women with psoriasis enter registries to better our understanding of pregnancy and psoriasis.[30]

Smoking

In the United States, the prevalence of smoking is greatest among adults 18 to 44 years old.[31] There is an increased smoking prevalence among psoriasis patients in Italy,[32,33] Finland,[34] the United Kingdom,[35,36] Norway,[37] China,[38] and the United States.[39] In a cross-sectional study using the Utah Psoriasis Initiative database, the prevalence of smoking among psoriasis patients aged 18 years or older was higher than that in the general Utah population (37% vs 13%; P<.001). The percent of psoriasis patients who smoke increases with age, whereas among the general Utah population, the percent decreases with age; in the group aged 18 and 34 years old, 32% of patients in the Utah Psoriasis Initiative database smoked compared with 13% of people in the general Utah population, and among those over 65 years old, 40% of psoriasis subjects smoked compared with 5% of the general Utah population. Although 22% of patients started smoking after the onset of psoriasis, 78% started smoking before the onset of psoriasis,[39] suggesting that smoking may contribute to psoriasis. The Nurses Health Study II found that past and current smoking was associated with psoriasis development in women.[40] Moreover, it has been reported that the risk of psoriasis is higher in former (relative risk [RR], 1.90) and current smokers (RR, 1.70) than in those who had never smoked.[32] Together, these data suggest that smoking may increase the risk of psoriasis and that psoriasis may contribute to the persistence of smoking habits.[39]

Alcohol

The prevalence of alcohol abuse and dependence in the United States among those aged 18 to 29 years old is 7.0% and 9.2% respectively, and 1.2% and 0.2% for those older than 65, demonstrating that alcohol abuse and dependence typically decrease with age.[41] Patients with psoriasis have a higher incidence of alcoholism compared with control populations.[42,43] Whether alcohol increases the risk of psoriasis or if patients with psoriasis are more likely to develop alcoholism has yet to be determined.

Several studies show that increased alcohol use and abuse are independent risk factors for psoriasis.[43,44] Psoriasis is found ten times more frequently in alcoholics compared with nonalcoholics.[45] When comparing young and middle-aged men with psoriasis (mean age, 35 years) with men with other skin diseases, psoriasis patients drank twice as much before disease onset.[44] Women (average age, 36 years) who drink 2.3 or more drinks per week were more likely to develop psoriasis; the risk of psoriasis is greatest with non–light beer intake.[46] Alcohol consumption has been linked to the onset of psoriasis, increased psoriasis severity, and decreased response to psoriasis therapies.[47]

Psoriasis may contribute to the development of problems with alcohol. Men with nonpsoriatic skin disease decreased alcohol use after their disease onset, whereas men with psoriasis had increased alcohol consumption after disease onset.[44] Psoriasis patients who experience psychosocial rejection have increased alcohol use,[17] suggesting that alcohol intake may be a result of the emotional distress associated with psoriasis.

The relationship of alcohol and psoriasis is significant; patients hospitalized for moderate-to-severe psoriasis were found to have excess mortality secondary to alcohol-related disease, including alcohol-related psychosis and liver disease.[48] Although the data suggest that one third of those with alcohol dependence or alcohol use disorders achieve remission,[49,50] the potential for relapse is a concern. As a result, the increased alcohol use in individuals with psoriasis may have a persistent medical, therapeutic (eg, methotrexate), psychological, and financial burden.

Psychiatric Disorders

Psoriasis is independently associated with depression, stress-related disorders, and behavior disorders.[51] The prevalence of depression in patients with psoriasis is 17% to 30%,[47,52,53] and up to 62% of patients report depressive symptoms.[54] Among psoriasis patients, men younger than 40 were more likely to report depressive symptoms than men older than 40.[54] A population-based cohort study demonstrated that those with psoriasis had higher rates of depression, anxiety and suicidality than those without psoriasis.[55] The hazard ratio for depression was greatest among males and those approximately 20 years old,[55] suggesting psoriasis patients may experience depression at a younger age than the general population, for which the greatest depression rates have been reported in those 45 to 54 years old.[56] Among 215 psoriasis patients, those 18 to 45 years old reported more frequent problems related to socialization, appearance, occupation and finances, in contrast with patients 45 to 65 years old, or those older than 65,[57] suggesting a possible explanation for why younger psoriasis patients experience depression. Although higher rates of depression have been seen with more severe psoriasis,[55] psychological distress does not always correlate with disease severity.[58]

It has been suggested that anti–tumor necrosis factor therapies may reduce depression in patients with psoriasis.[54,59] After treatment with adalimumab, the reduction in depressive symptoms significantly correlated with decreased psoriasis severity and improvement in HRQL.[59] Whether this is owing to disease improvement or an additive drug effect is not clear. Moreover, depression is associated with an increased risk of cardiovascular disease, suggesting that depression may contribute to the increased cardiovascular risk in patients with psoriasis.[60] These data emphasize the importance of dermatologists and all physicians to monitor for depressive symptoms in psoriasis patients.

Obesity

Patients with psoriasis tend to be overweight or obese when compared with patients without psoriasis.[39,61] In a cross-sectional study, obesity was 2 times more prevalent in psoriasis patients than in the general population[39] and in a Swedish population study, women with psoriasis had a higher prevalence of obesity.[61] In the Nurses Health Study II, females between 25 and 42 years old with increased adiposity and weight gain had a higher risk of psoriasis.[62] More specifically, weight gain from 18 years old, higher waist circumference, hip circumference, and waist–hip ratio were all associated with a higher risk of incident psoriasis.[62]

Although some studies conclude that obesity is a risk factor for psoriasis development,[32,62] a large, population-based study suggests that obesity is a consequence of psoriasis.[39] In this study, patients had a normal body mass index (BMI) at 18 years old and at the onset of psoriasis (mean age, 27.9 years), but 71% reported becoming overweight or obese after psoriasis was diagnosed,[39] raising the possibility that psoriasis may affect physical, social, and mental well-being, leading to inactivity and subsequent obesity. A systematic review and meta-analysis showed a pooled odds ratio of 1.66 for obesity in patients with psoriasis compared with those without psoriasis, with a greater risk for those with moderate-to-severe psoriasis compared with mild psoriasis.[63] Consistent with this, an International Psoriasis Council multicenter international review of 409 psoriatic children 5 to 17 years of age across America, Europe and Asia showed that excess adiposity and increased central adiposity (BMI $\geq$85th percentile) occurred in 37.9% of psoriatics compared with 20.5% of controls.[64]

Despite the association of obesity and psoriasis in childhood and young adulthood, this relationship persists through mid adulthood. In clinical trials for psoriasis, where the mean age at enrollment is approximately 45 years old, the mean weight of patients is approximately 90 kg.[65,66] A review of psoriasis clinical trials showed the average BMI for enrolled patients was 30.6 kg/m^2.[67] Similarly, in a retrospective study of psoriasis patients with a mean age of 44.1, 50% of the study population was obese.[68] In the systematic review that demonstrated an increased prevalence of obesity in psoriasis patients, the median age ranged from 36.5 to 68.6 years old,[63] suggesting the association between obesity and psoriasis can occur at any age and has the potential to persist for decades.

Although the relationship between obesity and psoriasis is still evolving, weight loss may have a role in the treatment of psoriasis; there are reports of remission of psoriasis after weight loss from gastric bypass surgery.[69–71] Additionally, weight loss has been shown to improve response to cyclosporine treatment in patients with chronic plaque psoriasis.[72] Obese children are more likely to be obese in adulthood, signifying that the effects of obesity remain throughout adulthood.[73]

Gastrointestinal Disease

There is a growing association between psoriasis and gastrointestinal diseases. The peak age of onset of inflammatory bowel disease, including ulcerative colitis or Crohn's disease, is 15 to 30 years old,[74] which approximates the age of onset of psoriasis. Reports in the literature have demonstrated an epidemiologic, genetic, and pathologic connection between psoriasis and Crohn's disease.[75,76] A recent case-control study found that psoriasis was associated with both ulcerative colitis (odds ratio, 1.64) and Crohn's disease (odds ratio, 2.49). The association with ulcerative colitis was statistically significant in 20- to 39-year-old males, whereas that for Crohn's disease was significant for males and females 20 to 59 years old.[77] Epidemiologic studies demonstrate that the frequencies of Crohn's disease and ulcerative colitis are increased in patients with psoriasis with prevalence ratios of 2.1 and 2.0, respectively.[8] Celiac disease has been reported to have an increased prevalence (4.3%) in patients with psoriasis[78] and there is an increased risk of psoriasis in individuals diagnosed with celiac disease with an increased risk across all age groups.[79] Celiac disease–associated antibodies have been linked with an increased severity of psoriasis.[80] Moreover, a small percentage of patients with psoriasis and antigliadin antibodies have shown improvement on a gluten-free diet.[81]

Nonmelanoma Skin Cancer

A nationwide, population-based study in Denmark found that patients with psoriasis are at a 1.4 increased risk of cancer than the general population.[82] A significantly elevated risk was seen most commonly with nonmelanoma skin cancer (NMSC). Women aged 20 to 40 years had the greatest risk of basal cell carcinoma and men aged 30 to 60 had the greatest risk of squamous cell carcinoma.[82] Although the incidence of NMSC is increasing in the population younger than 40, NMSC generally occurs in those older than 50 years,[83] suggesting that psoriasis patients may initially experience NMSC at a younger age than the general population. This effect, however, persists; in another study, psoriasis patients in the 50- to 59-year-old group were most likely to develop NMSC, and the risk was higher among patients with severe psoriasis.[84] Therapies such as Psoralen ultraviolet A and biologics have been shown to increase the NMSC incidence in the psoriatic population.[85]

MID ADULTHOOD (35–65 YEARS OLD)
Career

Psoriasis can impact careers by affecting job choice, the ability to perform well, and the length of time spent at work.[86] Patients with psoriasis report a greater number of work days missed and decreased work productivity when compared with healthy individuals.[86] Of patients with severe psoriasis, 35% describe that their careers had been affected, among whom 54% were not working or retired and 34% of those attributed not working to psoriasis.[87] In patients with severe psoriasis (median age, 54 years), 3% to 5% reported that psoriasis prevented them from getting a job,[88] and more than 4% of psoriasis patients go into early retirement between 40 and 62 years old because of their psoriasis.[89] Furthermore, 24.3% of patients with psoriasis had a reduced earning capacity owing to their psoriasis.[89] In a survey whose respondents had a mean age of 46 years old, a greater number of patients with severe psoriasis reported that psoriasis was their reason for not working when compared with those with mild psoriasis,[90] suggesting that the impact of psoriasis on career may be influenced by disease severity.

Psoriatic Arthritis

Psoriatic arthritis is often diagnosed 10 years after psoriatic skin manifestations develop, so it commonly affects people in mid adulthood, with an average age of onset of 36 years old.[91] By definition, psoriatic arthritis is an inflammation of the joints associated with psoriasis,[92] often presenting with pain and swelling of joints, but can progress to joint damage and long-term disability. The estimated prevalence of inflammatory arthritis in patients with psoriasis varies from 6% to 42%, with the accepted percentage being approximately 30%.[93]

The implications of psoriatic arthritis are not limited to joint disease. Patients with psoriatic arthritis are at a 59% and 65% increased risk of death in women and men, respectively, with cardiovascular disease being the most common cause of death.[94] When measuring HRQL indices in patients with psoriasis, joint pain correlated with significantly lower physical functioning.[7] Patients with psoriatic arthritis have a reduced quality of life and functional capacity when compared with those without joint disease.[93,95]

The Metabolic Syndrome

The metabolic syndrome is generally defined by the presence of 3 or more of the following conditions: Enlarged waist circumference, elevated fasting glucose, decreased high-density lipoprotein cholesterol, hypertriglyceridemia, and hypertension.[96] The prevalence increases with age as males and females over 60 years old are 4 and 6 times as likely to meet criteria for the metabolic syndrome than those under 40 years old.[97]

Psoriasis patients have an increased risk of developing the metabolic syndrome.[98,99] The increased risk begins at 40 to 49 years old, and persists with age.[99,100] These data suggest that psoriasis patients are more likely to develop the metabolic syndrome at a younger age than the general population. Metabolic syndrome increases the risk of coronary artery disease, stroke, and type 2 diabetes,[100] consequently increasing morbidity in patients with psoriasis.

Diabetes Mellitus

Multiple studies have demonstrated that psoriasis is independently associated with an increased risk of DM.[101,102] A systematic review and meta-analysis showed a 59% increased prevalence of DM in psoriasis patients and a 27% increased risk of developing DM among patients with psoriasis.[103] Those with severe psoriasis and younger patients may be at a higher risk of developing diabetes.[103] In a large population-based cohort study, psoriasis was associated with a 26% increased risk of type 2 diabetes in participants younger than 60 years.[104] Additionally, the risk of type 2 diabetes was higher for those diagnosed with psoriasis at an early age, greatest in those diagnosed younger than 40 years.[104] In another study, the incidence rate ratio for diabetes was greater for those with psoriasis than those without, highest in patients 0 to 29 years old but persisted through the 60- to 79-year-old group.[105] Similarly, another study showed the increased risk of DM

was present among those 40 to 49 years old.[42] Among psoriasis patients with a mean age of 42.7 years, diabetes was present in 13.8% compared with 7.3% of controls.[106] In 2008, the average age of onset of type 2 diabetes was 52.5 years of age,[107] suggesting that patients with psoriasis may develop diabetes at a younger age.

Dyslipidemia

Dyslipidemia is present in about 27.3% of psoriasis patients,[108] with psoriasis patients having a greater prevalence of hyperlipidemia when compared with the general population.[35] Significantly higher levels of total cholesterol, triglycerides, low-density lipoprotein and very low-density lipoprotein have been found in patients with psoriasis among whom the mean age was 41 years.[109] In psoriasis patients with a median age of 39 years old, males had significantly higher total cholesterol, triglyceride, and low-density lipoprotein levels, and females had significantly lower levels of high-density lipoprotein levels compared with a control population.[110] Dyslipidemia may be present at the onset of psoriasis,[111] suggesting that the lipid abnormalities in psoriasis patients may occur at an earlier age and not just related to obesity. As such, dyslipidemia in psoriasis may not be an acquired consequence of psoriasis.

Hypertension

Multiple studies and a systematic review have shown that hypertension occurs more often in patients with psoriasis than those without psoriasis,[42,61,112] with the increased prevalence beginning in the fourth or fifth decade and persisting throughout life.[42,61] A prospective study of female nurses, among whom the average age was 36 years, identified psoriasis as an independent risk factor for hypertension after adjusting for smoking status and BMI,[101] suggesting that psoriasis patients are at an increased risk for hypertension at an early age. On the contrary, after controlling for cardiovascular risk factors including age, hyperlipidemia, and BMI, a population-based study of more than 125,000 patients with severe psoriasis did not find a significant association between hypertension and psoriasis, suggesting that hypertension is not independently associated with severe psoriasis.[35] Further research is needed to better understand this relationship.

Myocardial Infarction

A prospective cohort study of psoriasis patients aged 20 to 90 years found that, after adjusting for hypertension, diabetes, history of myocardial infarction (MI), hyperlipidemia, age, sex, smoking, and BMI, psoriasis was an independent risk factor for MI.[113] The risk was greatest in younger patients, approximately 30 years of age, with severe psoriasis (RR, 3.10),[113] suggesting that psoriasis patients are at an increased risk of MI at an earlier age, because the prevalence in the general population is greatest among those over 55 years old.[114] Even after surviving an MI, individuals are at risk of reinfarction, sudden death, angina pectoris, cardiac failure, and stroke,[115] complications that can worsen morbidity and mortality.

Chronic Obstructive Pulmonary Disease

Chronic obstructive pulmonary disease (COPD) was reported in 5.7% of patients with psoriasis, among whom the mean age was 55.8 years old, compared with 3.6% of controls, demonstrating a higher prevalence of COPD in psoriasis patients.[116] Although the prevalence of COPD in the psoriasis group increased with age, there was a trend showing the strongest association between psoriasis and COPD in younger patients (ages 20–54), albeit not statistically significant, because the prevalence of COPD in the control group only increased after 55 years old.[116] Even after controlling for smoking, the association persisted.[116] In general, there is a higher prevalence of COPD in patients with psoriasis than expected based on the total US population data.[117] As the fourth leading cause of death worldwide[118] and a leading cause of hospitalizations,[119] COPD poses a substantial health and economic burden, only adding to that which already exists for psoriasis patients.

Hepatic Diseases

Nonalcoholic fatty liver disease (NAFLD) describes a spectrum of conditions ranging from benign fatty liver to nonalcoholic steatohepatitis, which can ultimately give rise to fibrosis, cirrhosis, and hepatocellular carcinoma.[120] The prevalence of NAFLD in patients with psoriasis with a mean age of 50 years old, has been reported as 47% to 59.2%,[120,121] whereas the reported prevalence in the general population is about 25%.[122]

Psoriatic patients with NAFLD are more likely to have the metabolic syndrome and greater levels of C-reactive protein than patients with psoriasis alone.[120] Insulin resistance is strongly associated with both NAFLD and the metabolic syndrome, and obesity, type 2 DM, and insulin resistance increase the risk of progression to liver fibrosis,[123] suggesting that the comorbid conditions associated with psoriasis increase the risk of liver fibrosis. Furthermore, fatty liver may increase the

likelihood of developing methotrexate-induced cirrhosis in psoriasis patients,[124] thereby complicating the treatment of psoriasis.

LATE ADULTHOOD (65 UNTIL DEATH)
Atherosclerosis and Cardiovascular Disease

The development of atherosclerosis has been associated with systemic inflammation.[125] Psoriasis is associated with elevated levels of C-reactive protein,[126] a marker of inflammation, which may be predictive of cardiovascular disease.[127] Additionally, psoriasis is an independent risk factor for coronary artery calcification.[128] When compared with nonpsoriatic patients, patients with psoriasis (mean age, 67.9 years) had a greater prevalence of coronary artery, cerebrovascular, and peripheral vascular disease.[129]

The prevalence of heart disease in psoriasis patients in the United States has been estimated at 14.3% compared with 11.3% for the general population.[117] Patients with psoriasis have an increased risk of coronary heart disease.[42] The increased prevalence of coronary heart disease in patients with psoriasis begins at 40 to 49 years of age and continues to increase with age.[42] In a Swedish study, hospitalized patients with severe psoriasis had an increased risk of cardiovascular mortality and the RR of cardiovascular mortality was highest in younger patients (<40 years old).[130]

Chronic Kidney Disease

Several studies suggest that patients with psoriasis may have an increased risk of chronic kidney disease or other renal abnormalities compared with patients without psoriasis.[131,132] In a population-based cohort study, psoriasis was an independent risk factor for moderate to advanced chronic kidney disease among patients with severe psoriasis, but not for individuals with mild psoriasis.[131] Furthermore, the age specific adjusted hazard ratio for individuals with chronic kidney disease was 3.82 (95% CI, 3.15–4.64) for patients aged 30 and 2.00 (95%CI, 1.86–2.17) for patients aged 60, demonstrating the greater risk among the younger age group compared with individuals without psoriasis in similar age groups, suggesting that individuals with psoriasis may be affected with chronic kidney disease at a younger age than those without psoriasis.[133] Importantly, patients with psoriasis are at an increased risk of death from kidney disease.[133] Although some studies suggest an association between psoriasis and renal failure,[134,135] other studies have not found an increased risk of renal failure or renal disease in patients with psoriasis.[117,136,137]

Cerebrovascular Disease (Stroke)

Stroke incidence in the general population increases with age, with the greatest incidence in individuals older than 65 years.[138] The association between psoriasis and stroke is currently evolving. A case-control study found that patients with severe psoriasis (mean age, 52.2 years) had a 44% increased risk of stroke compared with controls after adjusting for major risk factors, suggesting that psoriasis is an independent risk factor for stroke.[139] Although patients with mild psoriasis had an increased risk of stroke when compared with the general population, the risk increased with disease severity.[139] A retrospective study determined that the 10-year risk of stroke was 12% greater in patients with psoriasis when compared with the general population.[68]

Strokes have a considerable impact on one's life; it is a leading cause of mortality, but even with survival as many as 15% to 30% of patients are left permanently disabled, and 20% require institutional care after 3 months.[138] This impairment contributes to the overall disability psoriasis patients may experience with aging.

Parkinsonism

Parkinsonism is a neurologic syndrome characterized by postural instability, tremor, bradykinesia, and rigidity.[140] It has been suggested recently that individuals with psoriasis have an increased risk of parkinsonism (hazard ratio, 1.74).[140] The incidence was greatest in those over 69 years old, but there was an increased risk in the 50- to 59-year-old and 60- to 69-year-old groups as well.[140] Further studies are needed to better define the relationship between parkinsonism and psoriasis.

Malignancy

Although psoriasis patients experience NMSC at a younger age than the general population, there are multiple malignancies that warrant attention as patients age.[82] After following psoriasis patients (mean age, 50.1 years) for an average of 9.3 years, an increased risk of cancer was identified.[82] Noncutaneous malignancies that have been reported to be increased in psoriasis patients include cancers of the lung, larynx, pharynx, liver, pancreas, breast, kidney, colon, vulva, and penis.[82,141,142] In 1 study, the 7-year cumulative incidence of cancer among psoriasis patients was 4.8% and younger patients with psoriasis had the greatest risk of cancer.[143]

In a population-based study of approximately 67,761 patients, there was an overall greater incidence of cancer among psoriasis patients when compared with controls, with the greatest risk for pancreatic cancer and lymphohematopoietic malignancies.[144] A history of oral therapy and long duration of psoriasis increased the risk of malignancy.[144] The incidence of lymphoma, especially Hodgkin's lymphoma and cutaneous T-cell lymphoma, is increased in patients with psoriasis and this risk is greatest for those with more severe psoriasis.[145] Two studies have shown that the risk for lymphoma is greatest for older patients, particularly those over 60 to 65 years old.[146,147] Physicians should be aware of the risk of malignancy associated with psoriasis, particularly as it relates to systemic and biologic therapies with a gentle explanation to patients recommended.

Mortality

Prior studies[48,148] have shown an increased risk of death among patients hospitalized for psoriasis. In an observational study, there was a greater percentage of deaths among patients with psoriasis than those without psoriasis (19.6% vs 9.9%; $P<.01$), identifying psoriasis as an independent risk factor for all-cause mortality.[129] A population-based cohort study found an increased overall mortality risk in patients with severe psoriasis, but not with mild psoriasis.[149] Compared with patients without psoriasis, male and female patients with severe psoriasis died 3.5 and 4.4 years earlier, respectively.[149] Consistent with these results, patients with psoriasis die at a younger age than those without psoriasis; the mean age of death in 1 study for patients with psoriasis was 73 years old, and that for patients without psoriasis was 79 years old.[133] Patients with severe psoriasis were at increased risk of death from cardiovascular disease, malignancies, chronic lower respiratory disease, diabetes, infection, dementia, and kidney diseases.[133] The same study showed a trend for increased risk of death from intentional self-harm/suicide, accidents/unintentional injuries, and liver disease, although these results were not significant.[133]

Overall Well-Being

Approximately 75% of patients report that psoriasis has a moderate to large negative impact on their quality of life.[150] One study reported that 82.9% of patients felt the need to hide their psoriasis, and 74.3% described that their self-confidence was often affected by their psoriasis.[6] Moreover, 82.9% reported that they often or always avoided activities like swimming and sports owing to their psoriasis.[6] The reported quality-of-life responses were not influenced by disease severity.[6] Further studies suggest that disease severity does not influence the degree to which quality of life is affected.[25,151]

The impact of psoriasis on HRQL is similar to that of other major medical diseases, including cancer, arthritis, hypertension, heart disease, DM, and depression,[7] although some report psoriasis is more detrimental to life quality than angina or hypertension.[152] The impact of psoriasis is greatest on physical and mental functioning, and both psoriatic arthritis and the number of comorbidities have been shown to predict a greater impact on the physical component of HRQL.[7] Moreover, unlike previous studies, this study found that lesion severity was associated with HRQL.[7] On the Short Form 36, a self-report health status questionnaire, patients with psoriasis scored significantly lower than those without chronic disease and had a social functioning score significantly lower than those with other chronic diseases and those without chronic disease,[6] further demonstrating the effect of psoriasis on overall well-being.

Significance of Comorbidities

When compared with patients with psoriasis but without comorbidities, patients with psoriasis and comorbidities had significantly greater hospitalization rates (incidence rate ratio, 2.27) and outpatient visits (incidence rate ratio, 1.53).[108] Furthermore, patients with comorbidities incurred $2184 greater annual total costs.[108] Treatment of these comorbidities present an additional challenge; pharmacotherapy may interfere with the systemic therapies for psoriasis or worsen the disease itself.[153]

SUMMARY

The physical, psychosocial, and behavioral conditions associated with psoriasis impact all stages of life and ultimately contribute to the cumulative impairment associated with psoriasis. The purpose of this review was to map the deep impact of psoriasis, beyond skin disease, and the long-lasting effect of the comorbidities across ages. It is evident that many of these conditions affect psoriasis patients at an earlier age than in the general population, so it is our recommendation that dermatologists and general practitioners have a general awareness of this issue to better manage psoriasis patients and consider early intervention or referrals when appropriate.

REFERENCES

1. Henseler T, Christophers E. Psoriasis of early and late onset: characterization of two types of psoriasis vulgaris. J Am Acad Dermatol 1985;13:450–6.
2. Langley RG, Krueger GG, Griffiths CE. Psoriasis: epidemiology, clinical features, and quality of life. Ann Rheum Dis 2005;64(Suppl 2):ii18–23 [discussion: ii24–5].
3. Gottlieb AB, Dann F. Comorbidities in patients with psoriasis. Am J Med 2009;122:1150.e1–9.
4. Gottlieb AB, Chao C, Dann F. Psoriasis comorbidities. J Dermatolog Treat 2008;19:5–21.
5. Kimball AB, Gieler U, Linder D, et al. Psoriasis: is the impairment to a patient's life cumulative? J Eur Acad Dermatol Venereol 2010;24:989–1004.
6. Weiss SC, Kimball AB, Liewehr DJ, et al. Quantifying the harmful effect of psoriasis on health-related quality of life. J Am Acad Dermatol 2002;47:512–8.
7. Rapp SR, Feldman SR, Exum ML, et al. Psoriasis causes as much disability as other major medical diseases. J Am Acad Dermatol 1999;41:401–7.
8. Augustin M, Reich K, Glaeske G, et al. Co-morbidity and age-related prevalence of psoriasis: analysis of health insurance data in Germany. Acta Derm Venereol 2010;90:147–51.
9. Augustin M, Glaeske G, Radtke MA, et al. Epidemiology and comorbidity of psoriasis in children. Br J Dermatol 2010;162:633–6.
10. Seyhan M, Coskun BK, Saglam H, et al. Psoriasis in childhood and adolescence: evaluation of demographic and clinical features. Pediatr Int 2006;48: 525–30.
11. Kumar B, Jain R, Sandhu K, et al. Epidemiology of childhood psoriasis: a study of 419 patients from northern India. Int J Dermatol 2004;43:654–8.
12. Magin P, Adams J, Heading G, et al. Experiences of appearance-related teasing and bullying in skin diseases and their psychological sequelae: results of a qualitative study. Scand J Caring Sci 2008;22:430–6.
13. Forero R, McLellan L, Rissel C, et al. Bullying behaviour and psychosocial health among school students in New South Wales, Australia: cross sectional survey. BMJ 1999;319:344–8.
14. McCabe RE, Antony MM, Summerfeldt LJ, et al. Preliminary examination of the relationship between anxiety disorders in adults and self-reported history of teasing or bullying experiences. Cogn Behav Ther 2003;32:187–93.
15. Kimball AB, Wu EQ, Guerin A, et al. Risks of developing psychiatric disorders in pediatric patients with psoriasis. J Am Acad Dermatol 2012; 67:651–7.e1–2.
16. Colman I, Wadsworth ME, Croudace TJ, et al. Forty-year psychiatric outcomes following

assessment for internalizing disorder in adolescence. Am J Psychiatry 2007;164:126–33.

17. Ginsburg IH, Link BG. Psychosocial consequences of rejection and stigma feelings in psoriasis patients. Int J Dermatol 1993;32:587–91.

18. Vardy D, Besser A, Amir M, et al. Experiences of stigmatization play a role in mediating the impact of disease severity on quality of life in psoriasis patients. Br J Dermatol 2002;147:736–42.

19. Fortune DG, Main CJ, O'Sullivan TM, et al. Quality of life in patients with psoriasis: the contribution of clinical variables and psoriasis-specific stress. Br J Dermatol 1997;137:755–60.

20. Richards HL, Fortune DG, Griffiths CE, et al. The contribution of perceptions of stigmatisation to disability in patients with psoriasis. J Psychosom Res 2001;50:11–5.

21. Schmid-Ott G, Kunsebeck HW, Jager B, et al. Significance of the stigmatization experience of psoriasis patients: a 1-year follow-up of the illness and its psychosocial consequences in men and women. Acta Derm Venereol 2005;85:27–32.

22. Eghlileb AM, Davies EE, Finlay AY. Psoriasis has a major secondary impact on the lives of family members and partners. Br J Dermatol 2007; 156:1245–50.

23. Frangos JE, Kimball AB. Divorce/marriage ratio in patients with psoriasis compared to patients with other chronic medical conditions. J Invest Dermatol 2008;128(Suppl 1):S87.

24. Sampogna F, Gisondi P, Tabolli S, et al. Impairment of sexual life in patients with psoriasis. Dermatology 2007;214:144–50.

25. McKenna KE, Stern RS. The impact of psoriasis on the quality of life of patients from the 16-center PUVA follow-up cohort. J Am Acad Dermatol 1997;36:388–94.

26. Ben-David G, Sheiner E, Hallak M, et al. Pregnancy outcome in women with psoriasis. J Reprod Med 2008;53:183–7.

27. Lima XT, Janakiraman V, Hughes MD, et al. The impact of psoriasis on pregnancy outcomes. J Invest Dermatol 2012;132:85–91.

28. Seeger JD, Lanza LL, West WA, et al. Pregnancy and pregnancy outcome among women with inflammatory skin diseases. Dermatology 2007;214:32–9.

29. Bandoli G, Johnson DL, Jones KL, et al. Potentially modifiable risk factors for adverse pregnancy outcomes in women with psoriasis. Br J Dermatol 2010;163:334–9.

30. Horn EJ, Chambers CD, Menter A, et al. Pregnancy outcomes in psoriasis: why do we know so little? J Am Acad Dermatol 2009;61:e5–8.

31. US Centers for Disease Control and Prevention (CDC). Cigarette smoking among adults and trends in smoking cessation- United States. MMWR Morb Mortal Wkly Rep 2009;58(44):1227–32.

32. Naldi L, Chatenoud L, Linder D, et al. Cigarette smoking, body mass index, and stressful life events as risk factors for psoriasis: results from an Italian case-control study. J Invest Dermatol 2005;125:61–7.

33. Naldi L, Parazzini F, Brevi A, et al. Family history, smoking habits, alcohol consumption and risk of psoriasis. Br J Dermatol 1992;127:212–7.

34. Poikolainen K, Reunala T, Karvonen J. Smoking, alcohol and life events related to psoriasis among women. Br J Dermatol 1994;130:473–7.

35. Neimann AL, Shin DB, Wang X, et al. Prevalence of cardiovascular risk factors in patients with psoriasis. J Am Acad Dermatol 2006;55:829–35.

36. Mills CM, Srivastava ED, Harvey IM, et al. Smoking habits in psoriasis: a case control study. Br J Dermatol 1992;127:18–21.

37. Braathen LR, Botten G, Bjerkedal T. Psoriatics in Norway. A questionnaire study on health status, contact with paramedical professions, and alcohol and tobacco consumption. Acta Derm Venereol Suppl (Stockh) 1989;142:9–12.

38. Zhang X, Wang H, Te-Shao H, et al. Frequent use of tobacco and alcohol in Chinese psoriasis patients. Int J Dermatol 2002;41:659–62.

39. Herron MD, Hinckley M, Hoffman MS, et al. Impact of obesity and smoking on psoriasis presentation and management. Arch Dermatol 2005;141:1527–34.

40. Setty AR, Curhan G, Choi HK. Smoking and the risk of psoriasis in women: nurses' health study II. Am J Med 2007;120:953–9.

41. Grant BF, Dawson DA, Stinson FS, et al. The 12-month prevalence and trends in DSM-IV alcohol abuse and dependence: United States, 1991–1992 and 2001–2002. Drug Alcohol Depend 2004; 74:223–34.

42. Sommer DM, Jenisch S, Suchan M, et al. Increased prevalence of the metabolic syndrome in patients with moderate to severe psoriasis. Arch Dermatol Res 2006;298:321–8.

43. Higgins EM, Peters TJ, du Vivier AW. Smoking, drinking and psoriasis. Br J Dermatol 1993;129: 749–50.

44. Poikolainen K, Reunala T, Karvonen J, et al. Alcohol intake: a risk factor for psoriasis in young and middle aged men? BMJ 1990;300:780–3.

45. Evstaf'ev VV, Levin MM. Dermatologic pathology in chronic alcoholics. Vestn Dermatol Venerol 1989;(8):72–4 [in Russian].

46. Qureshi AA, Dominguez PL, Choi HK, et al. Alcohol intake and risk of incident psoriasis in US women: a prospective study. Arch Dermatol 2010;146: 1364–9.

47. Kimball AB, Gladman D, Gelfand JM, et al. National Psoriasis Foundation clinical consensus on psoriasis comorbidities and recommendations for screening. J Am Acad Dermatol 2008;58:1031–42.

48. Poikolainen K, Karvonen J, Pukkala E. Excess mortality related to alcohol and smoking among hospital-treated patients with psoriasis. Arch Dermatol 1999;135:1490–3.

49. Dawson DA, Grant BF, Stinson FS, et al. Recovery from DSM-IV alcohol dependence: United States, 2001–2002. Addiction 2005;100:281–92.

50. Schutte KK, Byrne FE, Brennan PL, et al. Successful remission of late-life drinking problems: a 10-year follow-up. J Stud Alcohol 2001;62:322–34.

51. Schmitt J, Ford DE. Psoriasis is independently associated with psychiatric morbidity and adverse cardiovascular risk factors, but not with cardiovascular events in a population-based sample. J Eur Acad Dermatol Venereol 2010;24:885–92.

52. Lynde CW, Poulin Y, Guenther L, et al. The burden of psoriasis in Canada: insights from the pSoriasis Knowledge IN Canada (SKIN) survey. J Cutan Med Surg 2009;13:235–52.

53. Waters CC, Piech CT, Annunziata K. The impact of psoriasis on psychological functioning and quality of life. J Am Acad Dermatol 2009;60(Suppl):AB183.

54. Esposito M, Saraceno R, Giunta A, et al. An Italian study on psoriasis and depression. Dermatology 2006;212:123–7.

55. Kurd SK, Troxel AB, Crits-Christoph P, et al. The risk of depression, anxiety, and suicidality in patients with psoriasis: a population-based cohort study. Arch Dermatol 2010;146:891–5.

56. Lindeman S, Hamalainen J, Isometsa E, et al. The 12-month prevalence and risk factors for major depressive episode in Finland: representative sample of 5993 adults. Acta Psychiatr Scand 2000;102:178–84.

57. Gupta MA, Gupta AK. Age and gender differences in the impact of psoriasis on quality of life. Int J Dermatol 1995;34:700–3.

58. Kirby B, Richards HL, Woo P, et al. Physical and psychologic measures are necessary to assess overall psoriasis severity. J Am Acad Dermatol 2001;45:72–6.

59. Menter A, Augustin M, Signorovitch J, et al. The effect of adalimumab on reducing depression symptoms in patients with moderate to severe psoriasis: a randomized clinical trial. J Am Acad Dermatol 2010;62:812–8.

60. Frasure-Smith N, Lesperance F. Recent evidence linking coronary heart disease and depression. Can J Psychiatry 2006;51:730–7.

61. Lindegard B. Diseases associated with psoriasis in a general population of 159,200 middle-aged, urban, native Swedes. Dermatologica 1986;172: 298–304.

62. Setty AR, Curhan G, Choi HK. Obesity, waist circumference, weight change, and the risk of psoriasis in women: nurses' health study II. Arch Intern Med 2007;167:1670–5.

63. Armstrong AW, Harskamp CT, Armstrong EJ. The association between psoriasis and obesity: a systematic review and meta-analysis of observational studies. Nutr Diabetes 2012;2:e54.

64. Paller AS, Mercy K, Kwasny MJ, et al. Association of pediatric psoriasis severity with excess and central adiposity: an international cross-sectional study. JAMA Dermatol 2013;149(2):166–76.

65. Krueger GG, Papp KA, Stough DB, et al. A randomized, double-blind, placebo-controlled phase III study evaluating efficacy and tolerability of 2 courses of alefacept in patients with chronic plaque psoriasis. J Am Acad Dermatol 2002;47: 821–33.

66. Mease PJ, Goffe BS, Metz J, et al. Etanercept in the treatment of psoriatic arthritis and psoriasis: a randomised trial. Lancet 2000;356:385–90.

67. Sterry W, Strober BE, Menter A, et al. Obesity in psoriasis: the metabolic, clinical and therapeutic implications. Report of an interdisciplinary conference and review. Br J Dermatol 2007;157:649–55.

68. Kimball AB, Guerin A, Latremouille-Viau D, et al. Coronary heart disease and stroke risk in patients with psoriasis: retrospective analysis. Am J Med 2010;123:350–7.

69. de Menezes Ettinger JE, Azaro E, de Souza CA, et al. Remission of psoriasis after open gastric bypass. Obes Surg 2006;16:94–7.

70. Higa-Sansone G, Szomstein S, Soto F, et al. Psoriasis remission after laparoscopic Roux-en-Y gastric bypass for morbid obesity. Obes Surg 2004;14:1132–4.

71. Hossler EW, Maroon MS, Mowad CM. Gastric bypass surgery improves psoriasis. J Am Acad Dermatol 2011;65:198–200.

72. Gisondi P, Del Giglio M, Di Francesco V, et al. Weight loss improves the response of obese patients with moderate-to-severe chronic plaque psoriasis to low-dose cyclosporine therapy: a randomized, controlled, investigator-blinded clinical trial. Am J Clin Nutr 2008;88:1242–7.

73. Guo SS, Chumlea WC. Tracking of body mass index in children in relation to overweight in adulthood. Am J Clin Nutr 1999;70:S145–8.

74. Loftus EV Jr. Clinical epidemiology of inflammatory bowel disease: incidence, prevalence, and environmental influences. Gastroenterology 2004;126: 1504–17.

75. Lee FI, Bellary SV, Francis C. Increased occurrence of psoriasis in patients with Crohn's disease and their relatives. Am J Gastroenterol 1990;85:962–3.

76. Najarian DJ, Gottlieb AB. Connections between psoriasis and Crohn's disease. J Am Acad Dermatol 2003;48:805–21.

77. Cohen AD, Dreiher J, Birkenfeld S. Psoriasis associated with ulcerative colitis and Crohn's disease. J Eur Acad Dermatol Venereol 2009;23:561–5.

78. Gisondi P, Del Giglio M, Cozzi A, et al. Psoriasis, the liver, and the gastrointestinal tract. Dermatol Ther 2010;23:155–9.

79. Ludvigsson JF, Lindelof B, Zingone F, et al. Psoriasis in a nationwide cohort study of patients with celiac disease. J Invest Dermatol 2011;131:2010–6.

80. Woo WK, McMillan SA, Watson RG, et al. Coeliac disease-associated antibodies correlate with psoriasis activity. Br J Dermatol 2004;151:891–4.

81. Michaelsson G, Gerden B, Hagforsen E, et al. Psoriasis patients with antibodies to gliadin can be improved by a gluten-free diet. Br J Dermatol 2000;142:44–51.

82. Frentz G, Olsen JH. Malignant tumours and psoriasis: a follow-up study. Br J Dermatol 1999;140:237–42.

83. Christenson LJ, Borrowman TA, Vachon CM, et al. Incidence of basal cell and squamous cell carcinomas in a population younger than 40 years. JAMA 2005;294:681–90.

84. Lee MS, Lin RY, Chang YT, et al. The risk of developing non-melanoma skin cancer, lymphoma and melanoma in patients with psoriasis in Taiwan: a 10-year, population-based cohort study. Int J Dermatol 2012;51:1454–60.

85. Lindelof B, Sigurgeirsson B, Tegner E, et al. PUVA and cancer risk: the Swedish follow-up study. Br J Dermatol 1999;141(1):108–12.

86. Schmitt JM, Ford DE. Work limitations and productivity loss are associated with health-related quality of life but not with clinical severity in patients with psoriasis. Dermatology 2006;213:102–10.

87. Finlay AY, Coles EC. The effect of severe psoriasis on the quality of life of 369 patients. Br J Dermatol 1995;132:236–44.

88. Krueger G, Koo J, Lebwohl M, et al. The impact of psoriasis on quality of life: results of a 1998 National Psoriasis Foundation patient-membership survey. Arch Dermatol 2001;137:280–4.

89. Sohn S, Schoeffski O, Prinz J, et al. Cost of moderate to severe plaque psoriasis in Germany: a multicenter cost-of-illness study. Dermatology 2006;212:137–44.

90. Horn EJ, Fox KM, Patel V, et al. Association of patient-reported psoriasis severity with income and employment. J Am Acad Dermatol 2007;57:963–71.

91. Gladman DD, Antoni C, Mease P, et al. Psoriatic arthritis: epidemiology, clinical features, course, and outcome. Ann Rheum Dis 2005;64(Suppl 2):ii14–7.

92. Moll JM, Wright V. Psoriatic arthritis. Semin Arthritis Rheum 1973;3:55–78.

93. Zachariae H, Zachariae R, Blomqvist K, et al. Quality of life and prevalence of arthritis reported by 5,795 members of the Nordic Psoriasis Associations. Data from the Nordic Quality of Life Study. Acta Derm Venereol 2002;82:108–13.

94. Wong K, Gladman DD, Husted J, et al. Mortality studies in psoriatic arthritis: results from a single outpatient clinic. I. Causes and risk of death. Arthritis Rheum 1997;40:1868–72.

95. Husted JA, Gladman DD, Farewell VT, et al. Validating the SF-36 health survey questionnaire in patients with psoriatic arthritis. J Rheumatol 1997;24:511–7.

96. Grundy SM, Cleeman JI, Daniels SR, et al. Diagnosis and management of the metabolic syndrome: an American Heart Association/National Heart, Lung, and Blood Institute Scientific Statement. Circulation 2005;112:2735–52.

97. Ervin RB. Prevalence of metabolic syndrome among adults 20 years of age and over, by sex, age, race and ethnicity, and body mass index: United States, 2003–2006. Natl Health Stat Report 2009;(13):1–7.

98. Armstrong AW, Harskamp CT, Armstrong EJ. Psoriasis and metabolic syndrome: a systematic review and meta-analysis of observational studies. J Am Acad Dermatol 2013;68:654–62.

99. Gisondi P, Tessari G, Conti A, et al. Prevalence of metabolic syndrome in patients with psoriasis: a hospital-based case-control study. Br J Dermatol 2007;157:68–73.

100. Alsufyani MA, Golant AK, Lebwohl M. Psoriasis and the metabolic syndrome. Dermatol Ther 2010;23:137–43.

101. Qureshi AA, Choi HK, Setty AR, et al. Psoriasis and the risk of diabetes and hypertension: a prospective study of US female nurses. Arch Dermatol 2009;145:379–82.

102. Azfar RS, Seminara NM, Shin DB, et al. Increased risk of diabetes mellitus and likelihood of receiving diabetes mellitus treatment in patients with psoriasis. Arch Dermatol 2012;148:995–1000.

103. Armstrong AW, Harskamp CT, Armstrong EJ. Psoriasis and the risk of diabetes mellitus: a systematic review and meta-analysis. JAMA Dermatol 2013;149:84–91.

104. Li WQ, Han JL, Manson JE, et al. Psoriasis and risk of nonfatal cardiovascular disease in U.S. women: a cohort study. Br J Dermatol 2012;166:811–8.

105. Brauchli YB, Jick SS, Meier CR. Psoriasis and the risk of incident diabetes mellitus: a population-based study. Br J Dermatol 2008;159:1331–7.

106. Cohen AD, Sherf M, Vidavsky L, et al. Association between psoriasis and the metabolic syndrome. A cross-sectional study. Dermatology 2008;216:152–5.

107. Centers for Disease Control and Prevention (CDC). CDC's diabetes program - data and trends - distribution of age at diagnosis of diabetes among adult incident cases aged 18–79 years, United States, 1980–2008. Available at: http://www.cdc.gov/diabetes/statistics/age/fig2.htm. Accessed December 10, 2012.

108. Kimball AB, Guerin A, Tsaneva M, et al. Economic burden of comorbidities in patients with psoriasis is substantial. J Eur Acad Dermatol Venereol 2011;25:157–63.

109. Akhyani M, Ehsani AH, Robati RM, et al. The lipid profile in psoriasis: a controlled study. J Eur Acad Dermatol Venereol 2007;21:1330–2.

110. Tekin NS, Tekin IO, Barut F, et al. Accumulation of oxidized low-density lipoprotein in psoriatic skin and changes of plasma lipid levels in psoriatic patients. Mediators Inflamm 2007;2007:78454.

111. Mallbris L, Granath F, Hamsten A, et al. Psoriasis is associated with lipid abnormalities at the onset of skin disease. J Am Acad Dermatol 2006;54:614–21.

112. Armstrong AW, Harskamp CT, Armstrong EJ. The association between psoriasis and hypertension: a systematic review and meta-analysis of observational studies. J Hypertens 2013;31:433–42 [discussion: 442–3].

113. Gelfand JM, Neimann AL, Shin DB, et al. Risk of myocardial infarction in patients with psoriasis. JAMA 2006;296:1735–41.

114. Goldberg RJ, McCormick D, Gurwitz JH, et al. Age-related trends in short- and long-term survival after acute myocardial infarction: a 20-year population-based perspective (1975–1995). Am J Cardiol 1998;82:1311–7.

115. Kannel WB, Sorlie P, McNamara PM. Prognosis after initial myocardial infarction: the Framingham study. Am J Cardiol 1979;44:53–9.

116. Dreiher J, Weitzman D, Shapiro J, et al. Psoriasis and chronic obstructive pulmonary disease: a case-control study. Br J Dermatol 2008;159:956–60.

117. Pearce DJ, Morrison AE, Higgins KB, et al. The comorbid state of psoriasis patients in a university dermatology practice. J Dermatolog Treat 2005;16:319–23.

118. World Health Organization (WHO). Top 10 causes of death. Available at: http://www.who.int/mediacentre/factsheets/fs310/en/. Accessed April 5, 2014.

119. Mannino DM. COPD: epidemiology, prevalence, morbidity and mortality, and disease heterogeneity. Chest 2002;121:121S–6S.

120. Gisondi P, Targher G, Zoppini G, et al. Non-alcoholic fatty liver disease in patients with chronic plaque psoriasis. J Hepatol 2009;51:758–64.

121. Miele L, Vallone S, Cefalo C, et al. Prevalence, characteristics and severity of non-alcoholic fatty liver disease in patients with chronic plaque psoriasis. J Hepatol 2009;51:778–86.

122. Loria P, Adinolfi LE, Bellentani S, et al. Practice guidelines for the diagnosis and management of nonalcoholic fatty liver disease. A decalogue from the Italian Association for the Study of the Liver (AISF) Expert Committee. Dig Liver Dis 2010;42:272–82.

123. Schuppan D, Gorrell MD, Klein T, et al. The challenge of developing novel pharmacological therapies for non-alcoholic steatohepatitis. Liver Int 2010;30:795–808.

124. Langman G, Hall PM, Todd G. Role of non-alcoholic steatohepatitis in methotrexate-induced liver injury. J Gastroenterol Hepatol 2001;16:1395–401.

125. Hansson GK. Inflammation, atherosclerosis, and coronary artery disease. N Engl J Med 2005;352:1685–95.

126. Chodorowska G, Wojnowska D, Juszkiewicz-Borowiec M. C-reactive protein and alpha2-macroglobulin plasma activity in medium-severe and severe psoriasis. J Eur Acad Dermatol Venereol 2004;18:180–3.

127. Ridker PM, Rifai N, Cook NR, et al. Non-HDL cholesterol, apolipoproteins A-I and B100, standard lipid measures, lipid ratios, and CRP as risk factors for cardiovascular disease in women. JAMA 2005;294:326–33.

128. Ludwig RJ, Herzog C, Rostock A, et al. Psoriasis: a possible risk factor for development of coronary artery calcification. Br J Dermatol 2007;156:271–6.

129. Prodanovich S, Kirsner RS, Kravetz JD, et al. Association of psoriasis with coronary artery, cerebrovascular, and peripheral vascular diseases and mortality. Arch Dermatol 2009;145:700–3.

130. Mallbris L, Akre O, Granath F, et al. Increased risk for cardiovascular mortality in psoriasis inpatients but not in outpatients. Eur J Epidemiol 2004;19:225–30.

131. Wan J, Wang S, Haynes K, et al. Risk of moderate to advanced kidney disease in patients with psoriasis: population based cohort study. BMJ 2013;347:f5961.

132. Dervisoglu E, Akturk AS, Yildiz K, et al. The spectrum of renal abnormalities in patients with psoriasis. Int Urol Nephrol 2012;44(2):509–14.

133. Abuabara K, Azfar RS, Shin DB, et al. Cause-specific mortality in patients with severe psoriasis: a population-based cohort study in the U.K. Br J Dermatol 2010;163(3):586–92.

134. Yang YW, Keller JJ, Lin HC. Medical comorbidity associated with psoriasis in adults: a population-based study. Br J Dermatol 2011;165:1037–43.

135. Yeung H, Takeshita J, Mehta NN, et al. Psoriasis severity and the prevalence of major medical comorbidity: a population-based study. JAMA Dermatol 2013;149(10):1173–9.

136. Kaftan O, Kaftan B, Toppare MF, et al. Renal involvement in psoriasis. Dermatology 1996;192:189–90.

137. Cassano N, Vestita M, Panaro M, et al. Renal function in psoriasis patients. Eur J Dermatol 2011;21:264–5.

138. Rosamond W, Flegal K, Furie K, et al. Heart disease and stroke statistics–2008 update: a report

from the American Heart Association Statistics Committee and Stroke Statistics Subcommittee. Circulation 2008;117:e25–146.

139. Gelfand JM, Dommasch ED, Shin DB, et al. The risk of stroke in patients with psoriasis. J Invest Dermatol 2009;129:2411–8.

140. Sheu JJ, Wang KH, Lin HC, et al. Psoriasis is associated with an increased risk of parkinsonism: a population-based 5-year follow-up study. J Am Acad Dermatol 2013;68:992–9.

141. Boffetta P, Gridley G, Lindelof B. Cancer risk in a population-based cohort of patients hospitalized for psoriasis in Sweden. J Invest Dermatol 2001; 117:1531–7.

142. Olsen JH, Moller H, Frentz G. Malignant tumors in patients with psoriasis. J Am Acad Dermatol 1992;27:716–22.

143. Chen YJ, Wu CY, Chen TJ, et al. The risk of cancer in patients with psoriasis: a population-based cohort study in Taiwan. J Am Acad Dermatol 2011;65:84–91.

144. Brauchli YB, Jick SS, Miret M, et al. Psoriasis and risk of incident cancer: an inception cohort study with a nested case-control analysis. J Invest Dermatol 2009;129:2604–12.

145. Gelfand JM, Shin DB, Neimann AL, et al. The risk of lymphoma in patients with psoriasis. J Invest Dermatol 2006;126:2194–201.

146. Tavani A, La Vecchia C, Franceschi S, et al. Medical history and risk of Hodgkin's and non-Hodgkin's lymphomas. Eur J Cancer Prev 2000;9:59–64.

147. Gelfand JM, Berlin J, Van Voorhees A, et al. Lymphoma rates are low but increased in patients with psoriasis: results from a population-based cohort study in the United Kingdom. Arch Dermatol 2003;139:1425–9.

148. Lindegard B. Mortality and causes of death among psoriatics. Dermatologica 1989;179:91–2.

149. Gelfand JM, Troxel AB, Lewis JD, et al. The risk of mortality in patients with psoriasis: results from a population-based study. Arch Dermatol 2007;143: 1493–9.

150. Bhosle MJ, Kulkarni A, Feldman SR, et al. Quality of life in patients with psoriasis. Health Qual Life Outcomes 2006;4:35.

151. Spuls PI, Lecluse LL, Poulsen ML, et al. How good are clinical severity and outcome measures for psoriasis? Quantitative evaluation in a systematic review. J Invest Dermatol 2010;130:933–43.

152. Finlay AY, Khan GK, Luscombe DK, et al. Validation of sickness impact profile and psoriasis disability index in psoriasis. Br J Dermatol 1990;123:751–6.

153. Gerdes S, Zahl VA, Knopf H, et al. Comedication related to comorbidities: a study in 1203 hospitalized patients with severe psoriasis. Br J Dermatol 2008;159:1116–23.

Psoriasis Is a Systemic Disease with Multiple Cardiovascular and Metabolic Comorbidities

Caitriona Ryan, MD[a],*, Brian Kirby, MD[b]

KEYWORDS

- Psoriasis • Comorbidities • Cardiovascular • Myocardial infarction • Obesity • Metabolic syndrome
- Diabetes • Smoking

KEY POINTS

- Patients with moderate to severe psoriasis have a reduced life expectancy of approximately 5 years because of cardiovascular disease.
- There is an increased prevalence of traditional cardiovascular risk factors in patients with moderate to severe psoriasis; these include hypertension, cigarette smoking, dyslipidemia, diabetes mellitus, and obesity.
- Alcohol misuse and depression are also increased in this population and may contribute to excess cardiovascular mortality.
- In diseases such as rheumatoid arthritis, systemic inflammation plays a role in the development of cardiovascular disease; this may also be the case in psoriasis.
- It is recommended that patients with moderate to severe psoriasis should be screened for cardiovascular risk factors and that these should be managed according to national guidelines.

INTRODUCTION

Once considered to be solely a cutaneous disease, there is now robust evidence that psoriasis is associated with systemic inflammation and a significantly increased risk of cardiovascular disease. Moderate to severe psoriasis is associated with a higher incidence of cardiovascular risk factors such as diabetes mellitus, obesity, smoking, and the metabolic syndrome.[1,2] It is now well established that patients with severe psoriasis have an excess mortality compared with the general population.[1] The spectrum of comorbidities observed in patients with psoriasis is described by Garshick and Kimball elsewhere in this issue. It has yet to be established whether these comorbidities occur as a direct result of the systemic inflammation associated with psoriasis, as a consequence of genetically determined selection, or whether other factors are involved.[3]

EPIDEMIOLOGY

Cardiovascular Risk in Patients with Psoriasis

Although the association of psoriasis with cardiovascular disease was first described more than

Funding: None.
Conflicts of Interest: Dr C. Ryan has acted as an advisor and speaker for Abbvie and Pfizer. Prof B. Kirby is in receipt of research grants from Merck-Sharpe-Dolme, Pfizer, and AbbVie. He has acted as an advisor for Pfizer, Janssen, Abbvie, Novartis, and Roche.
[a] Department of Dermatology, Baylor University Medical Center Dallas, 3900 Junius Street, Suite 145, Dallas, TX 75246, USA; [b] St Vincent's University Hospital, University College Dublin, Elm Park, Dublin 4, Ireland
* Corresponding author.
E-mail address: caitrionaryan80@gmail.com

40 years ago, the significance of the association between psoriasis and cardiovascular disease has only become apparent over the past decade.[4] A seminal, population-based cohort study using the United Kingdom General Practice Research Database (GPRD) showed that patients with psoriasis had an increased adjusted relative risk for myocardial infarction, after controlling for other cardiovascular risk factors. The relative risk increased with increasing psoriasis severity, with a 3-fold increase in the risk of myocardial infarction for male patients with psoriasis at the age of 30 years.[2] This increased risk was observed in all age groups, although it decreased with age. Patients with psoriasis at the age of 60 years still had an increased risk of cardiovascular disease even when the data were controlled for traditional cardiovascular risk factors. This finding suggests that psoriasis may be an independent risk factor for premature cardiovascular disease. Other studies have confirmed an increase in cardiovascular disease, peripheral vascular disease, stroke, and overall mortality, and these studies also show a correlation between the risk of cardiovascular morbidity and psoriasis severity.[1,2,5,6] Another study using the GPRD showed that the incidence of risk factors for cardiovascular disease, including incident diabetes, hypertension, obesity, and hyperlipidemia, were increased compared with the general population after a first recorded diagnosis of psoriasis.[5] A systematic review and meta-analysis of observational studies examining cardiovascular risk in 201,239 patients with mild psoriasis and 17,415 patients with severe psoriasis showed an estimated excess of 11,500 major adverse cardiovascular events each year.[7] A cohort study using the GPRD showed that patients with severe psoriasis have a 6-year reduction in life expectancy, with cardiovascular death accounting for the greatest proportion of excess mortality.[8]

In contrast, 2 large studies did not show an increase in cardiovascular risk.[9,10] A 30-year cohort study in 1376 patients concluded that only patients with exceptionally severe psoriasis had an increased risk of overall noncardiovascular mortality and that severe psoriasis was not an independent risk factor for cardiovascular disease.[10] These findings are unusual because no association was observed between obesity and cardiovascular mortality, or between severe psoriasis and obesity, despite robust evidence to the contrary in other populations. In an article refuting these findings, it was suggested that the epidemiologic study design was flawed.[11] However, most studies have reported a link between psoriasis and premature cardiovascular disease. The mechanisms underpinning this increased risk are unclear. Patients with psoriasis have an excess prevalence of cardiovascular risk factors. There is evidence of systemic inflammation in psoriasis. Systemic inflammation has been identified as causing excess cardiovascular disease in other immune-mediated diseases such as systemic lupus erythematosus and rheumatoid arthritis. Further long-term, population-based, epidemiologic studies are needed to define more accurately the risk of cardiovascular disease in patients with psoriasis. Inception cohort studies of patients with newly diagnosed psoriasis, which comprehensively record patient demographics, risk factors, and psoriasis history, will minimize survivorship bias and confounding caused by cardiovascular comorbidities.

The results from epidemiology studies have prompted smaller studies to try to address whether psoriasis is causal rather than associated with cardiovascular disease. A study of 39 patients with psoriasis compared with 38 healthy controls showed evidence of increased arterial stiffness, independent of other cardiovascular risk factors, and this stiffness increased with duration of disease.[12] Another study showed increased coronary artery calcification in 32 asymptomatic patients with psoriasis compared with healthy controls.[13] Epicardial fat thickness, measured by transthoracic echocardiography, is another risk factor for atherosclerosis. In a small case-control study, epicardial fat thickness was significantly higher in 31 patients with psoriasis compared with 32 controls, independently of other cardiometabolic risk factors.[14]

CARDIOVASCULAR RISK FACTORS AND PSORIASIS

Hypertension

Several studies have reported a strong association between hypertension and moderate to severe psoriasis. In a large meta-analysis examining the prevalence of hypertension in 309,469 patients with psoriasis, the odds ratio (OR) for hypertension in patients with mild psoriasis was 1.30 (95% confidence interval [CI], 1.15–1.47) and 1.49 (95% CI, 1.20–1.86) in those with severe psoriasis compared with healthy controls.[15] In a subgroup analysis, patients with psoriatic arthritis also had an increased prevalence of hypertension (OR, 2.07; 95% CI, 1.41–3.04).

Diabetes Mellitus

Psoriasis is associated with an increased prevalence and incidence of type II diabetes mellitus. A recent meta-analysis and systematic review concluded that the prevalence of diabetes was increased in patients with psoriasis with an OR of

1.53 (95% CI, 1.06–1.24) for mild disease and 1.97 (95% CI, 1.48–2.62) for severe disease.[16] The incidence of diabetes in patients with psoriasis had an OR of 1.27 (95% CI, 1.16–1.4).

Obesity and the Metabolic Syndrome

Although it has been well established that patients with psoriasis are more likely to be obese, it is unclear whether obesity antedates or occurs after the development of psoriasis.[3,17–19] A prospective study in 78,626 women followed for 14 years showed a biological gradient between increasing body mass index (BMI) and the risk of incident psoriasis, suggesting that obesity precedes the development of the disease.[17] Another study showed that patients with newly diagnosed psoriasis have lipid abnormalities at the onset of disease, compared with healthy controls.[18] In contrast, a large cross-sectional study using a self-reported questionnaire showed that patients became overweight after the onset of psoriasis and concluded that obesity was a consequence of psoriasis rather than a risk factor for development of the disease.[19] It has been shown more recently in a large international study that children and adolescents with psoriasis are more obese than age-marched and sex-matched controls, with a tendency toward central adiposity.[20,21]

Patients with moderate to severe psoriasis have an increased prevalence of the metabolic syndrome in a constellation of comorbidities that includes visceral obesity, insulin resistance, dyslipidemia, and hypertension (**Box 1**).[22–24] This association increases with increasing disease severity. In addition, the increased risk of individual components of the metabolic syndrome also shows a dose-response relationship with psoriasis severity, independently of other metabolic syndrome components.[25] Children with psoriasis have a significantly higher risk of developing the metabolic syndrome, with 30% of children meeting the criteria in one small study.[26]

There is substantial evidence of dyslipidemia in patients with psoriasis.[27] A study of 95,540 participants from the Nurses' Health Study II showed that hypercholesterolemia is associated with an increased risk of incident psoriasis, particularly in those who had a diagnosis of hypercholesterolemia for greater than 7 years.[27] There was no association between psoriasis and the use of lipid-lowering drugs. Important differences have also been observed in lipoprotein composition and particle size, and cholesterol efflux mechanisms in patients with psoriasis. Patients with psoriasis have lower levels of protective high-density lipoprotein (HDL), with an increased proportion of more atherogenic small low-density lipoprotein (LDL) and HDL particles, similar to that observed in diabetic patients.[28,29] It has been shown that abnormal HDL particle size is associated with aortic vascular inflammation in patients with psoriasis after correction for other cardiovascular risk factors, when measured by PET–computed tomography (CT), a validated surrogate marker of cardiovascular disease.[28] Compositional alterations of HDL in patients with psoriasis result in impaired ability to promote cholesterol efflux from macrophages, and this worsens with increasing psoriasis severity.[30] Note that successful treatment of psoriasis results in recovery of HDL particle size and cholesterol efflux capacity.[31]

Cigarette Smoking and Excessive Alcohol Use

The frequencies of smoking and excess alcohol consumption, which are independent risk factors for the development of cardiovascular disease,

---

Box 1
National Heart, Lung, and Blood Institute and the American Heart Association (AHA) guidelines for diagnosis of the metabolic syndrome

Patient has at least 3 of the following 5 conditions:

- Fasting glucose greater than or equal to 100 mg/dL (or receiving drug therapy for hyperglycemia)
- Blood pressure greater than or equal to 130/85 mm Hg (or receiving drug therapy for hypertension)
- Triglycerides greater than or equal to 150 mg/dL (or receiving drug therapy for hypertriglyceridemia)
- High-density lipoprotein C (HDL-C) less than 40 mg/dL in men or less than 50 mg/dL in women (or receiving drug therapy for reduced HDL-C)
- Waist circumference greater than or equal to 102 cm (40 inches) in men or greater than or equal to 88 cm (35 inches) in women; if Asian American, greater than or equal to 90 cm (35 inches) in men or greater than or equal to 80 cm (32 inches) in women

Adapted from Grundy SM, Brewer HB, Cleeman JI, et al, American Heart Association. Definition of metabolic syndrome: report of the National Heart, Lung, and Blood Institute/American Heart Association conference on scientific issues related to definition. Circulation 2004;109:435; with permission.

are increased in patients with psoriasis.[17,19,32–35] However, it remains unclear whether these lifestyle factors influence the development of psoriasis or occur as a result of disease-related psychological distress. A recent meta-analysis of 25 prevalence studies (146,934 patients with psoriasis) and 3 incidence studies showed an association between psoriasis and current or former smoking and suggested that smoking is an independent risk factor for the development of psoriasis.[36] Recent evidence has shown that cigarette smoke increases the percentage of circulating T helper 17 (Th17) cells in the peripheral blood of patients with psoriasis compared with nonsmokers.[37]

Excess alcohol intake has been reported in up to 30% of patients with psoriasis and is likely associated with psychological distress.[35] Excess alcohol intake can lead to a wide spectrum of cardiovascular complications, including alcoholic cardiomyopathy, atrial fibrillation, sudden death, and hemorrhagic stroke.[38] Alcohol-related diseases accounted for a significant proportion of excess mortality in a population of Finnish patients with psoriasis.[34]

Other associated comorbid conditions in patients with psoriasis may also contribute indirectly to cardiovascular disease. Obstructive sleep apnea and chronic obstructive pulmonary disease are associated with excessive cardiovascular disease and are commoner in patients with moderate to severe psoriasis.[39] Patients with psoriasis have also been shown to have increased levels of homocysteine, which is an independent risk factor for cardiovascular disease.[40] Moderate to severe psoriasis is associated with increased levels of depression, which is another independent risk factor for cardiovascular disease.[41,42] In summary, there seems to be an excess of lifestyle factors and medical conditions in patients with psoriasis that predispose to premature cardiovascular disease.

PATHOMECHANISMS UNDERLYING THE ASSOCIATION OF PSORIASIS WITH CARDIOMETABOLIC COMORBIDITES AND CARDIOVASCULAR RISK

Further research is needed to investigate the complex relationship between psoriasis and metabolic comorbidities at a clinical and molecular level. Multiple hypotheses have been suggested. Although it is possible that patients with psoriasis are genetically predisposed to develop obesity, diabetes, and premature atherosclerosis, genome-wide association scans of patients with psoriasis have not shown an increased inheritance of genes associated with metabolic comorbidities.[3]

Common inflammatory pathways are likely involved in the pathophysiology of psoriasis and cardiovascular inflammation, both of which are associated with a chronic proinflammatory, proangiogenic, and prothrombotic state.[43–46] The proinflammatory cytokine profile of psoriasis lesions is remarkably similar to that of atherosclerotic lesions, with a similar inflammatory cell infiltrate of T cells, macrophages, and monocytes observed in both conditions (**Fig. 1**).[44,47,48] Psoriasis plaques and unstable atherosclerotic plaques both have an increased frequency of activated T cells with both Th1 and Th17 patterns of cytokine production.[44,47–49] Th17 cells and their inflammatory mediators, including interleukin (IL)-17, IL-6, and IL-8, are also increased in the blood of patients with unstable coronary artery disease.[50–58] Increased expression of known cardiovascular biomarkers, such as monocyte chemoattractant protein-1 (MCP-1) and macrophage-derived chemokine, has been observed in the lesional skin and serum of patients with psoriasis compared with healthy controls, suggesting shared inflammatory pathways linking psoriasis and cardiometabolic disease.[59]

Although there is significant evidence that systemic inflammation drives the increased cardiovascular risk in psoriasis, it is unclear whether psoriatic inflammation primarily contributes to the development of cardiometabolic comorbidities, or whether preexisting metabolic dysfunction causes immunologic dysregulation that then leads to the development of psoriasis. The former explanation has been described as the metabolic march of psoriasis, in which systemic inflammation caused by psoriasis affects the function of other cells and tissues driving the metabolic dysregulation, dyslipidemia, obesity, and increase in cardiovascular risk observed in patients with psoriasis.[44,47] Release of skin-derived cytokines and inflammatory mediators from psoriasis lesions into the circulation and upregulation of cell adhesion molecules may result in compartmental shifts in inflammatory cells between lesional psoriatic skin, the peripheral circulation, and atheromatous plaques of the coronary vasculature.

Adipokines

Inflammation of adipose tissue caused by psoriasis-related systemic inflammation likely leads to metabolic dysregulation. Monocytes and macrophages infiltrating adipose tissue in obese patients create an inflammatory microenvironment through the production of proinflammatory cytokines such as tumor necrosis factor-alpha (TNF-α), IL-6, and MCP-1. When adipose tissue

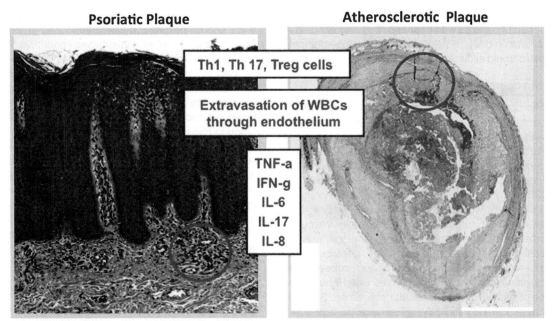

Psoriatic Plaque

Atherosclerotic Plaque

Th1, Th 17, Treg cells

Extravasation of WBCs through endothelium

TNF-a
IFN-g
IL-6
IL-17
IL-8

Fig. 1. Comparison of the inflammatory nature of a psoriasis lesion and an atherosclerotic plaque. IFN-g, interferon gamma; IL, interleukin; TNF-a, tumor necrosis factor-alpha; Treg, T regulatory cell; WBC, white blood cell.

becomes inflamed, adipokines, which are a family of inflammatory mediators, are released into the circulation. Adipokines, such as leptin and adiponectin, play an important role in the pathogenesis of the metabolic syndrome, which is a proinflammatory, prothrombotic state, characterized by an increase in C-reactive protein (CRP), TNF-α, IL-6, fibrinogen, and plasminogen activator inhibitor-1 (PAI-1) (**Box 2**).[44,60] Increased leptin levels and low adiponectin levels in patients with psoriasis are thought to contribute to the development of the metabolic syndrome, independently of BMI.[61–63]

Leptin has a proinflammatory effect, causing inflammatory cytokine production, angiogenesis, increased expression of activation markers on T cells and monocytes, and upregulation of adhesion molecules on endothelial cell walls.[64–67] Increased levels of leptin in patients with psoriasis have been shown to be independent of obesity, and correlate with disease severity and disease duration.[61,68] Some studies have suggested that increased levels of leptin contribute to the initial development of psoriasis through the release of proinflammatory mediators.[69–71]

Adiponectin inhibits the production of proinflammatory cytokines such as IL-6 and TNF-α, downregulates cell adhesion molecule expression in endothelial cells, and induces antiinflammatory cytokines IL-10 and IL-1 receptor antagonist in monocytes and macrophages.[60,72] Plasma levels of adiponectin are decreased in obesity and type 2 diabetes and studies have suggested that adiponectin plays an antiinflammatory role in cardiovascular disease.[62,73] Circulating levels of adiponectin are reduced in patients with psoriasis, even after adjusting for cardiometabolic risk factors, and negatively correlate with TNF-α and IL-6 levels.[74–78]

Resistin is another proinflammatory adipokine produced by macrophages in adipose tissue, which is associated with atherosclerosis and is increased in patients with psoriasis.[75,79–84] Adipocyte-derived retinol-binding protein 4 is thought to play

---

Box 2
Serum markers in the metabolic syndrome

- Proinflammatory state: increased levels of C-reactive protein, TNF-α, and IL-6

- Prothrombotic state: increased PAI-1 and fibrinogen

- Adipokines: increased levels of leptin, resistin, and retinol-binding protein 4, with lower level of adiponectin

Adapted from Grundy SM, Brewer HB, Cleeman JI, et al, American Heart Association. Definition of metabolic syndrome: report of the National Heart, Lung, and Blood Institute/American Heart Association conference on scientific issues related to definition. Circulation 2004;109:433–8; with permission.

a role in insulin resistance and is increased in the serum of patients with psoriasis.[85,86] Together, adipokines in obese patients with psoriasis perpetuate this chronic inflammatory state.

Microparticles

Microparticle formation has recently been shown to contribute to accelerated atherogenesis in patients with psoriasis and other inflammatory conditions.[87–89] Microparticles are membrane vesicles containing nucleic acids and inflammatory mediators, such as IL-1, Cluster of Differentiation 40 (CD40) ligand, and intercellular adhesion molecule 1 (ICAM-1), which are released following cell activation or apoptosis and contribute to vascular inflammation, thrombosis, and angiogenesis.[90] Leukocyte-derived microparticles contribute to atherosclerotic plaque rupture and subsequent cardiovascular events, and have been shown to be predictive of cardiovascular outcomes. Studies have shown significantly higher microparticle concentrations in the blood of patients with psoriasis, even after adjusting for cardiovascular risk factors.[87–89]

Hypercoagulability

Upregulation of platelets and coagulation factors may produce a hypercoagulable state contributing to an increase in thromboembolic events in psoriasis.[45] There is increased activation of platelets in patients with psoriasis compared with healthy controls, with increased levels of beta-thromboglobulin and platelet factor 4, increased platelet volume, and hyperaggregability, all of which normalize with resolution of disease.[91,92] There is an increase in platelet expression of p-selectin and increased release of platelet-derived microparticles in patients with psoriasis, which correlate with disease severity.[88,93] Circulating levels of PAI-1 are also increased in patients with psoriasis.[94]

Management of Cardiovascular Risk

Education and primary prevention
Until alternative evidence is available, the presence of severe psoriasis should be considered an independent cardiovascular risk factor. It is the responsibility of physicians and dermatologists to counsel patients with psoriasis regarding the increased risk of cardiometabolic conditions and the need for lifestyle modifications, including smoking cessation, weight reduction, and regular screening for diabetes and hypertension.[95,96] Patients with moderate to severe psoriasis should have annual monitoring of blood pressure, BMI, waist circumference, lipid profile, fasting glucose, glycosylated hemoglobin, and smoking status. In addition, appropriate weight-loss and lifestyle advice should be given by dermatologists in the routine management of patients with psoriasis.[96] This advice is of particular importance in the pediatric population, in which there is a high risk of both metabolic and psychosocial comorbidities, thus stressing the need for early monitoring for cardiac risk factors and aggressive lifestyle modification in this patient population.

In a cohort study using the GPRD, the presence of severe psoriasis (defined as patients receiving systemic therapy) conferred an additional 6.2% absolute risk of 10-year major adverse cardiac events, after adjusting for age, gender, diabetes, hypertension, tobacco use, and hyperlipidemia.[97] A further study showed that the Framingham Risk Score underestimated cardiovascular risk in patients with psoriasis, and, when the attributable risk associated with psoriasis was applied to calculate the risk, most patients were reclassified into a higher risk category. This finding has important implications for cardiovascular risk stratification and preventative strategies, further reinforcing the view that dermatologists are key to ensuring that both patients and their physicians are informed of this increased risk. Studies are required to ensure that patients are aware of these associated conditions and are making lifestyle modifications accordingly.

Further research to determine how to optimize primary prevention of cardiovascular events in patients with psoriasis is also required. It is of vital importance that standardized screening tools are developed to identify cardiometabolic comorbidities in routine clinical practice. Collaboration with primary care physicians, internists, cardiologists, endocrinologists, and dieticians is essential to optimally manage this increase in cardiometabolic risk in these patients.[96]

The impact of weight reduction on the clinical course of psoriasis and treatment response needs further investigation. Weight reduction may improve psoriasis and small case series have shown a beneficial effect of gastric bypass surgery on psoriasis severity.[98,99] Several studies have suggested that weight loss may supplement the response to psoriasis therapies. In a study of 303 overweight or obese patients with psoriasis on stable-dose systemic treatment randomized to receive a 20-week quantitative and qualitative dietary and exercise intervention or basic counseling at baseline, patients in the intervention group showed a significantly greater decrease in psoriasis severity.[100] In another study, obese patients with psoriasis showed a superior response when cyclosporine was combined with a low-calorie diet.[101] A small study of 10 patients showed an improved response to topical treatment in obese patients with psoriasis on a low-calorie diet.[102] These findings emphasize the need for more holistic management of patients with psoriasis and the incorporation of lifestyle interventions into treatment regimens.

BIOMARKERS

In recent years, much research has focused on identifying biomarkers of systemic inflammation and cardiovascular risk in patients with psoriasis. Although patients with more severe psoriasis seem to have an increased risk of cardiometabolic comorbidities, the degree of cutaneous involvement does not necessarily correlate with the level of systemic or cardiovascular inflammation. For example, patients with psoriatic arthritis may only have mild cutaneous involvement, despite significant extracutaneous tissue inflammation and increased inflammatory markers. Validated biomarkers would provide a more reliable means of screening for increased cardiovascular risk. For example, in a recent study, increases in known cardiovascular biomarkers, including soluble ICAM-1 (sICAM-1), soluble E (sE)-selectin, matrix metalloproteinase (MMP)-9, myeloperoxidase (MPO), and total PAI-1 (tPAI-1), did not correlate significantly with Psoriasis Area and Severity Index (PASI), and it was suggested that this represented increased systemic inflammation rather than increases resulting from local cutaneous inflammation.[103]

Because the pathomechanisms leading to increased cardiovascular risk in patients with psoriasis may differ from mechanisms in the nonpsoriatic population, it is not known whether conventional inflammatory biomarkers of atherosclerotic disease are reliable predictors of risk in patients with psoriasis. Studies have shown that conventional biomarkers of inflammation and cardiovascular disease, such as CRP, human soluble CD40 ligand (sCD40L), human matrix gla-protein, and fetuin-A, are significantly altered in patients with psoriasis after controlling for age and BMI.[104] CRP is a serum protein produced by the liver and is increased by infection and systemic inflammation.[105] Patients with immune-mediated diseases such as rheumatoid arthritis have increased levels of CRP compared with normal controls. CRP is increased in patients with psoriatic arthritis and to a lesser extent in those with cutaneous psoriasis alone.[106,107] High-sensitivity CRP is an independent risk factor for the development of coronary artery disease and is increased in patients with psoriasis.[106,107]

The use of activated myeloid cell–derived and neutrophil-derived biomarkers has also been examined in several studies. One study showed the neutrophil/lymphocyte ratio (NLR) to be the most reliable predictor of subclinical atherosclerosis in patients with psoriasis, as measured by the aortic velocity propagation and carotid intima media thickness, and NLR also correlated with PASI.[108] In several studies patients with psoriasis have shown significant increases in serum MPO, which is a known biomarker of cardiovascular inflammation that mediates its effects through lipid oxidation and endothelial dysfunction.[103,109] MPO is also highly expressed in psoriasis plaques. In one of these studies, serum levels of MPO correlated with coronary artery calcification, carotid plaque burden, carotid intima media thickness, and flow-mediated dilatation in patients with psoriasis but showed no association with psoriasis severity.[103,109]

The Effect of Systemic Treatments on Cardiovascular Risk and Treatment Recommendations

Systemic and biologic treatments used to treat psoriasis may modulate cardiovascular risk. Although certain traditional systemic drugs may have a negative impact on cardiovascular risk factors such as hyperlipidemia or hypertension, it has been suggested that the suppression of systemic inflammation may reduce cardiovascular risk. Careful evaluation of a patient's cardiovascular risk factor profile is needed when selecting individual therapies. When medication-related adverse effects such as hypertension and dyslipidemia occur, dermatologists should be adept at initiating antihypertensive and lipid-lowering agents for the optimal management of cardiovascular risk.

Although growing evidence suggests that the aggressive management of moderate to severe psoriasis may mitigate cardiovascular risk, it is still unclear whether this is caused by the effect of individual systemic treatments on circulating immune cells, or whether clearance of cutaneous disease by any means decreases the systemic inflammatory burden.[110] In a retrospective cohort study of 8845 patients in the Kaiser Permanente health care database followed for a median of 4.1 years, the use of either TNF inhibitors or oral agents/phototherapy was associated with statistically significant reductions (50% and 46%, respectively) in the risk of myocardial infarction risk, compared with patients treated with topical agents alone, suggesting that systemic treatment of psoriasis decreases systemic inflammation.[111] In a previously mentioned small study of 15 patients, successful treatment with either topical or systemic psoriasis therapies significantly improved HDL-cholesterol efflux capability and normalized HDL composition and function. This finding also suggested that the observed lipid abnormalities were secondary to systemic inflammation. In contrast, another study examining the effect of treatment on multiple biomarkers of cardiovascular risk showed considerable decreases in serum levels of these biomarkers following etanercept treatment but no change after phototherapy.[103]

Methotrexate

Methotrexate (MTX) has been the first-line systemic agent for psoriasis for more than 40 years. There is considerable evidence to support the beneficial effect of MTX on cardiovascular risk in both the psoriasis and rheumatoid arthritis populations.[110–112] In a retrospective cohort study of 7615 patients with psoriasis and 6707 patients with rheumatoid arthritis at the Veterans Integrated Service network, MTX significantly reduced the risk of vascular disease compared with those who were not treated with MTX, particularly in those treated with low-dose MTX and concomitant folic acid.[112]

As a result of the growing evidence suggesting the possible cardioprotective effect of MTX, the National Institutes of Health (NIH) are currently conducting the Cardiovascular Inflammation Reduction Trial (CIRT; clinicaltrials.gov identifier NCT01594333) to examine the effect of low-dose MTX on the rate of heart attacks, strokes, or death in 7000 patients with type 2 diabetes or metabolic syndrome who have known coronary artery disease.[113] The results of this study will be relevant to the psoriasis population.

Cyclosporine

Cyclosporine is a highly effective oral medication, but has an unfavorable side effect profile. In addition to nephrotoxicity, cyclosporine can adversely affect the cardiovascular risk factor profile by increasing the risk of hypertension and dyslipidemia.[114] The reported incidence of new-onset hypertension with short-course cyclosporine therapy typically ranges from 0% to 24%, and is generally reversible with dose reduction or the use of antihypertensives. The onset of hypertension did not seem to be dose related, suggesting that there may a subset of patients with increased individual sensitivity to cyclosporine.[114]

Hyperlipidemia, particularly hypertriglyceridemia, develops in approximately 15% of patients with psoriasis on cyclosporine therapy.[114] If hyperlipidemia develops, a lipid-lowering diet should be introduced, followed by dose reduction of cyclosporine or commencement of a lipid-lowering agent if dietary measures fail.[114] The use of cyclosporine in moderate to severe psoriasis is currently limited to short-term to medium-term interventional treatment courses in order to achieve rapid disease control before transitioning to another systemic therapy with a more favorable long-term toxicity profile. The potential adverse effects of cyclosporine on cardiovascular risk factors such as hypertension have to be balanced by the short duration of modern cyclosporine therapy regimens and the need to achieve rapid control of skin disease in appropriate patients.

Acitretin

Acitretin is a vitamin A derivative that has been used to treat psoriasis since the early 1980s. Although less effective than other traditional systemic agents when used as a monotherapy, acitretin can play a valuable role in patients with generalized pustular psoriasis and palmoplantar disease.[115] Chronic increase of triglyceride levels may increase the risk of atherosclerosis, so monitoring of hyperlipidemia is necessary, but this should not be considered a contraindication because it is usually readily managed with dietary modification and lipid-lowering agents.[116]

Fumaric Acid Esters

Fumaric acid esters are compounds derived from the unsaturated dicarbonic acid, fumaric acid, which have been used in Europe since the late 1970s for the treatment of psoriasis.[117] Patients with psoriasis treated with fumaric acid esters show a reduction in circulating CRP and an increase in adiponectin following treatment.[118] A similar study showed a beneficial effect of continuous treatment with fumaric acid esters on biomarkers of cardiovascular risk.[110]

Tumor Necrosis Factor-Alpha Inhibitors

A large body of evidence from psoriasis and rheumatoid arthritis populations suggests that TNF-α inhibitors have a beneficial effect on cardiovascular risk. In the previously mentioned retrospective cohort study using the Kaiser Permanente health care database in California, patients receiving TNF-α inhibitors had a 50% reduction in the risk of myocardial infarction compared with those treated with topical agents, but there was no significant difference in TNF-α inhibitor use compared with traditional systemic agents or phototherapy.[111] However, a study of 2400 patients with severe psoriasis in nationwide administrative databases in Denmark showed that patients treated with biologic agents or MTX had lower cardiovascular event rates compared with patients treated with other antipsoriatic therapies (cyclosporine, acitretin, and phototherapy).[119]

Larger studies in patients with rheumatoid arthritis also support the cardioprotective effect of TNF-α inhibition. In a longitudinal cohort study of 10,156 patients enrolled in the Consortium of Rheumatology Researchers of North America (CORRONA) rheumatoid arthritis registry, treatment with TNF-α inhibitors was associated with a reduced risk of cardiovascular events (hazard ratio, 0.39) compared with disease-modifying antirheumatic drugs, and MTX was not associated with a reduction in risk.

The effect of etanercept on inflammatory biomarkers in psoriasis has been evaluated in several studies.[103,120,121] In a previously mentioned study, etanercept treatment resulted in a highly significant reduction in all investigated biomarkers of cardiovascular risk including soluble vascular cell adhesion molecule-1, sICAM-1, sE-selectin, MMP-9, MPO, and tPAI-1, although these parameters did not improve in patients who had successful treatment with phototherapy.[103] Another study showed a significant decrease in CRP in patients with psoriasis and psoriatic arthritis treated with etanercept.[103,120,121] Significant reductions in fibrinogen, ferritin, high-sensitivity CRP, erythrocyte sedimentation rate, haptoglobin, ceruloplasmin, and alpha1-antitrypsin have also been observed after etanercept treatment.[121]

Another large-scale, retrospective cohort study of patients with rheumatoid arthritis or psoriasis showed that the adjusted risk of diabetes was lower for individuals starting TNF-α inhibitors and hydroxychloroquine compared with other nonbiologic disease-modifying agents, including MTX, suggesting that these agents may reduce the risk of metabolic dysfunction.[122]

Ustekinumab

There has been considerable controversy regarding the association between the use of anti–IL-12p40 agents in patients with psoriasis and major adverse cardiovascular events (MACE).[123–125] Ustekinumab has been approved for clinical use in psoriasis for more than 5 years, whereas briakinumab was withdrawn from clinical trials because of concerns over cardiovascular safety. Two meta-analyses examined the association of anti–IL-12p40 inhibitors and cardiovascular events in patients with psoriasis. The first compared the excess probability of MACE in 22 randomized controlled trials (RCTs) in patients receiving active treatment of anti–IL-12p40 agents (ustekinumab and briakinumab) and TNF-α

inhibitors.[123] Although the apparent increase in MACE observed with patients receiving anti–IL-12p40 antibodies was not statistically significant, the findings raised questions about the cardiovascular safety of the anti–IL-12p40 agents. A subsequent meta-analysis examining the rate of MACE in patients in RCTs of IL-12/23 antibodies using different statistical methods showed a significantly higher risk of MACE in patients treated with anti–IL-12p40 agents compared with placebo.[126] Note that these studies analyzed short-term use (up to 16 weeks) of anti–IL-12p40 agents in patients in clinical trials. However, a 5-year safety study conducted by the manufacturers of ustekinumab has shown no increase or decrease in the rate of MACE over time and compares favorably with population-based rates of MACE.[127]

There are several ongoing studies to assess the role of systemic inflammation in accelerated cardiovascular disease. These studies will further define the relationship between psoriasis, traditional cardiovascular risk factors, systemic inflammation, and accelerated coronary artery disease. Two large-scale, prospective cohort studies are currently underway at the National Institutes of Health in the United States. The first, entitled the Psoriasis, Atherosclerosis and Cardiometabolic Disease Initiative (NCT01778569), is a longitudinal cardiometabolic phenotyping program of 1800 patients who will be followed for up to 5 years. These patients will undergo comprehensive cardiovascular and metabolic risk assessment using high-level multimodal imaging (fluorodeoxyglucose PET-CT, PET-MRI, and cardiac CT angiography) to assess vascular inflammation (**Fig. 2**), along with comprehensive analysis of blood, skin, and adipose tissue samples. The second study, entitled A Trial to Determine the Effect of Psoriasis Treatment on Cardiometabolic Disease: Vascular Inflammation in Psoriasis Trial (clinicaltrials.gov identifier NCT01553058), is designed to assess the effects of biologic treatment and phototherapy on systemic inflammation and cardiovascular disease risk factors in patients with moderate to severe psoriasis. It is hoped that these studies will provide further insight into the mechanistic links between inflammation and the development of cardiometabolic disease in patients with psoriasis.

SUMMARY

There is strong evidence, both clinical and scientific, supporting an association between psoriasis and cardiovascular risk. Prospective, population-based, long-term studies of patients with newly diagnosed psoriasis will better examine the inherent increase of cardiometabolic risk factors

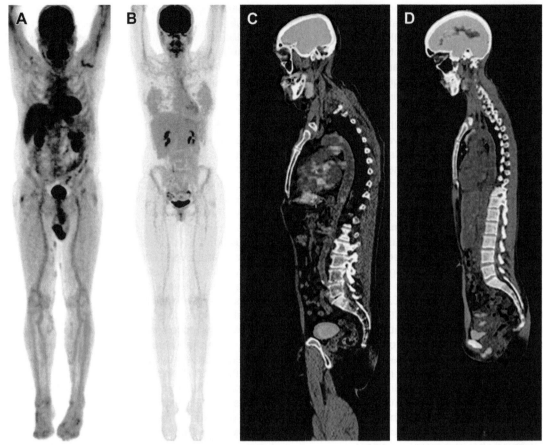

Fig. 2. Fluorodeoxyglucose-PET-CT imaging shows multifocal inflammation in a 37-year-old man with psoriasis (*A, C*) with no known cardiovascular risk factors, compared with a 26-year-old woman (*B, D*). Note the increased uptake within the aorta of the patient with psoriasis in the sagittal color-fused image (*C*) compared with that of the healthy control (*D*). (*Courtesy of* Dr Nehal Mehta, National Heart, Lung and Blood Institute, National Institutes of Health, Bethesda, MD.)

and cardiovascular events, the influence of objectively measured disease severity, and the effect of individual therapies on this risk. Reliable biomarkers of systemic inflammation or cardiovascular risk in patients with psoriasis have not yet been identified. Until further evidence is available, all patients with moderate to severe psoriasis and/or psoriatic arthritis should be considered to be at a higher risk of cardiovascular disease and managed accordingly. Further research and interventions to adequately screen for and optimally manage cardiovascular comorbidities are also warranted.

There are currently multiple newly developed psoriasis therapies undergoing clinical trials. It is essential that long-term cardiovascular safety data are collected in a comprehensive and systematic manner within these trials. RCTs are not currently designed to detect rare events such as major cardiovascular events. A systematic strategy needs to be implemented to ensure the

cardiovascular safety of new agents under development, using appropriate imaging, assessments of endothelial function, and carefully selected biomarkers of cardiovascular risk. Further understanding of the complex pathophysiology of psoriasis and the common mechanistic pathways shared with cardiovascular disease will likely facilitate the development of more innovative approaches to reducing cardiovascular inflammation while treating the complete spectrum of psoriasis.

REFERENCES

1. Gelfand JM, Troxel AB, Lewis JD, et al. The risk of mortality in patients with psoriasis: results from a population-based study. Arch Dermatol 2007;143: 1493–9.
2. Gelfand JM, Neimann AL, Shin DB, et al. Risk of myocardial infarction in patients with psoriasis. JAMA 2006;296:1735–41.

3. Henseler T, Christophers E. Disease concomitance in psoriasis. J Am Acad Dermatol 1995; 32:982–6.

4. McDonald CJ, Calabresi P. Occlusive vascular disease in psoriatic patients. N Engl J Med 1973;288: 912.

5. Kaye JA, Li L, Jick SS. Incidence of risk factors for myocardial infarction and other vascular diseases in patients with psoriasis. Br J Dermatol 2008; 159:895–902.

6. Mallbris L, Akre O, Granath F, et al. Increased risk for cardiovascular mortality in psoriasis inpatients but not in outpatients. Eur J Epidemiol 2004;19: 225–30.

7. Armstrong EJ, Harskamp CT, Armstrong AW. Psoriasis and major adverse cardiovascular events: a systematic review and meta-analysis of observational studies. J Am Heart Assoc 2013;2:e000062.

8. Abuabara K, Azfar RS, Shin DB, et al. Cause-specific mortality in patients with severe psoriasis: a population-based cohort study in the UK. Br J Dermatol 2010;163:586–92.

9. Wakkee M, Herings RM, Nijsten T. Psoriasis may not be an independent risk factor for acute ischemic heart disease hospitalizations: results of a large population-based Dutch cohort. J Invest Dermatol 2010;130:962–7.

10. Stern RS, Huibregtse A. Very severe psoriasis is associated with increased noncardiovascular mortality but not with increased cardiovascular risk. J Invest Dermatol 2011;131:1159–66.

11. Gelfand JM, Mehta NN, Langan SM. Psoriasis and cardiovascular risk: strength in numbers, part II. J Invest Dermatol 2011;131:1007–10.

12. Gisondi P, Fantin F, Del Giglio M, et al. Chronic plaque psoriasis is associated with increased arterial stiffness. Dermatology 2009;218:110–3.

13. Ludwig RJ, Herzog C, Rostock A, et al. Psoriasis: a possible risk factor for development of coronary artery calcification. Br J Dermatol 2007; 156:271–6.

14. Akyildiz ZI, Seremet S, Emren V, et al. Epicardial fat thickness is independently associated with psoriasis. Dermatology 2014;228:55–9.

15. Armstrong AW, Harskamp CT, Armstrong EJ. The association between psoriasis and hypertension: a systematic review and meta-analysis of observational studies. J Hypertens 2013;31:433–42 [discussion: 442–3].

16. Armstrong AW, Harskamp CT, Armstrong EJ. Psoriasis and the risk of diabetes mellitus: a systematic review and meta-analysis. JAMA Dermatol 2013; 149:84–91.

17. Setty AR, Curhan G, Choi HK. Obesity, waist circumference, weight change, and the risk of psoriasis in women: Nurses' Health Study II. Arch Intern Med 2007;167:1670–5.

18. Mallbris L, Granath F, Hamsten A, et al. Psoriasis is associated with lipid abnormalities at the onset of skin disease. J Am Acad Dermatol 2006;54:614–21.

19. Herron MD, Hinckley M, Hoffman MS, et al. Impact of obesity and smoking on psoriasis presentation and management. Arch Dermatol 2005; 141:1527–34.

20. Available at: http://www.clinicaltrials.gov/ct2/show/NCT00879944?term=pediatric+psoriasis&rank=3. Accesssed 29 June, 2014.

21. Paller AS, Mercy K, Kwasny MJ, et al. Association of pediatric psoriasis severity with excess and central adiposity: an international cross-sectional study. JAMA Dermatol 2013;149:166–76.

22. Eckel RH, Grundy SM, Zimmet PZ. The metabolic syndrome. Lancet 2005;365:1415–28.

23. Sommer DM, Jenisch S, Suchan M, et al. Increased prevalence of the metabolic syndrome in patients with moderate to severe psoriasis. Arch Dermatol Res 2006;298:321–8.

24. Grundy SM, Brewer HB, Cleeman JI, et al, American Heart Association. Definition of metabolic syndrome: report of the National Heart, Lung, and Blood Institute/American Heart Association conference on scientific issues related to definition. Circulation 2004;109:433–8.

25. Langan SM, Seminara NM, Shin DB, et al. Prevalence of metabolic syndrome in patients with psoriasis: a population-based study in the United Kingdom. J Invest Dermatol 2012;132:556–62.

26. Goldminz AM, Buzney CD, Kim N, et al. Prevalence of the metabolic syndrome in children with psoriatic disease. Pediatr Dermatol 2013;30:700–5.

27. Wu S, Li WQ, Han J, et al. Hypercholesterolemia and risk of incident psoriasis and psoriatic arthritis in US women. Arthritis Rheumatol 2014;66:304–10.

28. Yu Y, Sheth N, Krishnamoorthy P, et al. Aortic vascular inflammation in psoriasis is associated with HDL particle size and concentration: a pilot study. Am J Cardiovasc Dis 2012;2:285–92.

29. Mehta NN, Li R, Krishnamoorthy P, et al. Abnormal lipoprotein particles and cholesterol efflux capacity in patients with psoriasis. Atherosclerosis 2012; 224:218–21.

30. Holzer M, Wolf P, Curcic S, et al. Psoriasis alters HDL composition and cholesterol efflux capacity. J Lipid Res 2012;53:1618–24.

31. Holzer M, Wolf P, Inzinger M, et al. Anti-psoriatic therapy recovers high-density lipoprotein composition and function. J Invest Dermatol 2014;134: 635–42.

32. Behnam SM, Behnam SE, Koo JY. Smoking and psoriasis. Skinmed 2005;4:174–6.

33. Wolk K, Mallbris L, Larsson P, et al. Excessive body weight and smoking associates with a high risk of onset of plaque psoriasis. Acta Derm Venereol 2009;89:492–7.

34. Poikolainen K, Karvonen J, Pukkala E. Excess mortality related to alcohol and smoking among hospital-treated patients with psoriasis. Arch Dermatol 1999;135:1490–3.

35. McAleer MA, Mason DL, Cunningham S, et al. Alcohol misuse in patients with psoriasis: identification and relationship to disease severity and psychological distress. Br J Dermatol 2011;164: 1256–61.

36. Armstrong AW, Harskamp CT, Dhillon JS, et al. Psoriasis and smoking: a systematic review and meta-analysis. Br J Dermatol 2014;170:304–14.

37. Torii K, Saito C, Furuhashi T, et al. Tobacco smoke is related to Th17 generation with clinical implications for psoriasis patients. Exp Dermatol 2011; 20:371–3.

38. Matsumoto C, Miedema MD, Ofman P, et al. An expanding knowledge of the mechanisms and effects of alcohol consumption on cardiovascular disease. J Cardiopulm Rehabil Prev 2014;34(3):159–71.

39. Dreiher J, Weitzman D, Shapiro J, et al. Psoriasis and chronic obstructive pulmonary disease: a case-control study. Br J Dermatol 2008;159: 956–60.

40. Tobin AM, Hughes R, Hand EB, et al. Homocysteine status and cardiovascular risk factors in patients with psoriasis: a case-control study. Clin Exp Dermatol 2011;36:19–23.

41. Schmitt J, Ford DE. Understanding the relationship between objective disease severity, psoriatic symptoms, illness-related stress, health-related quality of life and depressive symptoms in patients with psoriasis - a structural equations modeling approach. Gen Hosp Psychiatry 2007; 29:134–40.

42. Charlson FJ, Moran AE, Freedman G, et al. The contribution of major depression to the global burden of ischemic heart disease: a comparative risk assessment. BMC Med 2013;11:250.

43. Ryan C, Menter A. Psoriasis and cardiovascular disorders. G Ital Dermatol Venereol 2012;147: 179–87.

44. Davidovici BB, Sattar N, Prinz JC, et al. Psoriasis and systemic inflammatory diseases: potential mechanistic links between skin disease and co-morbid conditions. J Invest Dermatol 2010;130: 1785–96.

45. Gisondi P, Girolomoni G. Psoriasis and athero-thrombotic diseases: disease-specific and non-disease-specific risk factors. Semin Thromb Hemost 2009;35:313–24.

46. Armstrong AW, Voyles SV, Armstrong EJ, et al. Angiogenesis and oxidative stress: common mechanisms linking psoriasis with atherosclerosis. J Dermatol Sci 2011;63:1–9.

47. Boehncke WH, Boehncke S, Tobin AM, et al. The 'psoriatic march': a concept of how severe psoriasis may drive cardiovascular comorbidity. Exp Dermatol 2011;20:303–7.

48. Hansson GK, Hermansson A. The immune system in atherosclerosis. Nat Immunol 2011;12:204–12.

49. Libby P, Ridker PM, Hansson GK. Progress and challenges in translating the biology of atherosclerosis. Nature 2011;473:317–25.

50. Hashmi S, Zeng QT. Role of interleukin-17 and interleukin-17-induced cytokines interleukin-6 and interleukin-8 in unstable coronary artery disease. Coron Artery Dis 2006;17:699–706.

51. Wang Z, Lee J, Zhang Y, et al. Increased Th17 cells in coronary artery disease are associated with neutrophilic inflammation. Scand Cardiovasc J 2011;45:54–61.

52. Wyss CA, Neidhart M, Altwegg L, et al. Cellular actors, Toll-like receptors, and local cytokine profile in acute coronary syndromes. Eur Heart J 2010;31: 1457–69.

53. Cheng X, Yu X, Ding YJ, et al. The Th17/Treg imbalance in patients with acute coronary syndrome. Clin Immunol 2008;127:89–97.

54. Chen S, Crother TR, Arditi M. Emerging role of IL-17 in atherosclerosis. J Innate Immun 2010;2: 325–33.

55. Xie JJ, Wang J, Tang TT, et al. The Th17/Treg functional imbalance during atherogenesis in ApoE(-/-) mice. Cytokine 2010;49:185–93.

56. Eid RE, Rao DA, Zhou J, et al. Interleukin-17 and interferon-gamma are produced concomitantly by human coronary artery-infiltrating T cells and act synergistically on vascular smooth muscle cells. Circulation 2009;119:1424–32.

57. Taleb S, Romain M, Ramkhelawon B, et al. Loss of SOCS3 expression in T cells reveals a regulatory role for interleukin-17 in atherosclerosis. J Exp Med 2009;206:2067–77.

58. Wang M, Zhang W, Crisostomo P, et al. Endothelial STAT3 plays a critical role in generalized myocardial proinflammatory and proapoptotic signaling. Am J Physiol Heart Circ Physiol 2007; 293:H2101–8.

59. Mehta NN, Li K, Szapary P, et al. Modulation of cardiometabolic pathways in skin and serum from patients with psoriasis. J Transl Med 2013;11:194.

60. Rasouli N, Kern PA. Adipocytokines and the metabolic complications of obesity. J Clin Endocrinol Metab 2008;93:S64–73.

61. Chen YJ, Wu CY, Shen JL, et al. Psoriasis independently associated with hyperleptinemia contributing to metabolic syndrome. Arch Dermatol 2008;144:1571–5.

62. Spranger J, Kroke A, Möhlig M, et al. Adiponectin and protection against type 2 diabetes mellitus. Lancet 2003;361:226–8.

63. Hulthe J, Hultén LM, Fagerberg B. Low adipocyte-derived plasma protein adiponectin concentrations

are associated with the metabolic syndrome and small dense low-density lipoprotein particles: atherosclerosis and insulin resistance study. Metabolism 2003;52:1612–4.

64. Zhang Y, Proenca R, Maffei M, et al. Positional cloning of the mouse obese gene and its human homologue. Nature 1994;372:425–32.

65. Tartaglia LA. The leptin receptor. J Biol Chem 1997; 272:6093–6.

66. Bouloumié A, Drexler HC, Lafontan M, et al. Leptin, the product of Ob gene, promotes angiogenesis. Circ Res 1998;83:1059–66.

67. Frank S, Stallmeyer B, Kämpfer H, et al. Leptin enhances wound re-epithelialization and constitutes a direct function of leptin in skin repair. J Clin Invest 2000;106:501–9.

68. Cerman AA, Bozkurt S, Sav A, et al. Serum leptin levels, skin leptin and leptin receptor expression in psoriasis. Br J Dermatol 2008;159:820–6.

69. Hamminga EA, van der Lely AJ, Neumann HA, et al. Chronic inflammation in psoriasis and obesity: implications for therapy. Med Hypotheses 2006;67: 768–73.

70. Trayhurn P. The biology of obesity. Proc Nutr Soc 2005;64:31–8.

71. Wang Y, Chen J, Zhao Y, et al. Psoriasis is associated with increased levels of serum leptin. Br J Dermatol 2008;158:1134–5.

72. Wulster-Radcliffe MC, Ajuwon KM, Wang J, et al. Adiponectin differentially regulates cytokines in porcine macrophages. Biochem Biophys Res Commun 2004;316:924–9.

73. Okamoto Y, Kihara S, Funahashi T, et al. Adiponectin: a key adipocytokine in metabolic syndrome. Clin Sci (Lond) 2006;110:267–78.

74. Kaur S, Zilmer K, Kairane C, et al. Clear differences in adiponectin level and glutathione redox status revealed in obese and normal-weight patients with psoriasis. Br J Dermatol 2008;159:1364–7.

75. Coimbra S, Oliveira H, Reis F, et al. Circulating levels of adiponectin, oxidized LDL and C-reactive protein in Portuguese patients with psoriasis vulgaris, according to body mass index, severity and duration of the disease. J Dermatol Sci 2009;55: 202–4.

76. Shibata S, Saeki H, Tada Y, et al. Serum high molecular weight adiponectin levels are decreased in psoriasis patients. J Dermatol Sci 2009;55:62–3.

77. Takahashi H, Tsuji H, Takahashi I, et al. Plasma adiponectin and leptin levels in Japanese patients with psoriasis. Br J Dermatol 2008;159:1207–8.

78. Li RC, Krishnamoorthy P, DerOhannessian S, et al. Psoriasis is associated with decreased plasma adiponectin levels independently of cardiometabolic risk factors. Clin Exp Dermatol 2014;39:19–24.

79. Curat CA, Wegner V, Sengenès C, et al. Macrophages in human visceral adipose tissue: increased accumulation in obesity and a source of resistin and visfatin. Diabetologia 2006;49: 744–7.

80. Filková M, Haluzík M, Gay S, et al. The role of resistin as a regulator of inflammation: implications for various human pathologies. Clin Immunol 2009; 133:157–70.

81. Chu S, Ding W, Li K, et al. Plasma resistin associated with myocardium injury in patients with acute coronary syndrome. Circ J 2008;72:1249–53.

82. Reilly MP, Lehrke M, Wolfe ML, et al. Resistin is an inflammatory marker of atherosclerosis in humans. Circulation 2005;111:932–9.

83. Johnston A, Arnadottir S, Gudjonsson JE, et al. Obesity in psoriasis: leptin and resistin as mediators of cutaneous inflammation. Br J Dermatol 2008;159:342–50.

84. Boehncke S, Thaci D, Beschmann H, et al. Psoriasis patients show signs of insulin resistance. Br J Dermatol 2007;157:1249–51.

85. Yang Q, Graham TE, Mody N, et al. Serum retinol binding protein 4 contributes to insulin resistance in obesity and type 2 diabetes. Nature 2005;436: 356–62.

86. Rollman O, Vahlquist A. Psoriasis and vitamin A. Plasma transport and skin content of retinol, dehydroretinol and carotenoids in adult patients versus healthy controls. Arch Dermatol Res 1985;278:17–24.

87. Takeshita J, Mohler ER, Krishnamoorthy P, et al. Endothelial cell-, platelet-, and monocyte/macrophage-derived microparticles are elevated in psoriasis beyond cardiometabolic risk factors. J Am Heart Assoc 2014;3:e000507.

88. Tamagawa-Mineoka R, Katoh N, Kishimoto S. Platelet activation in patients with psoriasis: increased plasma levels of platelet-derived microparticles and soluble P-selectin. J Am Acad Dermatol 2010;62:621–6.

89. Pelletier F, Garnache-Ottou F, Angelot F, et al. Increased levels of circulating endothelial-derived microparticles and small-size platelet-derived microparticles in psoriasis. J Invest Dermatol 2011; 131:1573–6.

90. Rautou PE, Leroyer AS, Ramkhelawon B, et al. Microparticles from human atherosclerotic plaques promote endothelial ICAM-1-dependent monocyte adhesion and transendothelial migration. Circ Res 2011;108:335–43.

91. Kasperska-Zajac A, Brzoza Z, Rogala B. Platelet function in cutaneous diseases. Platelets 2008;19: 317–21.

92. Hayashi S, Shimizu I, Miyauchi H, et al. Increased platelet aggregation in psoriasis. Acta Derm Venereol 1985;65:258–62.

93. Ludwig RJ, Schultz JE, Boehncke WH, et al. Activated, not resting, platelets increase leukocyte

rolling in murine skin utilizing a distinct set of adhesion molecules. J Invest Dermatol 2004;122:830–6.

94. Nielsen HJ, Christensen IJ, Svendsen MN, et al. Elevated plasma levels of vascular endothelial growth factor and plasminogen activator inhibitor-1 decrease during improvement of psoriasis. Inflamm Res 2002;51:563–7.

95. Friedewald VE, Cather JC, Gelfand JM, et al. AJC editor's consensus: psoriasis and coronary artery disease. Am J Cardiol 2008;102:1631–43.

96. Strohal R, Kirby B, Puig L, the Psoriasis Expert Panel (Girolomoni G, Kragballe K, Luger T, Nestle FO, Prinz JC, Ståhle M, Yawalkar N). Psoriasis beyond the skin: an expert group consensus on the management of psoriatic arthritis and common co-morbidities in patients with moderate-to-severe psoriasis. Eur J Dermatol 2014;305–11. [Epub ahead of print].

97. Mehta NN, Yu Y, Pinnelas R, et al. Attributable risk estimate of severe psoriasis on major cardiovascular events. Am J Med 2011;124:775.e1–6.

98. Higa-Sansone G, Szomstein S, Soto F, et al. Psoriasis remission after laparoscopic Roux-en-Y gastric bypass for morbid obesity. Obes Surg 2004;14:1132–4.

99. Wolters M. Diet and psoriasis: experimental data and clinical evidence. Br J Dermatol 2005;153:706–14.

100. Naldi L, Conti A, Cazzaniga S, et al. Diet and physical exercise in psoriasis. A randomized trial. Br J Dermatol 2013;170(3):634–42.

101. Gisondi P, Del Giglio M, Di Francesco V, et al. Weight loss improves the response of obese patients with moderate-to-severe chronic plaque psoriasis to low-dose cyclosporine therapy: a randomized, controlled, investigator-blinded clinical trial. Am J Clin Nutr 2008;88:1242–7.

102. Roongpisuthipong W, Pongpudpunth M, Roongpisuthipong C, et al. The effect of weight loss in obese patients with chronic stable plaque-type psoriasis. Dermatol Res Pract 2013;2013:795932.

103. Sigurdardottir G, Ekman AK, Ståhle M, et al. Systemic treatment and narrowband ultraviolet B differentially affect cardiovascular risk markers in psoriasis. J Am Acad Dermatol 2014;70(6):1067–75.

104. Gerdes S, Osadtschy S, Buhles N, et al. Cardiovascular biomarkers in patients with psoriasis. Exp Dermatol 2014;23(5):322–5.

105. Silva D, Pais de Lacerda A. High-sensitivity C-reactive protein as a biomarker of risk in coronary artery disease. Rev Port Cardiol 2012;31:733–45 [in Portuguese].

106. Chandran V, Cook RJ, Edwin J, et al. Soluble biomarkers differentiate patients with psoriatic arthritis from those with psoriasis without arthritis. Rheumatology (Oxford) 2010;49:1399–405.

107. Coimbra S, Oliveira H, Reis F, et al. C-reactive protein and leucocyte activation in psoriasis vulgaris according to severity and therapy. J Eur Acad Dermatol Venereol 2010;24:789–96.

108. Yurtdaş M, Yaylali YT, Kaya Y, et al. Neutrophil-to-lymphocyte ratio may predict subclinical atherosclerosis in patients with psoriasis. Echocardiography 2014;31(9):1095–104.

109. Cao LY, Soler DC, Debanne SM, et al. Psoriasis and cardiovascular risk factors: increased serum myeloperoxidase and corresponding immunocellular overexpression by Cd11b(+) CD68(+) macrophages in skin lesions. Am J Transl Res 2013;6:16–27.

110. Boehncke S, Salgo R, Garbaraviciene J, et al. Effective continuous systemic therapy of severe plaque-type psoriasis is accompanied by amelioration of biomarkers of cardiovascular risk: results of a prospective longitudinal observational study. J Eur Acad Dermatol Venereol 2011;25(10):1187–93.

111. Wu JJ, Poon KY, Channual JC, et al. Association between tumor necrosis factor inhibitor therapy and myocardial infarction risk in patients with psoriasis. Arch Dermatol 2012;148:1244–50.

112. Prodanovich S, Prodanowich S, Ma F, et al. Methotrexate reduces incidence of vascular diseases in veterans with psoriasis or rheumatoid arthritis. J Am Acad Dermatol 2005;52:262–7.

113. Available at: http://clinicaltrials.gov/ct2/show/NCT01594333?term=NCT01594333&rank=1. Accessed March 31, 2014.

114. Ryan C, Amor KT, Menter A. The use of cyclosporine in dermatology: part II. J Am Acad Dermatol 2010;63:949–72 [quiz: 973–4].

115. Menter A, Korman NJ, Elmets CA, et al. Guidelines of care for the management of psoriasis and psoriatic arthritis: section 4. Guidelines of care for the management and treatment of psoriasis with traditional systemic agents. J Am Acad Dermatol 2009;61:451–85.

116. Vahlquist A. Long-term safety of retinoid therapy. J Am Acad Dermatol 1992;27:S29–33.

117. Mrowietz U, Rostami-Yazdi M, Neureither M, et al. 15 years of fumaderm: fumaric acid esters for the systemic treatment of moderately severe and severe psoriasis vulgaris. J Dtsch Dermatol Ges 2009;7(Suppl 2):S3–16 [in German].

118. Boehncke S, Fichtlscherer S, Salgo R, et al. Systemic therapy of plaque-type psoriasis ameliorates endothelial cell function: results of a prospective longitudinal pilot trial. Arch Dermatol Res 2011;303:381–8.

119. Ahlehoff O, Skov L, Gislason G, et al. Cardiovascular disease event rates in patients with severe psoriasis treated with systemic anti-inflammatory0 drugs: a Danish real-world cohort study. J Intern Med 2013;273:197–204.

120. Strober B, Teller C, Yamauchi P, et al. Effects of etanercept on C-reactive protein levels in psoriasis and psoriatic arthritis. Br J Dermatol 2008;159:322–30.

121. Kanelleas A, Liapi C, Katoulis A, et al. The role of inflammatory markers in assessing disease severity and response to treatment in patients with psoriasis treated with etanercept. Clin Exp Dermatol 2011;36(8):845–50.

122. Solomon DH, Massarotti E, Garg R, et al. Association between disease-modifying antirheumatic drugs and diabetes risk in patients with rheumatoid arthritis and psoriasis. JAMA 2011;305:2525–31.

123. Ryan C, Leonardi CL, Krueger JG, et al. Association between biologic therapies for chronic plaque psoriasis and cardiovascular events: a meta-analysis of randomized controlled trials. JAMA 2011;306:864–71.

124. Tzellos T, Kyrgidis A, Zouboulis CC. Re-evaluation of the risk for major adverse cardiovascular events in patients treated with anti-IL-12/23 biological agents for chronic plaque psoriasis: a meta-analysis of randomized controlled trials. J Eur Acad Dermatol Venereol 2013;27:622–7.

125. Dommasch ED, Troxel AB, Gelfand JM. Major cardiovascular events associated with anti-IL 12/23 agents: a tale of two meta-analyses. J Am Acad Dermatol 2013;68:863–5.

126. Greenland S, Salvan A. Bias in the one-step method for pooling study results. Stat Med 1990; 9:247–52.

127. Papp KA, Griffiths CE, Gordon K, et al. Long-term safety of ustekinumab in patients with moderate-to-severe psoriasis: final results from 5 years of follow-up. Br J Dermatol 2013;168:844–54.

Assessing Psoriasis Severity and Outcomes for Clinical Trials and Routine Clinical Practice

Robert J.G. Chalmers, MB, FRCP

KEYWORDS

- Psoriasis • Psychosocial morbidity • Quality of life • Severity assessment • Outcome measures
- Self-assessment • PROM • COSMIN

KEY POINTS

- Psoriasis is a disease with the potential to be life ruining.
- To justify health expenditure on its management, it is vital to be able to show that interventions make a difference to a patient's skin disease and ability to function normally.
- With modern methods of validating health care measurement instruments, more appropriate tools are being developed for use in clinical trials and routine clinical practice.
- The place of long-established tools is examined in the light of new tools that have recently been promoted.

ASSESSMENT AND OUTCOMES

Historically, dermatologists and others looking after patients with psoriasis have tended to record response to treatment, if at all, with rather imprecise phrases such as "nearly clear," "a bit better," "slightly improved," "worse," or "flared up." This probably still holds true for the majority of consultations between psoriasis patients and health care professionals. If they have instituted a new therapy, there is almost certainly a tendency for them to write "slightly better" rather than "no change," even if there is no clear evidence of meaningful benefit: Such wishful thinking is understandable, but can lead to long delays in changing to more appropriate therapy. Furthermore, the views of the patient may either not be sought or alternatively be dismissed as insignificant. Until recently,

it has been rare for formal assessments of severity to be undertaken outside the setting of clinical trials. Doctors managing hypertension would expect to get their patients' blood pressure checked on a regular basis. It should be a routine for at least some form of formal assessment of psoriasis severity and impact to be recorded on a regular basis for all patients receiving active treatment for psoriasis. The situation is slowly changing for the better, largely as a result of the cost implications of instituting expensive new agents for psoriasis and the need to demonstrate that they are producing benefit. Guidance is available from a range of specialist societies, patient organizations, and national health care bodies.[1–3]

Psoriasis is a disease with multiple dimensions, each of which can contribute in a range of different ways to its overall impact on the individual. To be

Funding Sources: None.

Conflict of Interest: Dr R.J.G. Chalmers has been involved in the development of the Simplified Psoriasis Index, but has no financial interests in this or in other matters relating to psoriasis.

Department of Dermatology, Manchester Royal Infirmary, Dermatology Centre, Salford Royal NHS Foundation Trust, University of Manchester, 16 Oaker Avenue, West Didsbury, Manchester M20 2XH, UK

E-mail address: r.chalmers@man.ac.uk

able to demonstrate objectively that any intervention for psoriasis can successfully modify that impact, it is necessary firstly to have tools for capturing and measuring that impact meaningfully and reliably (severity assessment) and second to understand what any given changes in such assessments actually mean in terms of modifying that impact. Only then can a meaningful assessment of the outcome of that intervention be derived.

Measuring change without reference to baseline severity (eg, "worse," "no change," "better") is little different from the traditional approach used by doctors in routine practice. In a chronic condition such as psoriasis, such assessments are of limited value for charting an individual patient's long-term disease behavior, because recall of fluctuations in disease severity over time is unlikely to be reliable. Neither are they useful for evaluating outcomes across a cohort of patients with unknown and potentially widely varying initial disease severity, as in a clinical trial comparing different interventions. Severity assessment at least 2 time points is a prerequisite for adequate documentation of change and thus for assessing outcomes.

The difference between severity assessment and outcome assessment can be illustrated clearly using the best known instrument for assessing psoriasis, the Psoriasis Area and Severity Index (PASI)[4]: The PASI assesses severity whereas a 75% reduction in PASI score (PASI-75) assesses outcome. Unfortunately, the term "outcome" is all too often used indiscriminately to describe both types, particularly in relation to so-called patient-reported outcome measures (PROMs). For instance, NHS England (The UK National Health Service as it applies to England) states: "PROMs measure a patient's health status or health-related quality of life at a single point in time."[5] In similar vein, the US Food and Drug Administration states: "A PRO (patient-reported outcome) is any report of the status of a patient's health condition that comes directly from the patient, without interpretation of the patient's response by a clinician or anyone else. The outcome can be measured in absolute terms (eg, severity of a symptom, sign, or state of a disease) or as a change from a previous measure."[6] Outcome can be assessed only by examining change, whether the desired outcome be change, as in interventions to treat disease, or no change, as in interventions intended to halt disease progression.

In many fields of medicine, outcome is straightforward to assess. Where there are well understood and easily measurable risk factors for adverse health outcomes, such as hypertension or hyperglycemia, it is straightforward to define a

successful outcome as a change of the parameter in question from abnormal/unacceptable to normal/acceptable. Thus, the outcomes of interventions to reduce risk of developing overt type II diabetes in individuals found to have high glycosylated hemoglobin levels (hemoglobin $A1_c \geq 6.5\%$) can be assessed by measuring whether the intervention has resulted in change to levels (eg, hemoglobin $A1_c \leq 6.0\%$) known to confer a lower risk.[7]

With many inflammatory or mental health conditions, however, it is not possible to assess change with such simple means. In disorders such as psoriasis and arthritis, there is a complex interplay between the externally apparent manifestations of the disease, the symptoms experienced by the patient, and the gamut of possible further physical, social, and psychological consequences of them. Furthermore, the latter are not necessarily directly related to the objective severity of the condition. The medical profession has been rather slow to recognize this complexity, but over the past 20 years significant progress has been made. In fact, the new discipline of clinimetrics has grown up around developing and validating disease severity assessments and outcome measures. This topic is well reviewed by Fava and colleagues.[8]

PSORIASIS ASSESSMENT TOOLS: A HISTORICAL PERSPECTIVE

For the current generation of dermatologists brought up to consider randomized, controlled trials as the norm for investigating new therapies for skin disease, it is instructive to look back a few decades. Until the advent of potent topical corticosteroids in the late 1950s, very few comparative trials in the field of psoriasis were conducted. The mainstays of treatment up until then had been tar, anthralin (dithranol), and broadband UVB phototherapy. At that time, there was no accepted methodology for performing clinical trials in inflammatory skin disease. Systemic therapy was largely limited to arsenic: Methotrexate was first investigated for treating psoriasis in the 1950s, but it was not until 2003 that this use of the drug was subjected to a randomized, controlled trial.[9]

A study selected at random from among the small number of formal psoriasis trials conducted in the 1960s exemplifies how much has changed.[10] It is clear that the investigators thought carefully how to design their study comparing 2 topical corticosteroid preparations with topical tar. Looked at from our perspective, however, it seems crude, with small patient numbers entered into an unblinded, unrandomized within-patient, left-right comparison of the 2 corticosteroids, which are then also compared with the patient's historical response to tar. What the investigators did do, however, was make an attempt to define what they meant by each of their outcome categories (**Box 1**) and this is by no means always the case, even in much more recent psoriasis trials.

In studies of psoralen photochemotherapy, which began to appear in the 1970s and where treatment could be expected to produce, at least in the short term, total or near total remission, the concept of "clearance" was introduced as the outcome success criterion.[11] In a large, randomized study from 1979 with well over 100 patients in each treatment arm, clearance was defined explicitly as "when all the lesions were flat and free of scales"; this was achieved in 91% and 82% of those who received psoralen photochemotherapy and dithranol, respectively.[12] More recently, "clearance" has tended to be qualified with phrases such as "clear or nearly clear" and "clear or minimal residual activity" to cater for those patients who may be left with a small residuum of psoriasis.[13] The UK National Institute of Health and Care Excellence (NICE) has further defined "minimal residual activity" as equivalent to greater than 90% reduction in PASI score.[14]

With the development of new systemic agents such as the oral retinoids, which were rarely capable of producing such clear-cut outcomes, the need for alternative outcome criteria became clear. It was for a dose-ranging study of etretinate published in 1978 that the PASI was created.[4] The PASI was, however, just one of the proliferation of scoring systems for psoriasis that Naldi and colleagues[15] found among psoriasis trials published in major journals between 1977 and 2000: They identified 44 separate measures among the 249

trials they examined. Nevertheless, a systematic review of treatments for severe psoriasis published in 2000 showed that PASI had become as widely used as "clearance" for defining outcomes, with each being utilized to define outcomes in about one quarter of all randomized controlled trials judged to be of sufficient quality for inclusion in the review (**Table 1**).[16] In the absence of a suitable alternative instrument, PASI was promoted for clinical trials of cyclosporine for psoriasis in the 1980s. There are many problems with PASI (which are discussed elsewhere), but a global consensus on how best to assess psoriasis and its response to treatment remains elusive. Many of the regulatory bodies continue to demand some form of PASI-based response criterion but supplemented by a simpler measure such as a change in global assessment score.[17,18] The need for both has recently been questioned.[19]

It is only much more recently that it has been recognized that there may be much to be gained by getting patients to assess their own disease severity either to complement or to replace an "objective" observer-rated assessment by a health professional. In diseases in which symptoms rather than signs predominate (eg, chronic pain), it is only the patient who can judge severity. In such a visible disease as psoriasis, however, rather little thought has been given to the potential advantages of asking patients to score their own disease. Not only may it be time saving for health professionals, but it can also give patients greater ownership of and participation in the management of their psoriasis. An adaptation of the PASI for completion by patients was introduced in the mid 1990s as the Self-Administered PASI.[20,21] It replicates the drawbacks of PASI itself and requires a professional to convert the patient's shading on line drawings to percentage body surface area (BSA) involvement. More recently the self-assessment Simplified Psoriasis Index (saSPI) has been proposed for patient self-reporting of psoriasis severity.[22,23]

It has been recognized for at least 70 years that there is an intimate relationship between psoriasis and psychological distress.[24–26] It has now become standard practice to include some measure of psychosocial impact in clinical trials of interventions for psoriasis. Such measures may be generic (applicable to any disease state), skin disease specific, or psoriasis specific.

The advantage of using a generic measure is that it may then be possible to compare the impact of a skin disease such as psoriasis with that of completely different disorders, such as musculoskeletal or respiratory disease. The disadvantage is that such generic measures may not capture

---

Box 1
Example of outcome measure used in 1964

ISQ = No change in the lesions.

O = Worse, when lesions became redder, more scaly, and thicker.

+++ = Marked improvement, when lesions almost cleared up completely.

++ = Fair or moderate improvement as shown by less erythema, scaling, and thickness.

+ = Slight improvement.

From Khoo OT, Fung WP, Koh KY. Clinical trial of P-1742 topical or fluperolone (9 fluoro-21 methyl prednisolone) in psoriasis. Singapore Med J 1964;5:69–72; with permission.

Table 1
Outcome measures used in randomized, controlled trials for severe psoriasis up to 2000

Active Intervention(s)	No. of Studies	Clear/Almost Clear	Psoriasis Area and Severity Index	Other/NR
Phototherapy regimens	21	4	2	15
Phototherapy plus topicals	19	6	1	12
Phototherapy with retinoids	11	1	4	6
Retinoids without phototherapy[a]	17	6	2	9
Cyclosporine[a]	18	3	12	3
Fumaric acid esters	4	2	1	1
Total	90	22	22	46

Abbreviation: NR, not reported.
[a] Comparison of retinoid versus cyclosporine included under cyclosporine only.
Data from Griffiths CE, Clark CM, Chalmers RJ, et al. A systematic review of treatments for severe psoriasis. Health Technol Assess 2000;4(40):1–125.

the particular elements of skin disease satisfactorily, because they were not designed with skin disease in mind. Study of the impact of chronic disease (eg, chronic pain, arthritis, stroke) on psychological well-being and functioning, together with developing methods of quantifying it, has spawned its own society (International Society for Quality of Life Research), the mission of which is "to advance the scientific study of health-related quality of life and other patient-centered outcomes to identify effective interventions, enhance the quality of health care and promote the health of populations."[27] One of the first and still most widely used generic quality of life instruments is the Medical Outcomes Study 36-Item Short Form Survey (SF-36).[28] The SF-36 has been used widely for psoriasis trials, but its components do not capture well much of the psychosocial impact that derives from having psoriasis.

The SF-36 was preceded by some 7 years by the Psoriasis Disability Index (PDI), which was pioneering when it was published in 1985.[29] This has been used widely in clinical studies[30]; in more recent times, however, the PDI has been largely supplanted by the more generic and simpler Dermatology Life Quality Index (DLQI; **Box 2**) that, like the PDI, was developed by Professor Andrew Finlay.[31] There is a range of other skin disease-specific, quality-of-life instruments that have been promoted, the most important of which are discussed elsewhere in this article.

THE DIMENSIONS OF PSORIASIS

Psoriasis is a complex disease, is often lifelong, and, in severe cases, life ruining. There is much more to it than its outwardly visible manifestations. This has recently been neatly summarized in the

Box 2
The questions of the dermatology life quality index[a]

1. Over the last week, how *itchy, sore, painful,* or *stinging* has your skin been?

2. Over the last week, how *embarrassed or self-conscious* have you been because of your skin?

3. Over the last week, how much has your skin interfered with you going *shopping* or looking after your *home* or *garden*?

4. Over the last week, how much has your skin influenced the clothes you wear?

5. Over the last week, how much has your skin affected any *social* or *leisure* activities?

6. Over the last week, how much has your skin made it difficult for you to do any *sport*?

7. Over the last week, has your skin prevented you from *working* or *studying*? If "no," over the last week how much has your skin been a problem at *work* or *studying*?

8. Over the last week, how much has your skin created problems with your *partner* or any of your *close friends* or *relatives*?

9. Over the last week, how much has your skin caused any *sexual difficulties*?

10. Over the last week, how much of a problem has the *treatment* for your skin been, for example, by making your home messy or by taking up time?

[a] The 10 questions contribute ≤3 points each (maximum 30) in answer to the question: "How much has your skin problem affected your life over the last week?"
Copyright © Finlay AY, Khan GK, April 1992. Used with permission.

UK's NICE Guidance on the assessment and management of psoriasis[17]:

> Death directly due to psoriasis is rare, but the chronic, incurable nature of psoriasis means that associated morbidity is significant. People with psoriasis, like those with other major medical disorders, have reduced levels of employment and income as well as a decreased quality of life. The impact of psoriasis encompasses functional, psychological, and social dimensions. Factors that contribute to this include symptoms specifically related to the skin (eg, chronic itch, bleeding, scaling and nail involvement), problems related to treatments (mess, odor, inconvenience and time), psoriatic arthritis, and the effect of living with a highly visible, disfiguring skin disease (difficulties with relationships, difficulties with securing employment and poor self esteem). Even people with minimal involvement state that psoriasis has a major effect on their life. The combined costs of long-term therapy and social costs of the disease have a major impact on healthcare systems and on society in general. About a third of people with psoriasis experience major psychological distress, and the extent to which they feel socially stigmatised and excluded is substantial. Healthcare professionals, including dermatologists, often fail to appreciate the extent of this disability and even when it is correctly identified, some estimates suggest that less than a third of people with psoriasis receive appropriate psychological interventions.

In attempting to capture these different dimensions, it is important to recognize that limiting assessment of psoriasis to its outward signs may grossly misrepresent the impact of that disease on the individual with psoriasis. Dermatologists have worked hard to ensure that the major regulatory and health care funding authorities incorporate some measure of quality of life impact into their appraisal of treatments for psoriasis. The principle of the "Rule of Tens," in which scores greater than 10 of any 1 of 3 measures, percent BSA involvement, PASI, or DLQI, would constitute evidence of current severe psoriasis,[32] has been adopted with minor modifications in a number of guidelines for the management of psoriasis.[17,33–35] There are, however, other dimensions of psoriasis that may be equally relevant in helping patients and clinicians to make informed decisions about management but that may not be captured by these tools. These omissions may in part be attributed to the deficiencies of PASI itself as an assessment tool or to the absence of a number of important items from DLQI, such as sleep deprivation or the economic cost of having psoriasis. Neither the presence nor absence of psoriatic arthritis, nor information about the historical behavior of an individual's psoriasis feature in any of the 3 measures, although they may be very important in reaching appropriate management decisions. Nevertheless, the acceptance that both "objective" severity and quality of life must be considered when assessing overall psoriasis severity has been a major advance.

DESIDERATA FOR PSORIASIS ASSESSMENT AND OUTCOME MEASURES

When PASI was born, its creators had very little guidance on how to go about the task. PASI was then adopted with rather little critical thought about its suitability for the tasks it was expected to perform. Since that time, there have been considerable advances in developing and evaluating assessment tools.

It is important to recognize that it is impossible to produce a "one size fits all" measure for assessing all aspects of psoriasis. The requirements for a proof-of-concept study of a new drug for psoriasis may be quite different from those for a tool that is sufficiently straightforward that it will be accepted for use in everyday clinical practice. There needs to be clarity about what it is important to measure and in which circumstances. Appraisal of any tool demands that a number of simple questions are asked.

The following list is based on the recommendations of Alvin Feinstein from the 1980s[8,36]:

- What is it for? (Purpose)
- Is it readily understood? (Comprehensibility)
- Does it make sense? (Face validity)
- Is it measuring the right things? (Content validity)
- Is it reliable? (Replicability)
- Can it detect differences? (Sensitivity)
- Can it detect change? (Responsiveness)
- When and where should it be used? (Applicability)
- Is it practical to use? (Employability)

The international COSMIN (COnsensus-based Standards for the selection of health Measurement INstruments) group based at the University Medical Center, Amsterdam, has set the standards required of new instruments for use in health care measurement, especially in the field of health-related quality of life.[37] The group has developed a critical appraisal tool (a checklist) to assist not only in assessing the methodological quality of published studies in which such measures are used, but also to guide the development and validation of new health measurement instruments (eg, clinical rating scales and patient-reported quality of life measures; **Table 2**). For a new instrument to be accepted its quality should be tested against these criteria.

INSTRUMENTS FOR OBSERVER-RATED ASSESSMENT OF PSORIASIS SEVERITY

A large number of scoring systems for psoriasis have been devised, the majority of which can be classed as "objective" in the sense that the assessment is performed by someone other than the patient (observer-rated). The most well-known of these is the PASI.

The Psoriasis Area and Severity Index

The PASI has become the "gold standard" for psoriasis severity measurement despite major flaws. The PASI was devised on the premise that a plaque of psoriasis is of equal significance wherever its location, such that equal weight is given to a large plaque on the lower back as is given to the same-sized plaque covering the face. For each of 4 body sites (the head and neck, the trunk, the upper extremities, and the lower extremities), 3 components of the psoriatic plaques within it (erythema, induration, and desquamation) are graded from 0 ("complete lack of") to 4 ("severest possible"). An estimate is then made of the extent of psoriasis in that site by estimating the BSA with possible scores ranging from 0 to 6 (**Fig. 1**). A complex formula (**Fig. 2**) is then applied to derive a score which may theoretically range from 0 to 72, although in practice scores above 36 are rare.

Despite its widespread use, the PASI has never been formally validated. Its gradings have never been properly defined or standardized. Although the original publication[4] is used as the standard reference source, it is not desquamation (shedding of skin scales) but scale thickness that is generally scored. There is no agreement on how erythema should be scored when obscured by overlying adherent scale. It is not explicitly stated whether induration excludes scale thickness. Its complex

---

Table 2
Domains of importance in appraising measurement instruments

Domain	Measurement
Reliability	The degree to which the measurement is free from measurement error.
Test–retest reliability	The extent to which scores for patients who have not changed are the same when measured repeatedly under different conditions.
Intrarater reliability	The patient or examiner rating on different (but temporally closely related) occasions.
Interrater reliability	Different examiners rating the same patient on the same occasion.
Validity	The degree to which an instrument measures what it purports to measure (the construct).
Content validity	The degree to which the content of an instrument is an adequate reflection of the construct to be measured.
Face validity	The degree to which the items of an instrument indeed look as though they are an adequate reflection of the construct to be measured.
Construct validity	The degree to which the scores of an instrument are consistent with hypotheses based on the assumption that the instrument validly measures the construct to be measured.
Structural validity	The degree to which the scores of an instrument are an adequate reflection of the dimensionality ("size and shape") of the construct to be measured.
Criterion validity	The degree to which the scores of an instrument are an adequate reflection of a 'gold standard.'
Responsiveness	The ability of an instrument to detect changes in severity over time in the construct to be measured.
Interpretability	Interpretability is the degree to which one can assign qualitative meaning—that is, clinical or commonly understood connotations—to an instrument's quantitative scores or change in scores. Does it make sense?

Adapted from COSMIN. COnsensus-based Standards for the selection of health Measurement Instruments. Available at: http://www.cosmin.nl/cosmin_1_0.html. Accessed May 31, 2014; with permission.

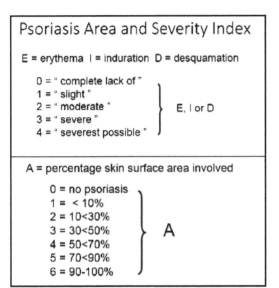

Fig. 1. Psoriasis Area and Severity Index (PASI) scoring guide.

arithmetical leaves it open to errors of calculation and its use of decimals for the final score gives it a false impression of precision.

These are not, however, its main drawbacks. The accuracy of BSA estimation by dermatologists is poor, with wide interrater variability and a tendency to overestimate. Studies have shown up to 4-fold differences between observers and up to 11-fold overestimate of BSA compared with measurement of plaque tracings, particularly with nummular (small plaque) psoriasis.[38,39] The estimates by 3 dermatologists and 1 experienced dermatology nurse of the BSA extent of psoriasis in the patient illustrated in **Fig. 3** ranged from 12% to 41%; plaque tracings and photographic analysis gave figures of 5% and 8%, respectively, for which the PASI extent score would be 1 (<10%).[38] Similar findings have been reported by others. From the point of view of the patient, however, his psoriasis is all over his body.

The PASI gives equal weight to psoriasis wherever it is located. From a patient's perspective, however, the impact of psoriasis is likely to be much greater if it involves the face, the hands, or the anogenital area than the back. Severe and disabling psoriasis of the hands and feet may result in the same score as a single large plaque on the lower back. The presence of a few scattered thick plaques can result in a PASI score equal to that from near erythrodermic psoriasis (**Table 3**).[40] There are, therefore, many reasons to criticize the PASI:

- Adopted without proper validation;
- Meanings not standardized and agreed
- Potential for wide interobserver variation
- Not linearly related to severity
- The upper half of the scale is rarely used
- Pseudoscientific precision has given it unjustified credence
- Often poorly correlated with patient perception of severity
- Insensitive to change for mild-to-moderate psoriasis
- Insensitive to involvement of "sensitive" sites (eg, face, genitalia, hands, and feet); and
- Cumbersome to use and prone to error in calculation.

There have been various attempts to overcome some of these problems including the Psoriasis Log-based Area and Severity Index,[41] the Psoriasis Exact Area and Severity Index,[41] and the Simplified Psoriasis Area Severity Index,[42] but none of these has found general favor.[43]

Physician Global Assessment Instruments for Psoriasis

There is no single physician global assessment (PGA) tool for psoriasis. The various versions of PGA have in common, however, much greater simplicity than PASI and usually employ a 5- to 7-point ranked scale from clear to severe. The differences relate to the number of points in the scale and the means by which each point is defined. This can be by very simple description ("clear," "mild," mild-to-moderate," etc) or may require comparison with images or with reference cards embossed with elevations to assist with estimation of plaque thickness.[44] In general, they do not take psoriasis extent into account. Changes in score may be more useful for documenting response to therapy than a static score to document severity.

Modified Physician Global Assessment Instruments

Investigators have recognized that the omission of scoring extent in PGA limits its usefulness.

Psoriasis Area and Severity Index

	head		trunk
	$0.1(E_h + I_h + D_h)A_h$ +		$0.3(E_t + I_t + D_t)A_t$ +
$PASI =$	upper extremities	+	lower extremities
	$0.2(E_u + I_u + D_u)A_u$		$0.4(E_l + I_l + D_l)A_l$

where E = erythema I = infiltration D = desquamation
A = percentage skin surface area involved

Maximum score = 72

Fig. 2. Psoriasis Area and Severity Index (PASI) formula.

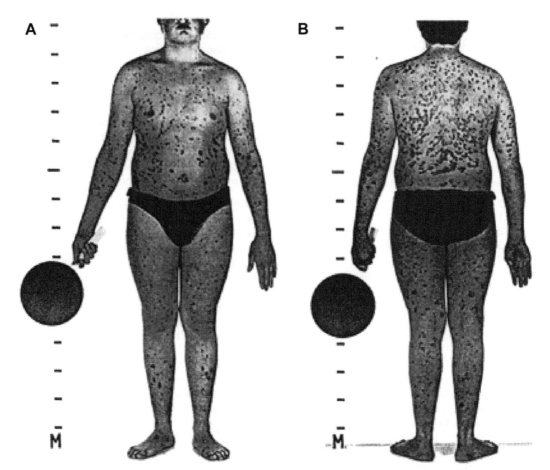

Fig. 3. Illustration of Psoriasis Area and Severity Index (PASI) extent score =1 (<10% body surface area). (*From* Ramsay B, Lawrence CM. Measurement of involved surface area in patients with psoriasis. Br J Dermatol 1991;124:565–70; with permission.)

Table 3
Examples of problems with Psoriasis Area and Severity Index (PASI) scoring

Distribution	BSA Affected (%)	Mean Area Score	Lesion Character	Lesion Score	PASI Score	Comment
A few plaques elbows and knees	4	1	Moderately thick, red, scaly plaques	2 + 2 + 2 = 6	3.6	Mild disease
Hands and feet only	3	1	Disabling confluent psoriasis	2 + 3 + 2 = 7	4.2	Severe and disabling psoriasis
One small plaque on scalp, 1 thigh, 1 arm, and on trunk	2	1	Very thick and scaly	4 + 4 + 4 = 12	12.0	Mild disease
Nearly half of body covered	40	3	Thin, quite red with slight scale	3 + 1 + 1 = 5	15.0	Very severe psoriasis
Near total body erythroderma	85	5	Quite red, but no thickness or scale	3 + 0 + 0 = 3	15.0	Severe, potentially life threatening

Data from Feldman SR. A quantitative definition of severe psoriasis for use in clinical trials. J Dermatolog Treat 2004;15:27–9.

There are 2 instruments that set out to combine extent with a PGA in an attempt to redress this. In the Lattice System Physician's Global Assessment (LS-PGA),[45] percent BSA involvement is categorized into 1 of 7 unequal ranges (0%, 1%–3%, 4%–9%, 10%–20%, 20%–29%, 30%–50%, and 50%–100%). Average overall plaque thickness (ignoring scale), erythema and scale are graded according to defined criteria into none, mild, moderate or marked. The single highest plaque quality score and the BSA are then entered into a lattice grid, which allots greater weight to plaque thickness than to scale or erythema, to derive a final severity score ranging from 0 (clear) to 7 (very severe) (**Fig. 4**). The extra weighting for plaque thickness was felt to be a better indicator of disease severity than erythema or scale, particularly because the latter can readily be removed by emollients and keratolytics without fundamentally altering the underlying severity of the psoriasis.

More recently, it has been proposed that the product of PGA and BSA (PGAxBSA) might provide a simpler alternative to PASI.[46] This provides

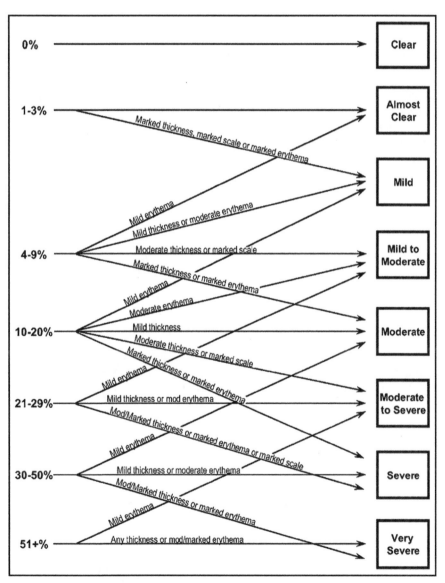

Fig. 4. Extract from lattice–Physician Global Assessment (PGA) score sheet. (*From* Langley RG, Ellis CN. Evaluating psoriasis with psoriasis area and severity index, psoriasis global assessment, and lattice system physician's global assessment. J Am Acad Dermatol 2004;51:563–9; with permission.)

a more continuous range of possible scores than the LS-PGA, but is conceptually similar. It has been tested mainly in patients with mild-to-moderate psoriasis with a median PASI score of only 3.2. Further validation is required. Both the LS-PGA and PGAxBSA have the disadvantage shared with PASI that they rely on an accurate estimation of BSA.

The Simplified Psoriasis Index

Simplified Psoriasis Index (SPI)[22] is a composite summary measure of psoriasis with separate components for current severity (SPI-s), psychosocial impact (SPI-p), and past history and interventions (SPI-i). It is available in 2 complementary versions, one for completion by health care professionals including dermatologists, dermatology nurses, and primary care physicians (proSPI) and a self-assessment version for completion by the patient (saSPI). The current severity component, SPI-s, dispenses with the need for estimation of BSA. Assessors are asked to judge psoriasis extent in 10 unequal body areas, weighted to reflect the impact of psoriasis affecting functionally or psychosocially important body sites. Thus, 50% of the total possible extent score is allotted to scalp, face, hands (+nails), feet (+nails), and anogenital area (**Fig. 5**). For each site the assessor has 3 options from which to choose:

- Clear or minimal with no more than a few scattered thin plaques (0)
- Obvious but still leaving plenty of normal skin (0.5); or
- Widespread and involving much of the affected area (1).

The maximum extent score is 10 with each site scored 0, 0.5, or 1. It thus differs from PASI in that dispersion of plaques in each given area is more important than actual BSA involvement. It also allows minimal psoriasis in any given site to be disregarded. Furthermore, nail disease can contribute up to 20% of the total extent score, even in the absence of skin involvement.

In common with LS-PGA and PGAxBSA, a single average is used for scoring plaque severity with a 6-point score ranging from 0 (essentially clear, with faint erythema or residual pigmentation

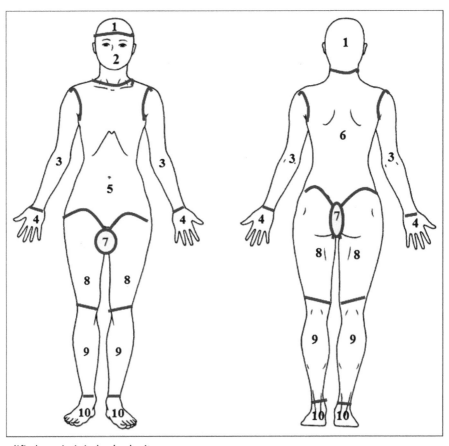

Fig. 5. Simplified psoriasis index body sites.

only) to 5 (intensely inflamed skin, with or without pustulation). A photographic key with thumbnail images is available in addition to the text descriptors to aid consistency in scoring each gradation. Separate scoring of scale, plaque thickness, and induration is not required.

The observer-rated psoriasis severity score (proSPI-s) has a maximum value of 10 × 5 = 50. The proSPI-s has been validated according to COSMIN criteria. In 100 patients with plaque psoriasis, there was a wide response distribution with close correlation between proSPI-s and PASI ($r = 0.91$). Strong intrarater and interrater reliability was demonstrated (intraclass correlation coefficients, >0.75). PASI-equivalent cutoff scores for mild (PASI <10) and severe (PASI >20) psoriasis were less than 9 and greater than 18, respectively (n = 300).

INSTRUMENTS FOR SELF-ASSESSMENT OF PSORIASIS SEVERITY BY PATIENTS

Despite focus in recent years on patient-reported assessments, there has been surprisingly little attempt to develop these for psoriasis.

Self-Administered Psoriasis Area and Severity Index

This instrument has already been described earlier in this article.[20,21] It is sufficiently similar to the PASI to inherit many of the latter's disadvantages. It has, however, been found to be a valid and reliable tool with reasonable correlation with PASI ($r^2 = 0.59$).[18,19] It does require a professional to estimate BSA from the patient's sketches.

Self-Assessment Simplified Psoriasis Index

The Self-Assessment Simplified Psoriasis Index (saSPI-s) is the counterpart of proSPI-s and apart from simplification of the language it is identical (Fig. 6).[22,23] It was shown to correlate more closely with DLQI ($r = 0.82$) and the psychosocial impact score of SPI (SPI-p; $r = 0.78$) than did either proSPI-s ($r = 0.59$) or PASI ($r = 0.60$), suggesting that it better reflected the patients' own perceptions of their disease severity than did the observer-rated scores.[20] There was nevertheless good correlation between the saSPI-s and both the PASI ($r = 0.70$) and the proSPI-s ($r = 0.70$). Furthermore, the saSPI-s had a wide response distribution. The authors reported that most patients have little difficulty in completing the proforma and recommended that it was suitable for use in the routine clinic as well as for clinical trials.

INSTRUMENTS FOR ASSESSING THE PSYCHOSOCIAL IMPACT OF PSORIASIS

These instruments have been systematically reviewed.[47] Eight scales were found to perform satisfactorily in terms of validity, reliability, sensitivity to change (responsiveness), and acceptability. By far the most widely used in psoriasis trials are the DLQI[29] and SF-36.[26] The other scales that were approved have been used much less frequently and included Skindex 29, Skindex 17, Dermatology Quality of life Scale PDI,[29] Impact of Psoriasis Questionnaire, and Psoriasis Index of Quality of Life. The SPI-p has been published too recently to have been considered in this review.

Dermatology Life Quality Index

This index was introduced earlier in this review. It consists of 10 questions (see Table 3), each of which can contribute up to 3 points toward a total of 30. It is not psoriasis specific, but has been used widely in psoriasis trials and for longer term monitoring of patients. It is simple to complete and can help health care professionals to understand better the ways in which psoriasis may be affecting a patient's life.

The Simplified Psoriasis Index

The SPI-p is one of the three domains of SPI. Patients are presented with a simple 10-cm visual analog scale and the instruction[20]: "Please make a mark on the line below to show us how much your psoriasis is affecting you in your day-to-day life today." They are given some guidance with the following examples of responses:

0 = my psoriasis is not affecting me at all.
5 = my psoriasis is affecting me quite a lot.
10 = my psoriasis is affecting me very much (I could not imagine it affecting me more).

Their responses are converted into an 11-point Likert score (0–10). In 100 patients who completed DLQI at the same time, there was a wide response distribution and a close correlation between SPI-p and DLQI ($r = 0.89$). Although the precise components contributing to psychosocial distress cannot be deduced from this simple measure, it can be used very readily and repeatedly within the setting of the routine clinic.

COMPOSITE INSTRUMENTS FOR THE ASSESSMENT OF PSORIASIS

In the field of rheumatology, a large number of composite assessment scores have been developed to

Simplified Psoriasis Index
Self-Assessment Form

Date:

LABEL or Record no: Sex:

First name:

Surname:

Thank you for completing this questionnaire which will help us understand more about you and your psoriasis. If you need help with filling in the form please ask the nurse or researcher present. The questions are in three parts and tell us a little about how your psoriasis is now, how it is affecting you personally and how it has behaved in the past.

Please mark how you think your psoriasis is today

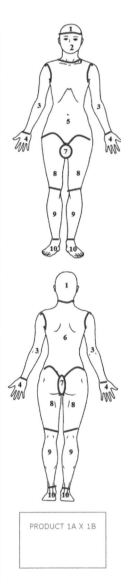

PART 1A For each of these 10 body areas please **circle** one choice which best describes your psoriasis **today**

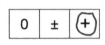

0	clear or so minor that it does not bother me (0)
±	obvious but still leaving plenty of normal skin (0.5)
+	widespread and involving much of the affected area (1.0)

1	Scalp & hairline	0	±	+
2	Face, neck & ears	0	±	+
3	Arms & armpits	0	±	+
4	Hands, fingers & fingernails*	0	±	+
5	Chest & abdomen (stomach)	0	±	+
6	Back & shoulders	0	±	+
7	Genital area and/or around anus (back passage)	0	±	+
8	Buttocks & thighs	0	±	+
9	Knees, lower legs & ankles	0	±	+
10	Feet, toes & toenails*	0	±	+

*PSORIASIS OF THE NAILS: even if the skin of the hands or feet is unaffected you can score ± for severe psoriasis of at least 2 and + for 6 or more finger or toenails

SUM

PART 1B Please **circle** whichever of these choices best describes the overall state of your psoriasis **today**. Your score should reflect the **average** of **all** of your psoriasis, not just the worst areas.

0	Clear or just slight redness or staining
1	Mild redness or scaling with no more than slight thickening
2	Definite redness, scaling or thickening
3	Moderately severe with obvious redness, scaling or thickening
4	Very red and inflamed, very scaly or very thick
5	Intensely inflamed skin with or without pustules (pus spots)

You may be given some photographic images to help you score your psoriasis.

PRODUCT 1A X 1B

Fig. 6. Self-assessment version of simplified psoriasis index (first side). (*From* Chularojanamontri L, Griffiths CE, Chalmers RJ. The simplified psoriasis index (SPI): a practical tool for assessing psoriasis. J Invest Dermatol 2013;133:1956–62; with permission.)

assist in defining response to interventions. For example, the American College of Rheumatologists/European League Against Rheumatism Core Data Set for rheumatoid arthritis studies includes 3 assessor-derived measures—tender joint count, swollen joint count, and PGA; 1 laboratory test—erythrocyte sedimentation rate or C-reactive protein level; and 3 patient self-reported questionnaires—on functional disability, pain, and overall assessment. The magnitude of improvement is then based on attaining a given percentage reduction both in tender and in swollen joint counts, as well as specified improvements in 3 of the 5 other measures, to achieve ACR20, ACR50, or ACR70 responses.[48]

Because of its visibility, psoriasis is fortunately simpler to measure than is rheumatoid arthritis, even though the ideal means of doing so have yet to be agreed. There is rightly a reluctance to combine very different types of data into a single composite, as is required for many of the rheumatology measures. Nevertheless, it can be informative to present summary information in an easily comprehensible format.

Salford Psoriasis Index

This instrument was developed in the late 1990s and was the prototype for SPI.[49] It introduced the concept of a triplet summary score comprising current severity, psychosocial impact, and psoriasis history. Although well-received by commentators, its wide adoption was hindered by the requirement for prior calculation of PASI and its complex history and interventions score.

The Simplified Psoriasis Index

The SPI was designed as a simple, 3-part summary measure including current psoriasis severity (SPI-s), psychosocial impact (SPI-p), and past history and interventions (SPI-i).[22,23] Most of its elements have been discussed previously. It is available in complementary observer-rated (proSPI) and patient self-assessed (saSPI) versions, which differ only in the means of scoring current psoriasis severity (proSPI-s and saSPI-s, respectively). The SPI-i includes information on interventions received and on age of onset and duration of psoriasis. Good correlation between proSPI-s and saSPI-s has been demonstrated ($r = 0.70$)[47] and, as mentioned, the correlation between saSPI-s and psychosocial impact (saSPI-p and SLQI) was greater for saSPI-s than for proSPI-s or PASI, suggesting that saSPI may provide a better indication of a patient's perception of psoriasis severity than proSPI-s or PASI.

OUTCOME MEASURES FOR PSORIASIS

Outcome measures involve either assessing the magnitude of change or the attainment of a particular goal, which in the case of psoriasis would normally be clearance or near clearance. There is a presumption that psoriasis was present when the intervention was instituted. It would be rare, however, for some measure of psoriasis severity not to have been recorded at enrollment into an interventional study for psoriasis.

Clearance or Minimal Residual Activity

This category involves change from an undefined prior severity to clearance and has largely been restricted to phototherapy trials.

Psoriasis Area and Severity Index-75 and -90

These measures record a reduction in PASI score by at least 75% and 90%, respectively. They have been widely used in clinical trials. The PASI-90 is similar to clearance or minimal residual activity and, with the development of more effective agents for psoriasis, there have been calls to make PASI-90 rather than the currently used PASI-75 the standard criterion of success.[50]

Physician Global Assessment 0 to 1

The attainment of a PGA score of 0 or 1 in a 6- or 7-point PGA scale may be regarded as equivalent to clearance or minimal residual activity.

Professionals Simplified Psoriasis Index and Self-Assessment Simplified Psoriasis Index

The SPI equivalents of PASI-75 were shown to be 85% and 95% reductions in proSPI-s and saSPI-s, respectively.[23]

SUMMARY

The advent of powerful new agents for treating psoriasis has put a spotlight on the need for reliable and practical tools for assessing psoriasis and its impact. Further work is still needed to validate existing instruments and to develop new ones, with the hope that PASI will no longer remain the mainstay of psoriasis severity assessment. The International Psoriasis Council recognizes the need for change and will continue to work to improve the tools at our disposal.

REFERENCES

1. UK National Clinical Guideline Centre (2012). Psoriasis: assessment and management of psoriasis. Available at: http://www.nice.org.uk/nicemedia/live/13938/61192/61192.pdf. Accessed May 22, 2014.

2. Kragballe K, Gniadecki R, Mørk NJ, et al. Implementing best practice in psoriasis: a Nordic expert group consensus. Acta Dermatovenerol 2014;94: 547–52. http://dx.doi.org/10.2340/00015555-1809.

3. Pathirana D, Ormerod AD, Saiag P, et al. European S3-guidelines on the systemic treatment of psoriasis vulgaris. J Eur Acad Dermatol Venereol 2009; 23(Suppl 2):1–70.

4. Fredriksson T, Pettersson U. Severe psoriasis-oral therapy with a new retinoid. Dermatologica 1978; 157:238–44.

5. NHS England. Patient Reported Outcome Measures (PROMs). Available at: http://www.england.nhs.uk/statistics/statistical-work-areas/proms/. Accessed May 22, 2014.

6. US Food and Drug Administration. Patient-reported outcome measures: use in medical product development to support labeling claims. Guidance for industry. 2009. Available at: http://www.fda.gov/downloads/Drugs/GuidanceComplianceRegulatoryInformation/Guidances/UCM071975.pdf. Accessed May 29, 2014.

7. UK National Institute for Health and Care Excellence (2012). PH38 preventing type 2 diabetes: risk identification and interventions for individuals at high risk. Available at: http://publications.nice.org.uk/preventing-type-2-diabetes-risk-identification-and-interventions-for-individuals-at-high-risk-ph38/. Accessed May 29, 2014.

8. Fava GA, Tomba E, Sonino N. Clinimetrics: the science of clinical measurements. Int J Clin Pract 2012;6:11–5.

9. Heydendael V, Spuls PI, Opmeer B, et al. Methotrexate versus cyclosporine in moderate-to-severe chronic plaque psoriasis. N Engl J Med 2003;349:658–65.

10. Khoo OT, Fung WP, Koh KY. Clinical trial of P-1742 topical or fluperolone (9 fluoro-21 methyl prednisolone) in psoriasis. Singapore Med J 1964;5:69–72.

11. Parrish JA, Fitzpatrick TB, Tanenbaum L, et al. Photochemotherapy of psoriasis with oral methoxsalen and longwave ultraviolet light. N Engl J Med 1974; 291:1207–11.

12. Rogers S, Marks J, Shuster S, et al. Comparison of photochemotherapy and dithranol in the treatment of chronic plaque psoriasis. Lancet 1979;8114: 455–8.

13. Yones SS, Palmer MA, Garibaldinos TT, et al. Randomized double-blind trial of the treatment of chronic plaque psoriasis: efficacy of psoralen–UV-A therapy vs narrowband UV-B therapy. Arch Dermatol 2006;142:836–42.

14. UK National Institute for Health and Care Excellence. Psoriasis: management of psoriasis - tools for assessing disease severity and impact. Available at: http://www.nice.org.uk/nicemedia/live/12344/58871/58871.pdf. Accessed May 24, 2014.

15. Naldi L, Svensson A, Diepgen T, et al. Randomized clinical trials for psoriasis 1977-2000: the EDEN survey. J Invest Dermatol 2003;120:738–41.

16. Griffiths CE, Clark CM, Chalmers RJ, et al. A systematic review of treatments for severe psoriasis. Health Technol Assess 2000;4(40):1–125.

17. European Medicines Agency. Guideline on clinical investigation of medicinal products indicated for the treatment of psoriasis. 2004. Available at: http://www.ema.europa.eu/docs/en_GB/document_library/Scientific_guideline/2009/09/WC500003329.pdf. Accessed May 30, 2014.

18. UK National Institute for Health and Care Excellence. Psoriasis - assessment and management of psoriasis - clinical guideline - methods, evidence and recommendations. 2012. Available at: http://www.nice.org.uk/nicemedia/live/13938/61192/61192.pdf. Accessed May 30, 2014.

19. Robinson A, Kardos M, Kimball AB. Physician Global Assessment (PGA) and Psoriasis Area and Severity Index (PASI): why do both? A systematic analysis of randomized controlled trials of biologic agents for moderate to severe plaque psoriasis. J Am Acad Dermatol 2012;66:369–75.

20. Fleischer AB, Rapp SR, Reboussin DM, et al. Patient measurement of psoriasis disease severity with a structured instrument. J Invest Dermatol 1994;102: 967–9.

21. Feldman SR, Fleischer AB Jr, Reboussin DM, et al. The self-administered psoriasis area and severity index is valid and reliable. J Invest Dermatol 1996; 106:183–6.

22. Chularojanamontri L, Griffiths CE, Chalmers RJ. The Simplified Psoriasis Index (SPI): a practical tool for assessing psoriasis. J Invest Dermatol 2013;133:1956–62.

23. Chularojanamontri L, Griffiths CE, Chalmers RJ. Responsiveness to change and interpretability of the simplified psoriasis index. J Invest Dermatol 2014;134:351–8.

24. Wittkower E. Psychological aspects of psoriasis. Lancet 1946;1:566–9.

25. Seville RH. Psoriasis and stress. Br J Dermatol 1977; 97:297–302.

26. Jobling R. Psoriasis—a preliminary questionnaire study of sufferers' subjective experience. Clin Exp Dermatol 1976;1:233–6.

27. International Society for Quality of Life Research. About ISOQOL. Available at: http://www.isoqol.org/about-isoqol. Accessed May 31, 2014.

28. Ware J, Sherbourne CD. The MOS 36-item short-form health survey (SF-36): I. Conceptual framework and item selection. Med Care 1992;30:473–83.

29. Finlay AY, Kelly SE. Psoriasis – an index of disability. Clin Exp Dermatol 1987;12:8–11.

30. Lewis VJ, Finlay AY. Two decades' experience of the psoriasis disability index. Dermatology 2005;210:261–8.

31. Finlay AY, Khan GK. Dermatology Life quality Index (DLQI): a simple practical measure for routine clinical use. Clin Exp Dermatol 1994;19:210–6.

32. Finlay AY. Current severe psoriasis and the Rule of Tens. Br J Dermatol 2005;152:861–7.

33. Smith CH, Anstey AV, Barker JN, et al. British Association of Dermatologists' guidelines for biologic interventions for psoriasis 2009. Br J Dermatol 2009; 161:987–1019.

34. Baker C, Mack A, Cooper A, et al. Treatment goals for moderate to severe psoriasis: an Australian consensus. Australas J Dermatol 2013;54:148–54.

35. Boehncke WH, Brasie RA, Barker J, et al. Recommendations for the use of etanercept in psoriasis: a European dermatology expert group consensus. J Eur Acad Dermatol Venereol 2006;20:988–98.

36. Feinstein AR. Clinimetrics. New Haven (CT): Yale University Press; 1987.

37. COSMIN. COnsensus-based Standards for the selection of health Measurement Instruments. Available at: http://www.cosmin.nl/cosmin_1_0.html. Accessed May 31, 2014.

38. Ramsay B, Lawrence CM. Measurement of involved surface area in patients with psoriasis. Br J Dermatol 1991;124:565–70.

39. Marks R, Barton SP, Shuttleworth D. Assessment of disease progress in psoriasis. Arch Dermatol 1989; 125:235–40.

40. Feldman SR. A quantitative definition of severe psoriasis for use in clinical trials. J Dermatolog Treat 2004;15:27–9.

41. Jacobson CC, Kimball AB. Rethinking the psoriasis area and severity index: the impact of area should be increased. Br J Dermatol 2004;151:381–7.

42. Louden BA, Pearce DJ, Lang W, et al. A Simplified Psoriasis Area Severity Index (SPASI) for rating psoriasis severity in clinic patients. Dermatol Online J 2004;10:7.

43. Henseler T, Schmitt-Rau KA. A comparison between BSA, PASI, PLASI and SAPASI as measures of disease severity and improvement by therapy in patients with psoriasis. Int J Dermatol 2008;47: 1019–23.

44. Feldman SR, Krueger GG. Psoriasis assessment tools in clinical trials. Ann Rheum Dis 2005;64:ii65–8.

45. Langley RG, Ellis CN. Evaluating psoriasis with psoriasis area and severity index, psoriasis global assessment, and lattice system physician's global assessment. J Am Acad Dermatol 2004;51:563–9.

46. Walsh JA, McFadden M, Woodcock J, et al. Product of the physician global assessment and body surface area: a simple static measure of psoriasis severity in a longitudinal cohort. J Am Acad Dermatol 2013;69:931–7.

47. Bronsard V, Paul C, Prey S, et al. What are the best outcome measures for assessing quality of life in plaque type psoriasis? a systematic review of the literature. J Eur Acad Dermatol Venereol 2010;24:17–22.

48. Pincus T, Strand V, Koch G, et al. An index of the three core data set patient questionnaire measures distinguishes efficacy of active treatment from that of placebo as effectively as the American College of Rheumatology 20% response criteria (ACR20) or the Disease Activity Score (DAS) in a rheumatoid arthritis clinical trial. Arthritis Rheum 2003;48: 625–30.

49. Kirby B, Fortune DG, Bhushan M, et al. The Salford Psoriasis Index: an holistic measure of psoriasis severity. Br J Dermatol 2000;142:728–32.

50. Puig L. Shortcomings of PASI75 and practical calculation of PASI area component. J Am Acad Dermatol 2013;68:180–1.

An Update on Topical Therapies for Mild-Moderate Psoriasis

Peter C.M. van de Kerkhof, MD, PhD

KEYWORDS

- Calcipotriol • Calcitriol • Corticosteroids • Ditranol • Small molecules • Tar • Tazarotene

KEY POINTS

- Current topical treatments are described in monotherapy and combination schedules.
- Evidence is available that the combination of calcipotriol and potent corticosteroids is more effective and has less side effects compared with monotherapies.
- Adherence is relevant for the success of a topical treatment.
- New small molecules provide opportunities for advances in new topical treatments of psoriasis.

GENERAL INTRODUCTION

Topical therapies are the first-line treatment in most patients with psoriasis.[1] In general treatments are given for short episodes. In patients who use systemic treatments or biologics, a topical treatment may be indicated for residual recalcitrant lesions. Combinations of several topicals or a topical and a systemic treatment is common practice.

Adherence to treatment may be a limitation of topicals. In particular if a treatment has a slow onset of efficacy or the treatment offers a practical problem, treatment adherence may seriously decrease the outcome.[2] Therefore, innovations in formulation of topicals may provide meaningful improvement in adherence.

The vehicle can have a therapeutic effect by itself. This is clearly shown in recent trials with the scalp lipogel containing calcipotriol and betamethasone dipropionate for scalp psoriasis, where response rates greater than 20% were achieved with the lipogel vehicle by itself without active ingredients.[3]

Evidence for efficacy is restricted for the classical topical treatments and more extensive for the first-line topical treatments.[4,5] Based on the best evidence and expert opinions treatment guidelines have been constructed.[6] This article highlights the current position of available topical agents and provides an insight into the future perspectives of small molecules.

THE CURRENT POSITION OF CLASSICAL TOPICAL AGENTS

The three classical topical therapies dithranol, tar, and salicylic acids have been used in the treatment of psoriasis for 50 to 100 years. Efficacy and safety studies at the highest level of evidence are sparse. Methods of classical treatments are not standardized and different protocols in different treatment settings are used. Therefore, the interpretation of studies comparing classical and more innovative topical results cannot be generalized.[7] When first-line topical treatments and systemic therapies are ineffective or contraindicated classical topicals may provide the solution.

Dithranol (anthralin, cignolin,1,8-dihydroxy-9-anthrone) has been available for nearly 100 years. It has a marked antihyperproliferative effect and inhibits mitogen-induced T-lymphocyte proliferation

Department of Dermatology, Radboud University Nijmegen Medical Centre, PO Box 9101, Nijmegen 6500HB, The Netherlands
E-mail address: Peter.vandekerkhof@radboudumc.nl

Dermatol Clin 33 (2015) 73–77
http://dx.doi.org/10.1016/j.det.2014.09.006
0733-8635/15/$ – see front matter © 2015 Elsevier Inc. All rights reserved.

and neutrophil chemotaxis. In Europe and other regions outside the United States, it is used most often in daycare centers and the inpatient setting.[8] Efficacy of dithranol in patients with moderate to severe psoriasis at inpatient departments and at daycare units has been reported to be 66% and 81.7%, respectively.[9]

Coal tar has a range of anti-inflammatory actions and is effective as an antipruritic agent. Coal tar activates the aryl hydrocarbon receptor, resulting in induction of epidermal differentiation. It also counteracts Th2 cytokine-mediated downregulation of skin barrier proteins.[10] Although tar has been shown to induce skin cancers in animal experiments, coal tar has not been shown to be a carcinogenic risk factor if provided as a specific antipsoriatic treatment.[11]

THE CURRENT POSITION OF FIRST-LINE TOPICAL AGENTS

The evidence-based approach to estimate efficacy and safety of topical treatments is hampered because few randomly controlled trials are available for the classical topical treatments. Evidence-based data for corticosteroids are less than for vitamin D–based treatments and tazarotene.[12] Strategies containing potent corticosteroids (alone or in combination with a vitamin D analogue) or very potent corticosteroids have dominated the treatment progress for psoriasis on the trunk, limbs, and scalp. For treatment of the face and flexures calcineurin inhibitors and weak topical corticosteroids are indicated.

Guidelines of care for the management and treatment of psoriasis with topical therapies have been developed by the American Academy of Dermatology.[6]

Vitamin D₃ Analogues

In the early 1990s, vitamin D_3 analogues became commercially available as a topical treatment for psoriasis. Vitamin D_3 inhibits excess epidermal proliferation, and enhances cornified envelope formation; it also inhibits several neutrophil functions. Because of their therapeutic efficacy and limited toxicity, calcipotriol, calcitriol, and tacalcitol have become a first-line treatment in psoriasis.

Calcipotriol monotherapy can result in a 59% reduction of psoriasis area and severity index (PASI) after 8 weeks of treatment.[13] In up to 5% of patients irritation of the skin necessitates discontinuation of vitamin D treatments. Calcitriol is now a widely accepted vitamin D treatment in psoriasis.[14] In view of the moderate efficacy and irritation vitamin D treatments are often combined with a topical corticosteroids.

Corticosteroids

Since their introduction in the early 1950s, topical corticosteroids have become a mainstay in the treatment of psoriasis. They are first-line therapy in mild to moderate psoriasis and are effective in low-potency sites, such as the flexures and genitalia, where other topical treatments can induce irritation.

Over the years, the anti-inflammatory properties of topical corticosteroids have been improved by increasing their lipophilicity. For example, fluticasone propionate is very lipophilic because of its highly esterified structure.[15,16]

Corticosteroids are manufactured in various vehicles, from ointments, creams, and lotions to gels, foams, sprays, and shampoo.[16–18] Novel formulations provide additional options for individuals. Clobetasol propionate 0.05% spray allows application of corticosteroids on areas that are difficult to reach[19] and has been shown to be even more potent than the ointment formulation.[20]

Clobetasol propionate and betamethasone valerate in foam formulations are well appreciated by patients because drying is rapid with minimal residue left on the skin after application. Significant efficacy has been shown in placebo-controlled studies.[20–22] These formulations are also well suited for the treatment of scalp psoriasis. Clobetasol in a shampoo formulation is now available for the treatment of scalp psoriasis and has been shown to be superior to a tar-blend shampoo.[23]

Long-term treatment with the shampoo formulation using twice weekly applications proved to be effective and safe, with 66% and 79% of the patients reporting treatment satisfaction and user convenience, respectively.[24] Innovations in corticosteroid formulation are also provided by nail lacquers. In a small study of 10 patients, 8% clobetasol nail lacquer resulted in reduced onycholysis, pitting, and salmon patches after only 4 weeks of treatment.[25] This formulation is safe, effective, and cosmetically acceptable for the treatment of nail bed and matrix psoriasis, locations that are difficult to treat because drug penetration is traditionally poor in these areas.

Corticosteroids are highly effective in psoriasis when used continuously for up to 8 weeks and intermittently for up to 52 weeks. There is a lack of long-term efficacy and safety data available on topical interventions used for psoriasis. Unfortunately, no efficacy data are available on prolonged treatment for more than 3 months. Because tachyphylaxis and/or rebound can occur fairly rapidly (ie, within a few days to weeks), intermittent treatment schedules (eg, once every 2 or 3 days or on weekends) are advised for more prolonged treatment courses. It should be kept in mind that decrease in treatment adherence may imitate tachyphylaxis.[26] Therefore, careful instruction to all patients initiating and being maintained on topical treatments is essential.

Topical Retinoids

All-*trans*-retinoic acid and 13-*cis*-retinoic acid, although effective in the treatment of acne, are not effective for psoriasis. However, topical tazarotene, an acetylene retinoid that selectively binds retinoic acid receptor-β and -γ, has been shown to be successful.[27] Tazarotene decreases epidermal proliferation and inhibits psoriasis-associated differentiation (eg, transglutaminase expression and keratin 16 expression).

After 6 weeks of treatment, at least 50% improvement (compared with baseline) was noted by 45% of the patients using twice-daily 0.05% tazarotene gel as compared with 13% of the patients using the placebo gel. In view of its modest efficacy and irritation in up to 23% of patients it is usually prescribed as a second-line therapy. For this reason, combination therapy with topical corticosteroids is useful. The maximal area that can be treated with tazarotene is 10% to 20% of the body surface. Safety data are available for up to 1 year of treatment.

Calcineurin inhibitors are used to treat facial and flexural psoriasis. Randomized, placebo-controlled studies have demonstrated efficacy and safety for this indication.[28,29]

BENEFICIAL COMBINATIONS

Combination of potent corticosteroids with calcipotriol has been studied most extensively and should be regarded as an efficacious and safe treatment option, with the two-compound single combination product shown to be a practical remedy.[30,31]

Other advantageous combinations, with limited evidence, are the combination of tazarotene gel with corticosteroid creams and the combination of dithranol and corticosteroids.

FUTURE PERSPECTIVES OF SMALL MOLECULES

In normal skin, molecules with a molecular weight higher than 500 Da are not capable of crossing the stratum corneum (the 500-Da rule) (**Table 1**).[30] The 500-Da rule is an important estimation as to whether a small molecule is small enough to be successful as a topical treatment.

WBI-1001 (2-isopropyl-5-[(E)-2-phenylethenyl] benzene-1,3-diol) is a nonsteroidal, anti-inflammatory, new chemical entity that was originally derived from the metabolites of a group of bacterial symbionts of entomopathogenic nematodes. WBI-1001 has been shown to affect T cells through the inhibition of multiple proinflammatory cytokines including tumor necrosis factor-α and by inhibiting T-cell viability and infiltration. A total of 61 patients were randomized (2:1) to receive either 1% WBI-1001 in a cream formulation or placebo, applied twice daily for 12 weeks.[32] At Week 12, the proportion of patients who achieved a PGA of clear or almost clear and the mean improvement in BSA were 67.5% and 79.1%, respectively, for patients randomized to WBI-1001 when compared with 4.8% (*P*<.0001) and an increase of 9.4% (*P*<.0001), respectively, for patients randomized to placebo. Mild to moderate site-adverse drug reactions were observed more frequently in patients randomized to WBI-1001 than in those randomized to placebo. Topical WBI-1001 induces rapid and significant improvement in patients with plaque psoriasis.

E804, an indirubin derivative, has been shown to block constitutive STAT3 signaling. Topical treatment with an ointment containing STA-21 successfully improved the psoriatic plaques in six out of eight patients.[33] Topical application of E804, like STA-21, attenuated the development of psoriasislike lesions of K5.Stat3C mice, probably through downmodulation of STAT3 activation.[33]

Table 1
Small molecules as potential future topicals for psoriasis

Target	Product	Response
T-cell signaling	WBI-1001	PGA clear or almost clear in 67% of patients
STAT3	E 804	Attenuated psoriasis-like lesions of K5.Stat3C mice
PDE4	AN-2728	40% of patients >2 grade improvement in plaque severity
JAK1/3	Tofacitinib	Target plaque score improved by 41%–54%
JAK1/2	INCB018424	Composite score decreased by 50%

Data from Refs.[32–36]

Cytokines are signaling molecules believed to be key factors in perpetuating the inflammatory process in psoriasis and atopic dermatitis. AN-2728 (Anacor Pharmaceuticals Inc) is a topically administered, boron-containing, anti-inflammatory compound that inhibits PDE4 activity and thereby suppresses the release of tumor necrosis factor-α, interleukin (IL)-12, IL-23, and other cytokines.[34] AN-2728 was reported to be well tolerated and to demonstrate significant effects on markers of efficacy, with results that were comparable with positive control subjects. AN-2728 seems to have good therapeutic potential, although further and larger trials are required to assess the long-term safety and characterize the broad utility of this drug.

Janus-associated kinases are involved in signal transduction from a variety of cytokines implicated in the pathogenesis of psoriasis, including IL-12, IL-23, and interferon-γ. Tofacitinib[35] is a small molecule inhibiting Janus-associated kinases (type 1 and 3). The primary end point of percentage change from baseline in the Target Plaque Severity Score at Week 4 demonstrated statistically significant improvement for two ointment formulations, ranging between 54.4% and 41.5% compared with 17.2%. Secondary end points (target plaque area and Itch Severity Item) improved similarly for tofacitinib ointment versus the corresponding vehicle. Adverse event occurrence was similar across treatment groups. All adverse events were mild or moderate and none were serious or led to subject discontinuation. Further studies of topical tofacitinib for psoriasis treatment are warranted.

INCB018424 is another Janus kinase (type 1 and 2) inhibitor.[36] Patients were dosed with vehicle, 0.5%, or 1.0% INCB018424 phosphate cream once a day or 1.5% twice a day for 28 days. Both the 1% and the 1.5% cream improved lesion thickness, erythema, and scaling and reduced lesion area compared with placebo. A composite lesion score decreased by greater than 50% with the efficacious doses of INCB018424 compared with 32% for vehicle control subjects. Topical application of INCB018424 was well tolerated with few mild adverse events noted.

SUMMARY

Topical treatment of psoriasis remains the mainstay for most patients. Vitamin D preparations in combination with corticosteroids of various potencies remain the most important active ingredients for maintenance of clinical response. New molecules have not been introduced for nearly two decades. Fortunately, there are several small molecules in various stages of clinical development that show promise as innovative new agents for the topical treatment of psoriasis.

REFERENCES

1. van de Kerkhof PC, Kragballe K, Segaert S, et al. International Psoriasis Council. Factors impacting the combination of topical corticosteroid therapies for psoriasis: perspectives from the International Psoriasis Council. J Eur Acad Dermatol Venereol 2011;25:1130–9.
2. Feldman SR, Horn EJ, Balkrishnan R, et al. Psoriasis: improving adherence to topical therapy. J Am Acad Dermatol 2008;59:1009–16.
3. van de Kerkhof PC, Hoffmann V, Anstey A, et al. A new scalp formulation of calcipotriol plus betamethasone dipropionate compared with each of its active ingredients in the same vehicle for the treatment of scalp psoriasis: a randomized, double-blind, controlled trial. Br J Dermatol 2009;160:170–6.
4. Mason AR, Mason J, Cork M, et al. Topical treatments for chronic plaque psoriasis: an abridged Cochrane systematic review. J Am Acad Dermatol 2013;69:799–807.
5. Samarasekera EA, Sawyer L, Wonderling D, et al. Topical therapies for the treatment of plaque psoriasis: systematic review and network meta-analyses. Br J Dermatol 2013;168:954–67.
6. Menter A, Korman NJ, Elmets CA, et al. Guidelines of care for the management of psoriasis and psoriatic arthritis. Section 3: guidelines of care for the management and treatment of psoriasis with topical therapies. J Am Acad Dermatol 2009;60:643–59.
7. Hendriks AG, Keijsers RR, de Jong EM, et al. Combinations of classical time-honoured topicals in plaque psoriasis: a systematic review. J Eur Acad Dermatol Venereol 2013;27:399–410.
8. van de Kerkhof PC. Dithranol treatment for psoriasis: after 75 years, still going strong. Eur J Dermatol 1991;1:79–88.
9. Swinkels OQ, Prins M, Veenhuis RT, et al. A care instruction programme of short contact dithranol in moderate to severe psoriasis. Eur J Dermatol 2004;14:159–65.
10. van den Bogaard EH, Bergboer JG, Vonk-Bergers M, et al. Coal tar induces AHR-dependent skin barrier repair in atopic dermatitis. J Clin Invest 2013;123:917–27.
11. Roelofzen JH, Aben KK, Oldenhof UT, et al. No increased risk of cancer after coal tar treatment in patients with psoriasis or eczema. J Invest Dermatol 2010;130:953–61.
12. Hendriks AG, Keijsers RR, de Jong EM, et al. Efficacy and safety of combinations of first-line topical treatments in chronic plaque psoriasis: a systematic literature review. J Eur Acad Dermatol Venereol 2013;27:931–51.

13. Kragballe K. Vitamin D in dermatology. New York: Marcel Dekker; 2000.

14. Kowalzick L. Clinical experience with topical calcitriol (1,25 dihydroxyvitamin D3) in psoriasis. Br J Dermatol 2001;144(Suppl 58):21–5.

15. Roeder A, Schaller M, Schafer-Korting M, et al. Safety and efficacy of fluticasone propionate in the topical treatment of skin diseases. Skin Pharmacol Physiol 2005;18:3–11.

16. Stein L. Clinical studies of a new vehicle formulation for topical corticosteroids in the treatment of psoriasis. J Am Acad Dermatol 2005;53:S39–49.

17. Feldman SR, Yentzer BA. Topical clobetasol propionate in the treatment of psoriasis: a review of newer formulations. Am J Clin Dermatol 2009;10:397–406.

18. Katz HI, Hien NT, Prower SE, et al. Betamethasone in optimized vehicle. Intermittent pulse dosing for extended maintenance treatment of psoriasis. Arch Dermatol 1987;123:1308–11.

19. Jarratt MT, Clark SD, Savin RC, et al. Evaluation of the efficacy and safety of clobetasol propionate spray in the treatment of plaque-type psoriasis. Cutis 2006;78:348–54.

20. Menter A. Topical monotherapy with clobetasol propionate spray0.05% in the COBRA trial. Cutis 2000;80:12–9.

21. Gottlieb AB, Ford RO, Spellman MC. The efficacy and tolerability of clobetasol propionate foam 0.05% in the treatment of mild to moderate plaque-type psoriasis of nonscalp regions. J Cutan Med Surg 2003;7:185–92.

22. Reid DC, Kimball AB. Clobetasol propionate foam in the treatment of psoriasis. Expert Opin Pharmacother 2005;6:1735–40.

23. Poulin Y, Papp K, Bissonnette R, et al. Clobetasol propionate shampoo 0.05% is efficacious and safe for long-term control of moderate scalp psoriasis. J Dermatolog Treat 2010;21:185–92.

24. Bovenschen H, Van de Kerkhof P. Treatment of scalp psoriasis with clobetasol-17 propionate 0.05% shampoo: a study on daily clinical practice. J Eur Acad Dermatol Venereol 2010;24:439–44.

25. Sanchez Regana M, Martin Ezquerra G, Umbert Millet P, et al. Treatment of nail psoriasis with 8% clobetasol nail lacquer: positive experience in 10 patients. J Eur Acad Dermatol Venereol 2005;19:573–7.

26. Feldman SR. Tachyphylaxis to topical corticosteroids: the more you use them, the less they work? Clin Dermatol 2006;24:229–30.

27. Lew-kaya DA, Sefton J, Krueger FF, et al. Safety and efficacy of a new retinoid gel in the treatment of psoriasis. J Invest Dermatol 1992;98:600.

28. Gribetz C, Ling M, Lebwohl M, et al. Pimecrolimus cream 1% in the treatment of intertriginous psoriasis: a double blind, randomized study. J Am Acad Dermatol 2004;51:731–8.

29. Kragballe K, Hoffmann V, Ortonne JP, et al. Efficacy and safety of calcipotriol plus betamethasone dipropionate scalp formulation compared with calcipotriol scalp solution in the treatment of scalp psoriasis: a randomized controlled trial. Br J Dermatol 2009; 161:159–66.

30. Luger TA, Cambazard F, Larsen FG, et al. A study of the safety and efficacy of calcipotriol and betamethasone dipropionate scalp formulation in the long-term management of scalp psoriasis. Dermatology 2008;217:321–8.

31. Bos JD, Meinardi MM. The 500 Dalton rule for the skin penetration of chemical compounds and drugs. Exp Dermatol 2000;9:165–9.

32. Bissonnette R, Bolduc C, Maari S, et al. Efficacy and safety of topical WBI-1001 in patients with mild to moderate psoriasis: results from a randomized double-blind placebo-controlled, phase II trial. J Eur Acad Dermatol Venereol 2012;26:1516–21.

33. Miyoshi K, Takaishi M, Nakajima KJ, et al. Stat3 as a therapeutic target for the treatment of psoriasis: a clinical feasibility study with STA-21, a Stat3 inhibitor. J Invest Dermatol 2011;131:108–17.

34. Moustafa F, Feldman SR. A review of phosphodiesterase-inhibition and the potential role for phosphodiesterase-E4 inhibitors in clinical dermatology. Dermatol Online J 2014;20:22608.

35. Ports WC, Khan S, Lan S, et al. A randomized phase 2a efficacy and safety trial of the topical Janus kinase inhibitor tofacitinib in the treatment of chronic plaque psoriasis. Br J Dermatol 2013;169: 137–45.

36. Punwani N, Scherle P, Flores R, et al. Preliminary clinical activity of a topical JAK1/2 inhibitor in the treatment of psoriasis. J Am Acad Dermatol 2012; 67:658–64.

Phototherapy and Photochemotherapy for Psoriasis

Emoke Racz, MD, PhD, Prof. Errol P. Prens, MD, PhD*

KEYWORDS

- UV-B • Narrow band • Broad band • PUVA • UV mode of action

KEY POINTS

- Phototherapy of psoriasis is efficacious.
- Phototherapy of psoriasis is relatively cost-effective.
- Phototherapy may be combined with topical agents and systemic therapies.
- More than 200 PUVA therapy treatments is associated with an increased risk of keratinocytic cancers.
- The mode of action of phototherapy is via inhibition of keratinocyte proliferation, induction of apoptosis in immunocytes, and inhibition of Th1 and Th17 cells and stimulation of Th2.

INTRODUCTION

Phototherapy is a standard treatment option for psoriasis, generally applied if topical treatment modalities fail or are contraindicated or not practical, such as in extensive guttate psoriasis. Phototherapy may lead to the clearance of psoriasis in 5 to 8 weeks and has one of the highest treatment satisfaction rates compared with other treatment modalities.[1] The development of phototherapy for psoriasis was based on the observation that sunlight improves the symptoms of the disease. Natural light in combination with herbal extracts has been in use for the treatment of skin disease from the era of the Ancient Egyptians. Artificial light sources have been used for the treatment of psoriasis since the 1920s. The most frequently applied regimen for psoriasis was the combination of topical coal tar and subsequent UV-B radiation, introduced by Göckerman in 1925.[2]

Broad-band (BB) UV-B alone (wavelengths between 280 and 320 nm) has been used since the 1970s.[3] Narrow-band (NB) UV-B phototherapy using Philips (Eindhoven, The Netherlands) TL-01 fluorescent lamps, emitting between 311 and 313 nm, was introduced in 1988 for the treatment of psoriasis. BB-UV-B and NB-UV-B were shown to have common, but also different biologic effects, because NB-UV-B radiation did not suppress contact hypersensitivity responses in mice, even at seven times higher doses than effective BB-UV-B doses.[3]

In the 1970s psoralen–UV-A therapy (PUVA; 320–400 nm) was introduced. Psoralens, plant-derived photosensitizers, can be applied topically or taken orally. Subsequent UV-A irradiation causes a therapeutically beneficial phototoxic reaction in the skin.[4] PUVA therapy has anti-inflammatory and antiproliferative effects, and is highly efficacious in the treatment of psoriasis, inducing response rates from 74% to 100%.[5] PUVA is thereby one of the most effective treatment options in psoriasis; however, it is less well tolerated than UV-B phototherapy, and there is more evidence on its carcinogenic potential.

The authors declare to have no relevant conflict of interest.
Department of Dermatology, Erasmus University Medical Center Rotterdam, PO Box 2040, Rotterdam 3000 CA, The Netherlands
* Corresponding author.
E-mail address: e.prens@erasmusmc.nl

Dermatol Clin 33 (2015) 79–89
http://dx.doi.org/10.1016/j.det.2014.09.007
0733-8635/15/$ – see front matter © 2015 Elsevier Inc. All rights reserved.

derm.theclinics.com

Further forms of UV phototherapy for psoriasis are climatotherapy and balneotherapy. Climatotherapy involves daily bathing in Dead Sea water and graduated exposure to natural sunlight. Treatment is usually for 4 weeks and results in reductions in Psoriasis Area and Severity Index (PASI) scores by 75% or more. Most of the benefit of climatotherapy at the Dead Sea has been attributed to the specific sunlight spectrum at the Dead Sea.[6] Balneophototherapy, which involves salt water baths and artificial UV radiation, can be used as an alternative to climatotherapy at the Dead Sea.[6] However, the clinical effect of adding salt water to BB-UV-B was negligible.[7] Therefore, because of the heavy burden of salt on sewage and the environment, salt water baths are not recommended for home use.

For the treatment of chronic localized psoriatic plaques, localized phototherapy is available in the form of hand-held nonlaser UV-B (light-emitting diode) lamps, and the 308-nm excimer laser. The excimer laser emits monochromatic light equivalent to that of NB-UV-B with similar biologic and clinical effects.[8] Localized phototherapy was shown to be less efficacious than total body irradiation,[9] but is a practical solution for adjunctive home treatment of localized psoriasis, such as scalp, hand, or foot psoriasis.

Photochemotherapy can also be applied locally by using psoralen-containing gels or solutions (topical PUVA); this form of treatment is most often used for the treatment of psoriasis of the palms and soles.

Discussed next are the practical aspects of phototherapy of psoriasis and the mode of action as currently understood.

TREATMENT REGIMENS

Phototherapy is mostly applied in a clinical setting, in light cabinets where patients stand from a few seconds to a few minutes, two to five times a week. The starting dose of phototherapy is ideally based on the minimal erythema dose (MED) in the case of UV-B treatment, or the minimal phototoxic dose in the case of PUVA (**Table 1**).

MED is defined as the lowest radiation dose that produces just perceptible erythema on exposed skin after 24 hours. Common MEDs reported for NB-UV-B and BB-UV-B are shown in **Table 2**. Thus, at least five-times higher doses of NB-UV-B, compared with BB-UV-B, are needed for the induction of erythema. NB-UV-B doses required for the induction of hyperplasia, edema, sunburn cell formation, and Langerhans cell depletion are 5 to 10 times higher than equally effective BB-UV-B doses.[10] A more convenient approach is to base the starting dose on the skin type of the patient, although MED-based therapy is thought to be the safest regimen for the patient.

Maintenance of a slight, asymptomatic erythema throughout the treatment results in optimal clinical efficacy.[11] Treatments are continued until total remission is reached or until no further improvement can be obtained with continued phototherapy. The median number of treatments needed for clearance with UV-B is between 25 and 30 and for PUVA between 17 and 19.[12]

EFFICACY, DURATION OF REMISSION

The European S3 guideline on the treatment of psoriasis presents clearance rates for the different

Table 1
Treatment regimens

	UV-B	PUVA	
		Oral	Bath
Initial dose determination	Reading after 24 h	Reading after 72–96 h	Reading after 96–120 h
Initial dose	70% of MED	75% of minimal phototoxic dose	30% of minimal phototoxic dose
Treatment frequency	2–5 times weekly	2–4 times weekly	
Dose adjustment during treatment	No erythema — Increase by 30%–40%	Increase by 30% max. 2 times weekly	
	Minimal erythema — Increase by 20%	No increase	
	Persistent asymptomatic erythema — No increase	No increase	
	Painful erythema — Break in therapy	Break in therapy	
Resume therapy after symptoms fade	Reduce last dose by 50%, further increase by 10%		

Adapted from Pathirana D, Ormerod AD, Saiag P, et al. European S3-guidelines on the systemic treatment of psoriasis vulgaris. J Eur Acad Dermatol Venereol 2009;23(Suppl 2):52–5; with permission.

Table 2 Minimal erythema dose with narrow-band and broad-band UV-B			
Study	Skin Type	MED BB-UV-B (mJ/cm^2)	MED NB-UV-B (mJ/cm^2)
Van Weelden et al,[87] 1988	II	76	410
Johnson et al,[88] 1988	II	100	500
Karvonen et al,[89] 1989	II	230	970
Storbeck et al,[17] 1993	II	114	1034
Srinivas,[90] 2002	IV	21	300
Tejasvi et al,[91] 2007	III–V	—	1000
Youn et al,[92] 2003	III–V	—	750–1075
Morita et al,[93] 2009	IV	—	700

Data from Refs.[17,87–93]

types of phototherapy (**Table 3**).[13] A few studies reported a superior clinical efficacy of NB-UV-B compared with BB-UV-B[14–17]; however, other studies found that BB-UV-B and NB-UV-B were equally effective.[18,19] A recent Cochrane review reports on only one randomized controlled trial (RCT) comparing NB-UV-B with selective BB-UV-B (none that compares NB-UV-B with conventional BB-UV-B), showing no significant differences between these two treatments in terms of clearance rate and withdrawals because of adverse events.[20]

The Cochrane review also compared the efficacy of NB-UV-B with oral PUVA for psoriasis.[12] The three RCTs they found show inconsistent results on the clearance rate, with one RCT showing equal efficacy and two a statistically significant higher clearance rate of oral PUVA. In terms of PASI 75 and withdrawals caused by adverse events no significant differences were found.

A recent European systematic review concluded that PUVA cleared psoriasis more often and in fewer treatment sessions than NB-UV-B alone, and that PUVA also resulted in longer lasting remission of the disease.[21] The number of sessions to clear was lower for PUVA (17 sessions) than for NB-UV-B (approximately 25 sessions); these conclusions are in accordance with those of the Cochrane review. The median duration of remission was studied by Markham and colleagues[22]; this study reported 288.5 days for NB-UV-B group, and 231 days for PUVA. However, according to the European systematic review, more patients are still in remission 6 months after completing PUVA therapy than after NB-UV-B therapy.[21] The duration of remission correlates with the PASI score at the end of the treatment.[23]

CONTRAINDICATIONS AND PRECAUTIONS

Before treatment with phototherapy it is necessary to evaluate the skin type of the patient and his or her reaction to sunlight, and the age and the history of skin cancer (**Box 1**). A total body check and an objective evaluation of psoriasis using the PASI should be performed before starting treatment. The contraindications for phototherapy are summarized in **Box 2** (based on the European S3 Guideline and the American Academy of Dermatology Guideline on the treatment of psoriasis[24,25]).

ADVERSE EFFECTS AND THEIR MANAGEMENT

Acute adverse effects of UV-B therapy include redness, itch, and blistering, all symptoms of sunburn reaction. These effects are temporary and generally manageable with adjustment of the frequency and dose of irradiation. A frequent adverse effect of PUVA therapy is nausea. Carcinogenicity is the most concerning long-term serious adverse effect of phototherapy and photochemotherapy. Sufficient evidence supports the increased risk of nonmelanoma skin cancer after more than 200 sessions of PUVA therapy. The risk is most

Table 3 Efficacy of phototherapy and photochemotherapy expressed as the percentage achieving Psoriasis Area and Severity Index 75					
	BB-UV-B	NB-UV-B	Balneotherapy	Oral PUVA	Bath PUVA
Psoriasis Area and Severity Index 75	50–75	38–100	73–83	75–100	64–100

Data from Nast A, Boehncke WH, Mrowietz U, et al. S3-Guidelines on the treatment of psoriasis vulgaris (English version). Update. J Dtsch Dermatol Ges 2012;10(Suppl 2):S1–95.

pronounced for squamous cell carcinomas, which may develop also on low exposures and on nonexposed skin, including penile tumors. The risk of basal cell carcinoma is also increased in patients

receiving more than 100 PUVA sessions.[26] A large US prospective follow-up study also identified an at least doubled incidence of melanoma (invasive and in situ) among patients exposed to at least 200 PUVA sessions. This increased risk began 15 years after first exposure to PUVA.[27,28] This has not been shown in European studies.

Although in mice NB-UV-B was more carcinogenic than BB-UV-B at equally erythemogenic doses,[29] follow-up of patients receiving extensive UV-B treatments did not demonstrate an increase in skin cancer incidence.[30,31] However, most of the available studies had an observation time shorter than 5.6 years, which might be too short to detect skin cancer as a long-term risk of phototherapy.[26] It is essential that the total number of treatments and the cumulative UV dose is recorded, because these are the factors that influence the skin cancer risk. Most commercially available UV cabinets are equipped with software for registration of the number of treatments and the cumulative dose.

Photoaging is induced by long-term phototherapy of patients with psoriasis, exacerbating the injury caused by natural sunlight.[32] An increased risk of cataract can be expected in patients undergoing PUVA or NB-UV-B therapy based on animal studies.[33] Therefore, eye protection is essential during irradiation, and additional UV-blocking glasses are recommended during daytime in patients who take oral psoralens. However, a recent systematic review found no evidence for an increased incidence of cataract in patients who have been treated with PUVA or NB-UV-B.[34] Box 3 outlines the prevention of complications.

SPECIAL PATIENT GROUPS

The advantage of phototherapy is that it may be used in almost any patient regardless of comorbidity, including children and pregnant women. NB-UV-B therapy can be considered first-line treatment in pregnant women who require a systemic approach. Because of the lack of data on the long-term risk of skin cancer, caution is required when UV-B is used in children. In a recent guideline, age younger than 18 was considered a relative contraindication for PUVA therapy.[35] Anxiety can be a limiting factor, especially when treating younger children. However, phototherapy should still be considered as a second-line therapy for children with psoriasis when topical treatments fail.

COMBINATION TREATMENTS
Combination of Phototherapy with Topical Treatments

Coal tar and anthralin
Coal tar and suberythemogenic doses of UV-B are superior to either agent alone, but tar has no benefit to emollients in clearing psoriasis when erythemogenic doses of UV-B are used.[36,37] Although the Göckerman regimen (involving treatment with UV-B light after pretreatment with 2%–10% topical crude coal tar) is rarely used today, recent reports have shown high efficacy in patients resistant to biologics, based on retrospective chart evaluation.[38,39] The Göckerman regimen may be combined with application of anthralin after UV-B exposure (the Ingram regimen).

Vitamin D derivatives
Calcipotriol increases the effectiveness (resulting in a faster clearance of the lesions) of both NB-UV-B phototherapy (when applied three times a week) and PUVA.[40]

Corticosteroid preparations
Topical corticosteroid preparations are not beneficial during NB-UV-B therapy.[40] They may accelerate the clinical response to PUVA, although relapse might also be more rapid.[41]

Combination with Traditional Systemic Treatments

Combination of NB-UV-B phototherapy with retinoids is a highly effective treatment of extensive psoriasis, and has been shown to result in a shorter time to remission than either of the two treatments alone.[42,43]

NB-UV-B plus retinoid and PUVA plus retinoid therapies were shown to have similar effects in terms of clearance rate in chronic plaque and guttate psoriasis, as shown by two RCTs reviewed in a recent Cochrane review.[12] Combination of phototherapy with methotrexate has been shown to increase the efficacy of NB-UV-B treatment. Methotrexate was started 3 weeks before the start of phototherapy, in a dose of 15 mg/week.[44] The combination of methotrexate with PUVA is not recommended because of an increased risk of skin cancer.

The combination of cyclosporine with phototherapy is contraindicated because of the increased future risk of skin cancer.

Combination with Biologics

A synergistic effect has been noted when NB-UV-B or BB-UV-B is combined with adalimumab, etanercept, and ustekinumab.[45–50] However, the combination with biologics carries the risk of induction of photocarcinogenesis, because of inhibition of the immunosurveillance of the skin. A higher incidence of skin cancer was reported in patients with rheumatoid arthritis on biologics, who only had been exposed to natural sunlight.[51] Theoretically biologics may enhance the risk of skin cancer in patients who receive a combination of biologics and UV-B, although this has not yet been well demonstrated in patients with psoriasis. Therefore, according to the British and Dutch guidelines UV-B phototherapy is a relative contraindication for treatment with biologics.[52]

LOCALIZED PHOTOTHERAPY

Forms of localized phototherapy include targeted UV-B therapy (nonlaser or the excimer laser) and topical PUVA therapy. These treatment modalities can be used for the treatment of localized recalcitrant psoriasis without adverse effects on the unaffected skin. Recent reports show clearance of recalcitrant psoriasis plaques after addition of targeted phototherapy during long-term treatment with systemic therapies.[53] A recent systematic review estimated the efficacy of targeted UV-B at 61% and that of topical PUVA at 77%,[9] which is lower than that of total body treatment.

COST-EFFECTIVENESS UV-B THERAPY

Outpatient office-based phototherapy is more cost-effective than systemic treatment with biologics, although phototherapy can be inconvenient for patients because of travel time and costs, and the costs of absence from work. In the United States high copayments for each treatment can cause considerable financial difficulties for patients. Home UV-B therapy can solve these problems for many patients. A Dutch study demonstrated equal efficacy and tolerability of hospital and home-based NB-UV-B phototherapy.[54,55] In this study home phototherapy was not more expensive than hospital-based phototherapy, and was preferred by patients.

MECHANISM OF ACTION
Primary Molecular Targets

The epidermis is the primary target of UV-B radiation. UV-B radiation is absorbed to the greatest extent by chromophores (light absorbing molecules) in the upper layers of the skin, mostly in the epidermis.[56] Light absorption by chromophores induces structural changes, thereby changing their functionality. Molecules that undergo light-induced structural modifications are called photoproducts.

DNA damage
When DNA absorbs UV-B radiation, different types of photoproducts are formed, the most frequent being cyclobutyl pyrimidine dimers (CPD) and (6-4)-photoproducts.[57] These UV-B signature molecules have been demonstrated in keratinocytes and Langerhans cells on UV-B radiation.[57] CPD were shown to be involved in UV-B–induced apoptosis, inflammation, immunosuppression, and photocarcinogenesis.[58] Interestingly, UV-induced tumor formation could be prevented by repair of CPD in the basal keratinocytes only, but this was not the case for UV-induced immunosuppression, demonstrating that different cell types mediate different biologic effects of UV radiation.[58]

Reactive oxygen species
Active cellular metabolism in the presence of oxygen results in the formation of reactive oxygen species, such as superoxide anion, hydrogen peroxide, and singlet oxygen. Reactive oxygen species are extremely unstable; react with other molecules; and cause a variety of damages in the cell, such as lipid peroxidation, DNA breaks, and DNA-protein cross-links.[59] To counteract oxidative damage, cells have an antioxidative defense system, comprised of natural radical scavengers (eg, tocopherol, vitamin A) and different enzymes (eg, superoxide dismutase, glutathione peroxidase, and catalase). UV-B radiation induces enhanced reactive oxygen species production. Cells respond with upregulation of scavenger enzyme activity and synthesis. As a result UV-B radiation drives the cells into a complex stress response, with consequences for the immune response and inflammation.[59]

Cell membrane alterations
UV-B radiation leads to clustering and internalization of cell membrane receptors for epidermal growth factor, tumor necrosis factor, and interleukin (IL)-1, resulting in ligand-independent activation of members of the MAPK family.[60] Furthermore, CD95 or FAS, another cell surface receptor, is also activated by UV-B radiation on a ligand-independent manner, playing a role in UV-B–induced apoptosis.[61]

Urocanic acid
Urocanic acid (UCA) is generated in the skin from histidine, and accumulates in the stratum corneum of the epidermis. The major source of UCA in the epidermis is filaggrin, a histidine-rich basic protein. Cleavage of filaggrin by caspase 14 produces UCA, which absorbs UV radiation, and carboxylic-pyrrolidone acid, which support cutaneous hydration. On UV radiation the naturally occurring trans-UCA isoform converts to cis-UCA. UCA was first identified as a chromophore responsible for UV-B–induced suppression of contact hypersensitivity.[62] On UV-B radiation in humans, cis-UCA is detectable in the skin and in the urine.[63]

The involvement of UCA and DNA damage with UV-B has been evaluated in psoriasis in addition to expression of cytoprotective enzymes. The epidermal cis-UCA concentration was found to be increased by heliotherapy of psoriasis, from a mean initial value of 0.2 nmol/cm^2 to a mean final value of 2.9 nmol/cm^2. Clinical response of psoriasis to heliotherapy, however, was independent of UCA isomer levels.[64]

The amount of DNA mutations during phototherapy was assessed to evaluate its carcinogenic potential and compare it with that of BB-UV-B.[65,66] NB-UV-B induced equal amounts of DNA photoproducts as BB-UV-B at equally erythemogenic doses, indicating that NB-UV-B is not more carcinogenic than BB-UV-B.[65] The amount of CPD increased in the psoriatic skin during the first three treatment sessions, but not hereafter, whereas clinical improvement is usually only noted after several weeks of treatment.[66]

T-Cell and Keratinocyte Apoptosis

NB-UV-B phototherapy reverses several pathologic alterations in psoriasis lesions. Keratinocyte proliferation decreases.[67] The key role of keratinocyte apoptosis in the therapeutic effect of NB-UV-B in psoriasis was recently highlighted by Weatherhead and colleagues.[68,69] Using computational modeling and human studies they demonstrated that keratinocyte apoptosis was sufficient for the clearance of psoriatic plaques.

The number of T lymphocytes in the epidermis and dermis has also been shown to decrease, likely caused by UV-B–induced apoptosis.[70,71] Although the decrease in epidermal T cells correlated well with clinical improvement, this was not shown for dermal T-cell numbers.[67] Epidermal and dermal T-cell numbers were significantly more reduced by NB-UV-B than by BB-UV-B.[70] T lymphocytes in vitro are 10-fold more sensitive to the cytotoxic effects of UV-B than keratino-cytes, which explains their depletion from the epidermis on UV-B phototherapy.[67] In addition, whereas hyperplastic keratinocytes in untreated psoriatic plaques do not express CD95L/FASL on their plasma membrane, after NB-UV-B treatment there is strong and diffuse keratinocyte FASL/CD95L expression that coincided in a temporal fashion with depletion of intraepidermal T cells, indicating a role for FASL in epidermal T-cell apoptosis.[72] Keratinocyte and lymphocyte apoptosis also plays a critical role in the mode of action of PUVA in psoriasis.[73]

T cells that remain in the lesions after 4 weeks of NB-UV-B treatment produce less interferon-γ and IL-12 and more IL-4.[71,74,75] A single dose of BB-UV-B radiation resulted in decreased interferon-γ production and increased IL-4 production in psoriatic skin; interestingly, neutrophils were found to be the source of the increased IL-4 production.[76] NB-UV-B treatment also affects the function of dendritic cells in lesional psoriatic skin. Triggering receptor expressed on myeloid cells type-1 on inflammatory dendritic cells was found to be a possible molecular target of effective antipsoriatic treatments, including NB-UV-B.[77] Clearance of psoriasis by NB-UV-B is associated with suppression of type I and type II interferon signaling and downregulation of the Th17 pathway in the lesional epidermis. NB-UV-B inhibits the phosphorylation of signal transducer and activator of transcription 3, resulting in reduced expression of its transcriptional targets (eg, the antimicrobial peptide human β-defensin 2).[78]

Phototherapy also affects circulating T lymphocytes in patients with psoriasis. Both NB-UV-B therapy and PUVA reduced the number of circulating Th17 cells, and restored the impaired regulatory T-cell function in psoriasis.[79]

Cytokine secretion of in vitro stimulated peripheral blood mononuclear cells isolated from patients with psoriasis before and during UV-B phototherapy was investigated by several groups. T helper cell activity of CD4+ lymphocytes of patients with psoriasis at the end of phototherapy was decreased compared with that of cells from healthy control subjects, as measured by a graft-versus-host response induced by these cells.[80] When peripheral blood mononuclear cells of patients with psoriasis, isolated before NB-UV-B therapy and weekly thereafter, were stimulated with superantigen in vitro, reduced production of IL-1β, IL-2, IL-5, and IL-6 and increased production of IL-10 was detected.[81] Furthermore, NB-UV-B treatment (and treatment with PUVA and BB-UV-B) resulted in reduced cytotoxic activity of circulating natural killer cells,[82] whereas the number of circulating natural killer cells remained unchanged.[83] In contrast, local coal tar treatment did not affect the cytotoxic activity of natural killer cells.[82]

After phototherapy, vitamin D levels were dramatically increased by UV-B (but not by PUVA) in patients with psoriasis and in control subjects.[84] Serum vitamin D levels in patients with psoriasis showed less increase with NB-UV-B than with BB-UV-B phototherapy.[85] This difference between BB-UV-B and NB-UV-B on vitamin D synthesis indicates that vitamin D synthesis does not correlate with the clinical efficacy, because NB-UV-B is at least as effective in treating psoriasis as BB-UV-B. Interestingly, a single nucleotide polymorphism in the vitamin D receptor gene was found to be a predictive factor for responsiveness to NB-UV-B treatment.[86]

SUMMARY

Phototherapy is considered a first-line, cost-effective option for the treatment of moderate to severe psoriasis, in particular in pregnant women. Patients are usually highly satisfied by treatment convenience and efficacy. Systematic reviews have shown divergent findings relating to the efficacy of various forms of phototherapy in psoriasis. They conclude that oral PUVA and bath PUVA are at least equally effective as NB-UV-B. Clearance rates may be higher if phototherapy is combined with topical coal tar, anthralin, vitamin D derivatives, oral retinoids, methotrexate, or biologics. Localized phototherapy can be used as monotherapy or as an adjunctive treatment of recalcitrant plaques during systemic treatment of psoriasis.

It is widely accepted that more than 200 sessions of PUVA therapy is associated with an increased risk of nonmelanoma skin cancer, whereas no increased risk has been demonstrated for NB-UV-B therapy. The risk of melanoma with PUVA therapy is controversial. Caution is required when phototherapy is combined with immunosuppressive treatments because of a further increase in skin cancer risk.

The main known mechanism of action of phototherapy in psoriasis is thought to be via inhibition of keratinocyte proliferation, induction of apoptosis in keratinocytes and intraepidermal bone marrow–derived cells, such as dendritic cells, (natural killer) T cells, and skewing of T cell differentiation from Th1 and Th17 toward the Th2 phenotype. Better understanding of the molecular mechanisms will likely contribute to the development of more effective and selective phototherapy and a reduction of unwanted adverse effects.

REFERENCES

1. Callis Duffin K, Yeung H, Takeshita J, et al. Patient satisfaction with treatments for moderate-to-severe plaque psoriasis in clinical practice. Br J Dermatol 2014;170(3):672–80.
2. Goeckerman WH. The treatment of psoriasis. Northwest Med 1925;24:229–31.
3. Bolognia J, Jorizzo J, Rapini R. Dermatology, vol. 2. St Louis (MO): Mosby; 2003.
4. Averbeck D. Recent advances in psoralen phototoxicity mechanism. Photochem Photobiol 1989;50(6):859–82.
5. Stern R. Psoralen and ultraviolet a light therapy for psoriasis. N Engl J Med 2007;357(7):682–90.
6. Halverstam C, Lebwohl M. Nonstandard and off-label therapies for psoriasis. Clin Dermatol 2008;26(5):546–53.
7. Boer J, Schothorst AA, Boom B, et al. Influence of water and salt solutions on UVB irradiation of normal skin and psoriasis. Arch Dermatol Res 1982;273(3–4):247–59.
8. Gerber W, Arheilger B, Ha TA, et al. 308-nm excimer laser treatment of psoriasis: a new phototherapeutic approach. Br J Dermatol 2003;149(6):1250–8.
9. Almutawa F, Thalib L, Hekman D, et al. Efficacy of localized phototherapy and photodynamic therapy for psoriasis: a systematic review and meta-analysis. Photodermatol Photoimmunol Photomed 2013. [Epub ahead of print].
10. el-Ghorr AA, Norval M. Biological effects of narrow-band (311 nm TL01) UVB irradiation: a review. J Photochem Photobiol B 1997;38(2–3):99–106.
11. Lapolla W, Yentzer BA, Bagel J, et al. A review of phototherapy protocols for psoriasis treatment. J Am Acad Dermatol 2011;64(5):936–49.
12. Chen X, Yang M, Cheng Y, et al. Narrow-band ultraviolet B phototherapy versus broad-band ultraviolet B or psoralen-ultraviolet A photochemotherapy for psoriasis. Cochrane Database Syst Rev 2013;(10):CD009481.
13. Pathirana D, Ormerod AD, Saiag P, et al. European S3-guidelines on the systemic treatment of psoriasis vulgaris. J Eur Acad Dermatol Venereol 2009;23(Suppl 2):1–70.
14. Coven TR, Burack LH, Gilleaudeau R, et al. Narrow-band UV-B produces superior clinical and histopathological resolution of moderate-to-severe psoriasis in patients compared with broadband UV-B. Arch Dermatol 1997;133(12):1514–22.
15. Walters IB, Burack LH, Coven TR, et al. Suberythemogenic narrow-band UVB is markedly more effective than conventional UVB in treatment of psoriasis vulgaris. J Am Acad Dermatol 1999;40(6 Pt 1):893–900.
16. Picot E, Meunier L, Picot-Debeze MC, et al. Treatment of psoriasis with a 311-nm UVB lamp. Br J Dermatol 1992;127(5):509–12.
17. Storbeck K, Holzle E, Schurer N, et al. Narrow-band UVB (311 nm) versus conventional broad-band UVB with and without dithranol in phototherapy for psoriasis. J Am Acad Dermatol 1993;28(2 Pt 1):227–31.
18. Green C, Ferguson J, Lakshmipathi T, et al. 311 nm UVB phototherapy: an effective treatment for psoriasis. Br J Dermatol 1988;119(6):691–6.
19. Larko O. Treatment of psoriasis with a new UVB-lamp. Acta Derm Venereol 1989;69(4):357–9.
20. Kirke SM, Lowder S, Lloyd JJ, et al. A randomized comparison of selective broadband UVB and narrowband UVB in the treatment of psoriasis. J Invest Dermatol 2007;127(7):1641–6.
21. Archier E, Devaux S, Castela E, et al. Efficacy of psoralen UV-A therapy vs. narrowband UV-B therapy in chronic plaque psoriasis: a systematic literature review. J Eur Acad Dermatol Venereol 2012;26(Suppl 3):11–21.
22. Markham T, Rogers S, Collins P. Narrowband UV-B (TL-01) phototherapy vs oral 8-methoxypsoralen psoralen-UV-A for the treatment of chronic plaque psoriasis. Arch Dermatol 2003;139(3):325–8.
23. Coimbra S, Oliveira H, Belo L, et al. Principal determinants of the length of remission of psoriasis vulgaris after topical, NB-UVB, and PUVA therapy: a follow-up study. Am J Clin Dermatol 2013;14(1):49–53.
24. Nast A, Boehncke WH, Mrowietz U, et al. S3-Guidelines on the treatment of psoriasis vulgaris (English version). Update. J Dtsch Dermatol Ges 2012;10(Suppl 2):S1–95.
25. Menter A, Korman NJ, Elmets CA, et al. Guidelines of care for the management of psoriasis and psoriatic arthritis: section 5. Guidelines of care for the treatment of psoriasis with phototherapy and photochemotherapy. J Am Acad Dermatol 2010;62(1):114–35.
26. Archier E, Devaux S, Castela E, et al. Carcinogenic risks of psoralen UV-A therapy and narrowband UV-B therapy in chronic plaque psoriasis: a systematic literature review. J Eur Acad Dermatol Venereol 2012;26(Suppl 3):22–31.
27. Stern RS, PUVA Follow up Study. The risk of melanoma in association with long-term exposure to PUVA. J Am Acad Dermatol 2001;44(5):755–61.
28. Stern RS, Nichols KT, Vakeva LH. Malignant melanoma in patients treated for psoriasis with methoxsalen (psoralen) and ultraviolet A radiation (PUVA). The PUVA Follow-Up Study. N Engl J Med 1997;336(15):1041–5.
29. Gibbs N, Traynor N, MacKie R, et al. The phototumorigenic potential of broad-band (270-350 nm) and narrow-band (311-313 nm) phototherapy sources cannot be predicted by their edematogenic potential in hairless mouse skin. J Invest Dermatol 1995;104:359–63.
30. Weischer M, Blum A, Eberhard F, et al. No evidence for increased skin cancer risk in psoriasis patients

treated with broadband or narrowband UVB phototherapy: a first retrospective study. Acta Derm Venereol 2004;84(5):370–4.

31. Hearn R, Kerr A, Rahim K, et al. Incidence of skin cancers in 3867 patients treated with narrow-band ultraviolet B phototherapy. Br J Dermatol 2008;159: 931–5.

32. Sator PG, Schmidt JB, Honigsmann H. Objective assessment of photoageing effects using high-frequency ultrasound in PUVA-treated psoriasis patients. Br J Dermatol 2002;147(2):291–8.

33. Andley UP, Chylack LT Jr. Recent studies on photo-damage to the eye with special reference to clinical phototherapeutic procedures. Photodermatol Photo-immunol Photomed 1990;7(3):98–105.

34. Archier E, Devaux S, Castela E, et al. Ocular damage in patients with psoriasis treated by psoralen UV-A therapy or narrow band UVB therapy: a systematic literature review. J Eur Acad Dermatol Venereol 2012;26(Suppl 3):32–5.

35. Samarasekera E, Sawyer L, Parnham J, et al, Guideline Development Group. Assessment and management of psoriasis: summary of NICE guidance. BMJ 2012;345:e6712.

36. Frost P, Horwitz SN, Caputo RV, et al. Tar gel-phototherapy for psoriasis. Combined therapy with suberythemogenic doses of fluorescent sunlamp ultraviolet radiation. Arch Dermatol 1979;115(7): 840–6.

37. Lowe NJ, Wortzman MS, Breeding J, et al. Coal tar phototherapy for psoriasis reevaluated: erythemo-genic versus suberythemogenic ultraviolet with a tar extract in oil and crude coal tar. J Am Acad Dermatol 1983;8(6):781–9.

38. Serrao R, Davis MD. Goeckerman treatment for remission of psoriasis refractory to biologic therapy. J Am Acad Dermatol 2009;60(2):348–9.

39. Fitzmaurice S, Bhutani T, Koo J. Goeckerman regimen for management of psoriasis refractory to biologic therapy: the University of California San Francisco experience. J Am Acad Dermatol 2013; 69(4):648–9.

40. Nast A, Boehncke WH, Mrowietz U, et al. German S3-guidelines on the treatment of psoriasis vulgaris (short version). Arch Dermatol Res 2012; 304(2):87–113.

41. Morison WL, Parrish JA, Fitzpatrick TB. Controlled study of PUVA and adjunctive topical therapy in the management of psoriasis. Br J Dermatol 1978; 98(2):125–32.

42. Tanew A, Guggenbichler A, Honigsmann H, et al. Photochemotherapy for severe psoriasis without or in combination with acitretin: a randomized, double-blind comparison study. J Am Acad Dermatol 1991;25:682–4.

43. Ruzicka T, Sommerburg C, Braun-Falco O, et al. Efficacy of acitretin in combination with UVB in the treatment of severe psoriasis. Arch Dermatol 1990; 126:482–6.

44. Asawanonda P, Nateetongrungsak Y. Methotrexate plus narrowband UVB phototherapy versus narrowband phototherapy alone in the treatment of plaque-type psoriasis: a randomized, placebo-controlled study. J Am Acad Dermatol 2006;54: 1013–8.

45. Calzavara-Pinton PG, Sala R, Arisi M, et al. Synergism between narrowband ultraviolet B phototherapy and etanercept for the treatment of plaque-type psoriasis. Br J Dermatol 2013;169(1):130–6.

46. Legat FJ, Hofer A, Wackernagel A, et al. Narrowband UV-B phototherapy, alefacept, and clearance of psoriasis. Arch Dermatol 2007;143(8):1016–22.

47. Wolf P, Hofer A, Legat FJ, et al. Treatment with 311-nm ultraviolet B accelerates and improves the clearance of psoriatic lesions in patients treated with etanercept. Br J Dermatol 2009;160(1):186–9.

48. Wolf P, Weger W, Legat FJ, et al. Treatment with 311-nm ultraviolet B-enhanced response of psoriatic lesions in ustekinumab-treated patients: a randomized intraindividual trial. Br J Dermatol 2012;166: 147–53.

49. Wolf P, Hofer A, Weger W, et al. 311 nm ultraviolet B-accelerated response of psoriatic lesions in adalimumab-treated patients. Photodermatol Photo-immunol Photomed 2011;27(4):186–9.

50. Kircik L, Bagel J, Korman N, et al. Utilization of narrow-band ultraviolet light B therapy and etanercept for the treatment of psoriasis (UNITE): efficacy, safety, and patient-reported outcomes. J Drugs Dermatol 2008;7(3):245–53.

51. Wolfe F, Michaud K. Biologic treatment of rheumatoid arthritis and the risk of malignancy: analyses from a large US observational study. Arthritis Rheum 2007;56(9):2886–95.

52. Smith CH, Anstey AV, Barker JN, et al. British Association of Dermatologists' guidelines for biologic interventions for psoriasis 2009. Br J Dermatol 2009;161(5):987–1019.

53. Park KK, Swan J, Koo J. Effective treatment of etanercept and phototherapy-resistant psoriasis using the excimer laser. Dermatol Online J 2012; 18(3):2.

54. Koek MB, Buskens E, van Weelden H, et al. Home versus outpatient ultraviolet B phototherapy for mild to severe psoriasis: pragmatic multicentre randomised controlled non-inferiority trial (PLUTO study). BMJ 2009;338:b1542.

55. Koek MB, Sigurdsson V, van Weelden H, et al. Cost effectiveness of home ultraviolet B phototherapy for psoriasis: economic evaluation of a randomised controlled trial (PLUTO study). BMJ 2010;340: c1490.

56. McGregor J, Hawk J. Acute effects of ultraviolet radiation on the skin. In: Freedberg I, Eisen A,

Wolff K, et al, editors. Fitzpatrick's dermatology in general medicine. 5th Edition. New York: The McGraw-Hill Companies, Inc; 2003. p. 1555–61.

57. Maccubbin AE, Przybyszewski J, Evans MS, et al. DNA damage in UVB-irradiated keratinocytes. Carcinogenesis 1995;16(7):1659–60.

58. Jans J, Garinis G, Schul W, et al. Differential role of basal keratinocytes in UV-induced immunosuppression and skin cancer. Mol Cell Biol 2006;26(22):8515–26.

59. Schade N, Esser C, Krutmann J. Ultraviolet B radiation-induced immunosuppression: molecular mechanisms and cellular alterations. Photochem Photobiol Sci 2005;4(9):699–708.

60. Rosette C, Karin M. Ultraviolet light and osmotic stress: activation of the JNK cascade through multiple growth factor and cytokine receptors. Science 1996;274(5290):1194–7.

61. Aragane Y, Kulms D, Metze D, et al. Ultraviolet light induces apoptosis via direct activation of CD95 (Fas/APO-1) independently of its ligand CD95L. J Cell Biol 1998;140(1):171–82.

62. De Fabo EC, Noonan FP. Mechanism of immune suppression by ultraviolet irradiation in vivo. I. Evidence for the existence of a unique photoreceptor in skin and its role in photoimmunology. J Exp Med 1983;158(1):84–98.

63. Kammeyer A, Pavel S, Asghar SS, et al. Prolonged increase of cis-urocanic acid levels in human skin and urine after single total-body ultraviolet exposures. Photochem Photobiol 1997;65(3):593–8.

64. Snellman E, Koulu L, Pasanen P, et al. Effect of psoriasis heliotherapy on epidermal urocanic acid isomer concentrations. Acta Derm Venereol 1992;72(3):231–3.

65. Snellman E, Strozyk M, Segerbäck D, et al. Effect of the spectral range of a UV lamp on the production of cyclobutane pyrimidine dimers in human skin in situ. Photodermatol Photoimmunol Photomed 2003;19(6):281–6.

66. Bataille V, Bykov VJ, Sasieni P, et al. Photoadaptation to ultraviolet (UV) radiation in vivo: photoproducts in epidermal cells following UVB therapy for psoriasis. Br J Dermatol 2000;143(3):477–83.

67. Krueger JG, Wolfe JT, Nabeya RT, et al. Successful ultraviolet B treatment of psoriasis is accompanied by a reversal of keratinocyte pathology and by selective depletion of intraepidermal T cells. J Exp Med 1995;182(6):2057–68.

68. Weatherhead SC, Farr PM, Jamieson D, et al. Keratinocyte apoptosis in epidermal remodeling and clearance of psoriasis induced by UV radiation. J Invest Dermatol 2011;131(9):1916–26.

69. Weatherhead SC, Farr PM, Reynolds NJ. Spectral effects of UV on psoriasis. Photochem Photobiol Sci 2013;12(1):47–53.

70. Ozawa M, Ferenczi K, Kikuchi T, et al. 312-nanometer ultraviolet B light (narrow-band UVB) induces apoptosis of T cells within psoriatic lesions. J Exp Med 1999;189(4):711–8.

71. Walters IB, Ozawa M, Cardinale I, et al. Narrowband (312-nm) UV-B suppresses interferon gamma and interleukin (IL) 12 and increases IL-4 transcripts: differential regulation of cytokines at the single-cell level. Arch Dermatol 2003;139(2):155–61.

72. Gutierrez-Steil C, Wrone-Smith T, Sun X, et al. Sunlight-induced basal cell carcinoma tumor cells and ultraviolet-B-irradiated psoriatic plaques express Fas ligand (CD95L). J Clin Invest 1998;101(1):33–9.

73. El-Domyati M, Moftah NH, Nasif GA, et al. Evaluation of apoptosis regulatory proteins in response to PUVA therapy for psoriasis. Photodermatol Photoimmunol Photomed 2013;29(1):18–26.

74. Piskin G, Koomen CW, Picavet D, et al. Ultraviolet-B irradiation decreases IFN-gamma and increases IL-4 expression in psoriatic lesional skin in situ and in cultured dermal T cells derived from these lesions. Exp Dermatol 2003;12(2):172–80.

75. Piskin G, Sylva-Steenland RM, Bos JD, et al. T cells in psoriatic lesional skin that survive conventional therapy with NB-UVB radiation display reduced IFN-gamma expression. Arch Dermatol Res 2004;295(12):509–16.

76. Piskin G, Tursen U, Bos JD, et al. IL-4 expression by neutrophils in psoriasis lesional skin upon high-dose UVB exposure. Dermatology 2003;207(1):51–3.

77. Hyder LA, Gonzalez J, Harden JL, et al. TREM-1 as a potential therapeutic target in psoriasis. J Invest Dermatol 2013;133(7):1742–51.

78. Racz E, Prens EP, Kurek D, et al. Effective treatment of psoriasis with narrow-band UVB phototherapy is linked to suppression of the IFN and Th17 pathways. J Invest Dermatol 2011;131(7):1547–58.

79. Furuhashi T, Saito C, Torii K, et al. Photo(chemo)therapy reduces circulating Th17 cells and restores circulating regulatory T cells in psoriasis. PLoS one 2013;8(1):e54895.

80. Shohat B, Kozenitzki L, David M, et al. Effect of UVB and AS101 on interleukin-2 production and helper activity in psoriatic patients. Nat Immun 1993;12(1):50–5.

81. Sigmundsdottir H, Johnston A, Gudjonsson JE, et al. Narrowband-UVB irradiation decreases the production of pro-inflammatory cytokines by stimulated T cells. Arch Dermatol Res 2005;297:39–42.

82. Gilmour JW, Vestey JP, George S, et al. Effect of phototherapy and urocanic acid isomers on natural killer cell function. J Invest Dermatol 1993;101(2):169–74.

83. Tobin AM, Maguire B, Enright H, et al. The effects of phototherapy on the numbers of circulating

natural killer cells and T lymphocytes in psoriasis. Photodermatol Photoimmunol Photomed 2009; 25(2):109–10.

84. Guilhou J, Colette C, Monpoint S, et al. Vitamin D metabolism in psoriasis before and after phototherapy. Acta Derm Venereol 1990;70(4):351–4.

85. Osmancevic A, Landin-Wilhelmsen K, Larkö O, et al. Vitamin D production in psoriasis patients increases less with narrowband than with broadband ultraviolet B phototherapy. Photodermatol Photoimmunol Photomed 2009;25(3):119–23.

86. Ryan C, Renfro L, Collins P, et al. Clinical and genetic predictors of response to narrowband ultraviolet B for the treatment of chronic plaque psoriasis. Br J Dermatol 2010;163(5):1056–63.

87. Van Weelden H, Baart de la Faille H, Young E, et al. A new development in UVB phototherapy of psoriasis. Br J Dermatol 1988;119:11–9.

88. Johnson B, Green C, Lakshmipathi T, et al. Ultraviolet radiation phototherapy for psoriasis; the use of a new narrow band UVB fluorescent lamp. In: Douglas R, Moan J, Dall'Acqua F, editors. Light in biology and medicine, vol. 1. Oxford (United Kingdom): Plenum; 1988. p. 173–9.

89. Karvonen J, Kokkonen LE, Routsalainen E. 311 nm UVB lamps in the treatment of psoriasis with the Ingram regimen. Acta Derm Venereol 1989;69:82–5.

90. Srinivas C. Minimal erythema dose (MED) to narrow band ultraviolet-B (NB-UVB) broad band ultraviolet-B (BB-UVB)–a pilot study. Indian J Dermatol Venereol Leprol 2002;68(2):63–4.

91. Tejasvi T, Sharma V, Kaur J. Determination of minimal erythemal dose for narrow band-ultraviolet B radiation in north Indian patients: comparison of visual and Dermaspectrometer readings. Indian J Dermatol Venereol Leprol 2007;73(2):97–9.

92. Youn J, Park J, Jo S, et al. Assessment of the usefulness of skin phototype and skin color as the parameter of cutaneous narrow band UVB sensitivity in psoriasis patients. Photodermatol Photoimmunol Photomed 2003;19(5):261–4.

93. Morita A, Shintani Y, Nishida E, et al. Feasibility and accuracy of a newly developed hand-held device with a flat-type fluorescent lamp for measuring the minimal erythema dose for narrow-band UVB therapy. Photodermatol Photoimmunol Photomed 2009; 25(1):41–4.

Current and Future Oral Systemic Therapies for Psoriasis

John B. Kelly III, MD, PhD[a], Peter Foley, MD[b],
Bruce E. Strober, MD, PhD[a,c],*

KEYWORDS

- Psoriasis • Methotrexate • Cyclosporine • Acitretin • Apremilast • Tofacitinib
- Mycophenolate mofetil

KEY POINTS

- Methotrexate is a relatively safe, long-term treatment of appropriately screened and monitored patients who can be expected to achieve a 75% reduction in the Psoriasis Area and Severity Index in approximately 40% of cases.
- For patients without any contraindications, cyclosporine in most cases is a rapidly effective, short-term medication frequently used as a bridge to longer term maintenance approaches to the control of psoriasis.
- Carefully selected and monitored patients, especially those with the pustular, palmoplantar or erythrodermic forms of psoriasis, may derive significant benefit from acitretin therapy.
- Apremilast (approved in the US for both psoriasis and psoriatic arthritis) and tofacitinib (approved in the US for rheumatoid arthritis) are novel oral medications that have shown effectiveness in clinical trials; these medications are likely to be approved for use in patients with moderate to severe psoriasis within the near future.
- Mycophenolate mofetil, 6-thioguanine, leflunomide, and other oral agents remain reasonable alternatives, but various aspects of their efficacy, monitoring requirements, and adverse event profiles relegate these drugs to patients who have failed both oral and biologic medications.

Psoriasis is a chronic, immunodysregulatory disease with significant prevalence and a range of severity in its dermatologic and rheumatologic signs and symptoms. Topical agents remain the first-line treatments for mild disease. For patients with greater percent body surface area (BSA) of involvement, or with disease that has significant quality of life impact, systemic therapy or phototherapy is indicated.[1] Strong evidence indicates that psoriasis is an independent risk factor for cardiovascular risk and that the inflammatory co-morbidities of psoriasis merit systemic therapy even in the absence of joint disease, though prospective data to assess whether there is a morbidity or mortality benefit to doing so are in their infancy.[2–4]

Systemic medication for psoriasis can be broadly divided into small molecules, which are usually given orally, and biologics, which are large molecules that must be delivered by injection or infusion. Systemic medications are often used as monotherapy but, in many, instances are combined or used with phototherapy to increase or maintain efficacy; decrease undesired effects; or,

Disclosure: See last page of article.
[a] Department of Dermatology, University of Connecticut Health Center, Farmington, CT, USA; [b] St Vincent's Hospital Melbourne, The University of Melbourne, Victoria, Australia; [c] Probity Medical Research, Waterloo, Ontario, Canada
* Corresponding author. Department of Dermatology, University of Connecticut Health Center, 21 South Road, 2nd Floor, Farmington, CT 06032, USA
E-mail address: strober@uchc.edu

Dermatol Clin 33 (2015) 91–109
http://dx.doi.org/10.1016/j.det.2014.09.008
0733-8635/15/$ – see front matter © 2015 Elsevier Inc. All rights reserved.

out of necessity, for refractory disease.[5] In some cases oral systemics are given in combination with biologics for synergistic effects or to forestall the development of biologic immunogenicity.

The small molecules used in therapy for psoriasis include mature drugs, such as methotrexate, cyclosporine, and acitretin, as well as newer compounds discovered through targeted development and understanding of molecular pathways, such as tofacitinib and apremilast.[6] This article focuses on the, small molecule systemic therapies with clinical data supporting their efficacy.

PATIENT ASSESSMENT

A thorough medical history, prior treatment history and focused physical examination should be the starting point from which systemic therapy for psoriasis is considered, with a review of systems that covers the cutaneous, immune, hematologic, cardiac, gastrointestinal, musculoskeletal, neurologic, reproductive, and family and social history. Concerns of the patient regarding mode of administration and risk aversion need to be considered (**Table 1**). This evaluation should include laboratory investigations, and it is prudent to include baseline studies necessary for the whole spectrum of possible systemic treatments. A suggested list of these tests is included in **Table 2**. A complete picture of the patient's disease severity, impact on their quality of life, overall health and comorbidities, and their willingness to attempt available treatment should coalesce, and a patient-centered, mutually agreeable therapeutic approach enacted. The nonbiologic, nonphototherapy options for modern systemic treatment of psoriasis are as follows.

METHOTREXATE

Methotrexate is the oldest systemic therapy for moderate to severe psoriasis having been approved over 40 years ago. Its anti-inflammatory effects are primarily mediated through its metabolism to polyglutamate derivatives that are potent inhibitors of 5-aminoimidazole-4-carboxamide ribonucleotide transformylase.[7] In so doing, methotrexate increases the endogenous levels of adenosine, a potent anti-inflammatory compound.[8] Methotrexate also has been shown to decrease primary and secondary antibody responses.[7–10] Generally, it is available in 2.5 mg tablets and is typically prescribed at 7.5 to 25 mg, taken once weekly; higher doses produce better response.[9] Older dosing schemes were split between 3 administrations, every 12 hours, but this is unnecessary from an efficacy or side-effect standpoint. Additionally, subcutaneous methotrexate dosed once weekly has displayed better bioavailability, efficacy, and tolerability relative to the oral formulation in studies of patients with rheumatoid arthritis.[10–18] Daily or weekly folic or folinic acid supplements are recommended to decrease side effects (particularly bone marrow suppression) and improve gastrointestinal tolerability.[19,20]

Because methotrexate use for psoriasis predates the modern drug approval process, there have been, until the last decade, a lack of robust clinical data regarding its efficacy. This, however, is no longer the case. A multicenter, prospective, randomized, double-blind, placebo-controlled study involved 110 subjects receiving methotrexate doses from 7.5 to 25 mg/wk (plus folate 5 mg 2 days after the methotrexate dose). At 16 weeks, using the Psoriasis Area and Severity

Table 1
Selected patient considerations in systemic psoriasis therapy

Parameter	Consideration
Extent or severity of psoriasis	Typically >10% BSA, or involved areas significantly impede quality of life
Presence of psoriatic arthritis	Consider systemic, disease-modifying therapy regardless of level of skin involvement
Woman of childbearing potential	Not a good candidate for most oral psoriasis medications
Man attempting to conceive a child	Not a good candidate for methotrexate
Chronic or binge alcohol user	Avoid concomitant therapies with significant risk of hepatotoxicity
History of hepatitis	Avoid therapies with significant risk of hepatotoxicity
History of hematologic malignancy	Use immunosuppressants with caution
Immunodeficiency	Avoid immunosuppressants
Smoker	Counsel on quitting

Table 2
Suggested baseline laboratory workup before systemic psoriasis therapy

Frequent	Less Frequent
Comprehensive metabolic panel	Magnesium, phosphate
Complete blood count	β-human chorionic gonadotropin
	HIV serology
	Lipid panel
	Hepatitis B serology
	Hepatitis C serology
	Interferon-gamma releasing assay for the detection of latent tuberculosis or purified protein derivative tuberculin

Index (PASI), 35.5% of subjects achieved a 75% reduction in PASI (PASI 75).[21] A similar response rate, PASI 75 of 39.9% at 24 weeks, was seen in a comparison study of methotrexate and briakinumab.[22] These results parallel the largest single study involving methotrexate, in which 41.9% of the 215 subjects taking methotrexate (in an open-label, nonblinded manner) achieved PASI 75 at 16 weeks.[23] Although these PASI 75 response rates are somewhat lower than reported in other clinical trials, they represent the best quality data, and a reasonable expectation of oral methotrexate efficacy is that approximately 40% will achieve PASI 75. The advent of pharmacogenomics and identification of gene polymorphisms conferring a better response to methotrexate may facilitate patient screening and increase the percentage achieving optimal control, once such testing becomes more readily available.[24]

The most common clinical side effects of methotrexate at the low doses used for psoriasis are nausea, diarrhea, fatigue, and headache. Supplementation with folic and/or folinic acid may either mitigate or eliminate these adverse effects, which tend to become less severe with time.[19] Monitoring for rarer and more severe side effects is an integral part of every follow-up appointment. Liver function tests (LFTs) should be checked every 4 to 12 weeks because the first signs of hepatotoxicity may manifest as an elevation in transaminases. For long-term monitoring of hepatotoxicity, the general movement has been away from routine liver biopsy and toward noninvasive measurement of classic and newly validated serum biomarkers, such as type III procollagen amino terminal propeptide, which is currently standard in most European countries.[25,26] In some jurisdictions, liver biopsy may be recommended before methotrexate initiation in patients with hepatic disease risk factors, and by American Academy of Dermatology (AAD) guidelines once a cumulative dose of 3.5 to 4 g is reached.[25] Particular vigilance to hepatic monitoring is necessary because psoriasis has been identified as an independent risk factor for nonalcoholic fatty liver disease[27] and the comorbidities often found in psoriatic patients can place them at higher risk of methotrexate-induced hepatic injury.[28]

A complete blood count is necessary to warn of myelosuppression, whereas adequate kidney function must be verified because most methotrexate is renally excreted. Dose adjustments can be made for decreased glomerular filtration rate, but this should be done with care because these patients are at increased risk of cytopenia. Screening for any changes in pulmonary status, including breathing difficulty or persistent cough, is a requirement because of the rare side-effect of idiosyncratic pneumonitis or pulmonary fibrosis. Other adverse effects include alopecia (higher or, inadvertently, daily doses), mouth ulcers (particularly in the setting of neutropenia), and (rarely) radiation recall and/or acral erythema. In patients with rheumatoid arthritis, an increased frequency of melanoma, non-Hodgkin lymphoma and lung cancer has been reported[29]; however, these findings have not been well-substantiated.

Methotrexate has numerous potential interactions with other drugs. Care should be taken with concurrent salicylates, regular use and overuse of nonsteroidal anti-inflammatory drugs, and certain types of antibiotic use (particularly sulfonamides), and it is recommended to check a current interaction database before initiating new therapy.

Methotrexate is pregnancy category X; pregnancy and lactation are absolute contraindications. Individual accounts of accidental in utero exposure without any observed sequelae exist, but all patients (male and female) should discontinue methotrexate 3 months before any planned attempts at pregnancy, and those pregnancies conceived while on methotrexate should be considered high-risk until proven otherwise.

Methotrexate often is combined with other systemic therapies or phototherapy to achieve either additive or synergistic effects. Combination allows lower doses; minimized toxicity; augmented efficacy; and, via the reduction in immunogenicity, the preservation of the activity of biologic therapies. Combination may involve cyclosporine, acitretin (with careful liver monitoring, in appropriate patients), TNF-α inhibitors, and ustekinumab. The combination of methotrexate with another therapy frequently leads to superior and longer lasting efficacy than with either therapy alone.[29,30]

CYCLOSPORINE

Cyclosporine is a calcineurin inhibitor that is approved to treat moderate to severe psoriasis.[31–33] Its mechanism of action is to form a complex with cyclophilin, resulting in reduced activity of the nuclear transcription factor, nuclear factor of activated T cells, thus lowering the production of IL-2 and other proinflammatory cytokines, and, consequently, inhibiting T cell activation. In addition cyclosporine inhibits interferon-γ production. At typical doses (2.5–5.5 mg/kg/d) cyclosporine is highly effective for rapidly and consistently treating severe disease. Cyclosporine therapy may be used with many different approaches: (1) intermittently as a short-course (12–16 week) therapy with minimal renal and hypertensive toxicity, (2) continuously to maintain remission in a minority of patients with refractory disease, (3) as a crisis intervention (4–8 weeks) to reduce flare or treat severe disease, and (4) as a part of sequential and rotational therapy to help minimize toxicity and optimize efficacy. The treatment regimen should be tailored to the needs and medical history of the individual patient.[34]

Unlike methotrexate, cyclosporine has not been used as a comparator in any modern, large, multicenter, randomized, placebo-controlled clinical trials. There are, however, several moderate-size clinical trials that demonstrate the drug's high efficacy (**Tables 3** and **4**). Studies have established a clear dose-response curve in which 5 mg/kg/d is the inflection point that balances safety and side effects with impressive clearance; cyclosporine at this dose reliably results in average PASI 75 rates of 70%.[29,43,44] Further, there seems to be improved benefit in starting at this dose, then titrating down as the disease is controlled.[45]

Cyclosporine toxicities are related to dose and length of treatment, both of which should be kept to a minimum effective magnitude. In addition to baseline laboratory tests (see **Table 2**), monitoring includes weekly blood pressure readings and monthly comprehensive panel (including serum creatinine), lipids, magnesium and potassium. Sustained hypertension that is not responsive to pharmacologic intervention (eg, amlodipine) or increase in serum creatinine greater than 30% of baseline requires cyclosporine dose-reduction or cessation of therapy. Hypomagnesemia, hyperkalemia, and hyperlipidemia are potential laboratory abnormalities of which development, depending on the severity, could necessitate a therapeutic change of course.

Cyclosporine has many relative contraindications, including hypertension, renal insufficiency, history of extensive ultraviolet exposure, especially psoralen-UV-A (PUVA), or nonmelanoma skin cancer, or a history of lymphoproliferative disorder. Cyclosporine should not be administered in patients with active or chronic infections. With its extensive metabolism through the cytochrome P-450 3A4 enzyme system in the liver, and the potentially nephrotoxic effects, a comprehensive medication reconciliation should be performed before initiating cyclosporine therapy.

Relatively common side effects include hypertension, headache, hypertrichosis, gingival hyperplasia, nausea, and increased susceptibility to infections. Tremor, myalgias, paresthesia, and sensitivity to temperature may also develop. Despite the long list of potential adverse effects, cyclosporine has been found safe during pregnancy[48,49] and may be considered in both men and women attempting conception.

Because cyclosporine is not a long-term solution, it is often combined with other systemic medications early in a treatment course, then titrated down as an overlapping therapy until either methotrexate or acitretin takes effect. Like methotrexate, cyclosporine can be used before or coinciding with the initiation of biologic therapy or for flares during biologic therapy, in appropriate patients, and can enhance efficacy.

ACITRETIN

Systemic retinoids have been in use as psoriasis treatments since the 1970s, beginning with etretinate. Acitretin, the active acid metabolite of etretinate, is hypothesized to treat psoriasis through antiproliferative effects on keratinocytes, immunomodulatory effects, and antiangiogenic effects by binding to nuclear retinoic acid receptors and/or retinoid X receptors.[50] Unlike other systemic treatments for psoriasis, retinoids are not found to be immunosuppressive, a distinct advantage for certain patients. Acitretin generally is started at low doses (10–25 mg/d), and increased as tolerated, except in the case of generalized pustular psoriasis, where it should be started high and titrated down to the lowest effective dose.[50] A study of subjects treated with 50 mg daily of acitretin over 8 weeks reported 23% achieving PASI 75.[51] In another study, after 12 weeks of treatment with acitretin, the mean PASI improvement was 70% to 75%.[52] Clearance or marked improvement was achieved by 41% of 59 subjects treated with 20 mg/d acitretin, with dose increases of 10 mg every 2 weeks up to a final dose of 70 mg; however, 36% of subjects dropped out of the

Table 3
Select clinical studies evaluating oral methotrexate

Study, Year	Agent	Number of Subjects Evaluated	Study Type	Outcome Measure	Results	P	Comments
Heydendael et al,[29] 2003	MTX vs CsA	85 (43 MTX)	RCT, assessor blinded	PASI 75	At 16 wk MTX 15–22.5 mg/wk: 60% CsA 3–5 mg/kg: 71%	P = .29 comparing 2 groups receiving MTX and CsA	No placebo arm; doses of both MTX and CsA could be increased to achieve response; no folate supplementation in MTX arm. Treatment had to be discontinued in 12 subjects in the methotrexate group because of elevated liver enzyme levels
Flyström et al,[35] 2008	MTX vs CsA	68 (37 MTX)	MRCT	PASI reduction; calculated PASI 75	At 12 wk MTX PASI 75 21.6%; CsA 3–5 mg/kg 64%	P = .0028	5 mg daily folate in MTX arm; 7.5–15 mg/wk MTX
Ho et al,[36] 2010	MTX vs Traditional Chinese Medicine vs placebo	50 (19 MTX)	RPCT	PASI 75	At 24 wk MTX PASI 75 63%, placebo PASI 75 18%	P<.01	5 mg daily folate in MTX arm; 10–30 mg/wk MTX
Akhyani et al,[37] 2010	MTX vs MMF	38 (18 MTX)	Open label RCT	PASI 75	At 12 wk MTX PASI 75 73.3%, MMF PASI 75 58.8%	P>.05	1 mg folate daily (except MTX day); MTX titrated up to 20 mg/wk
Saurat et al,[21] 2008	MTX vs adalimumab vs placebo	271 (110 MTX)	MRDPCT	PASI 75	At 16 wk, MTX PASI 75 35.5%; adalimumab PASI 75 79.6%	P<.001	~5 mg folate/wk; MTX dose escalation 7.5–25 mg/wk
Barker et al,[23] 2011	MTX vs infliximab	868 (215 MTX)	Open-label RCT	PASI 75	At 16 wk MTX PASI 75 41.9%; infliximab PASI 75 77.8%	P<.001	Folate recommended but not mandated; dose escalation to 20 mg MTX permitted at week 6

(continued on next page)

Table 3
(continued)

Study, Year	Agent	Number of Subjects Evaluated	Study Type	Outcome Measure	Results	P	Comments
Radmanesh et al,[38] 2011	MTX daily vs weekly	202 (101 each daily or weekly)	RCT	PASI 75	At 16 wk: daily PASI 75 60%, weekly PASI 75 81%	P<.001	No placebo arm; no folate supplements; no topical or other systemic therapy. increased nausea/vomiting/ fatigue in weekly group
Dogra et al,[9] 2012	MTX 10 or 25 mg/wk	51 (25 at 10, 26 at 25 mg/wk)	RDCT	PASI 75	At 12 wk, 10 mg PASI 75 72%; 25 mg PASI 75 92%	P>.05	Folate 5 mg twice each week; excluded subjects with body mass index >30
Baranauskaite et al,[39] 2012	MTX 15 mg/wk vs MTX 15 mg/wk + infliximab	94 (47 MTX)	Open-label RCT	PASI 75 (in those with baseline PASI >2.5)	At 16 wk MTX alone PASI 75 54.3%; infliximab + MTX PASI 75 97.1%	P<.0001	More adverse events with dual therapy; no comment on folate supplementation
Ranjan et al,[40] 2007	MTX vs hydroxyurea	30 (15 MTX)	Open-label RCT	PASI 75	At 12 wk, MTX PASI 75 66.7%, hydroxyurea PASI 75 13.3%		Weekly dosing of hydroxyurea; less adverse events than reported with daily dosing
Mahbub et al,[41] 2013	MTX vs hydroxyurea	24 (13 MTX)	Case or control	PASI reduction	At 8 wk, MTX had 85% PASI reduction; hydroxyurea had 78%	P>.05	—
Fallah Arani et al,[42] 2011	MTX vs fumarates	51 (26 MTX)	RCT	PASI 75	At 16 wk MTX PASI 75 42%; fumarates PASI 75 38%	P>.65	MTX dose-escalated up to 15 mg/wk; folate used
Reich et al,[22] 2011	MTX vs briakinumab	317 (163 MTX)	MRDPCT	PASI 75	At 24 wk, MTX PASI 75 39.9%, briakinumab PASI 75 81.8%	P<.001	95/163 MTX discontinued study due to lack of efficacy; folate 5 mg/wk

Abbreviations: CsA, cyclosporine; MMF, mycophenolate mofetil; MRCT, multicenter, randomized clinical trial; MRDPCT, multicenter, randomized, double-blind, placebo-controlled clinical trial; MTX, methotrexate; NA, not available; RCT, randomized clinical trial; RDCT, randomized, double-blind clinical trial; RPCT, randomized, placebo-controlled clinical trial.
Data from Refs.[21–23,29,35–42]

Table 4
Select additional clinical studies evaluating cyclosporine

Study, Year	Agent	Number of Subjects Evaluated	Study Type	Outcome Measure	Results	P	Comments
Ellis et al,[43] 1991	CsA (2.5–7.5 mg/kg/d) vs placebo	85	RDPCT	PGA and Global Severity Score	At 8 wk, 36%, 65%, and 85% were clear or almost clear on doses of 2.5 mg/kg/d, 5 mg/kg/d, or 7.5 mg/kg/d, respectively	P<.0001	Higher doses associated with more renal toxicity, hypertension, intolerance
Reitamo et al,[44] 2001	CsA	34	RDPCT	PASI improvement	At 16 wk, CsA 1.25 mg/kg 33%; CsA 5 mg/kg 71%	P<.001	—
Yoon & Youn,[45] 2007	CsA	61	Open-label	PASI 75	At 12 wk, 75% of step-down subjects and 51.5% of standard subjects achieved PASI 75	P<.05	Standard regimen 2.5 mg/kg/d titrated up vs step-down regimen of 5 mg/kg/d titrated down
Pedraz et al,[46] 2006	CsA vs MMF	8	Sequential	PASI improvement	At 16 wk CsA PASI 75 85%, MMF PASI 75 50%	NA	CsA 4 mg/kg/d, MMF 30 mg/kg/d
Beissart et al,[47] 2009	CsA vs MMF	37 (21 CsA)	Multicenter open-label RCT	PASI 75	At 12 wk CsA PASI 75 58%, MMF PASI 75 18%	P<.01	2.5 mg/kg CsA 2 g/d MMF; dose escalation at 6 wk if <25% improvement in PASI

Abbreviations: CsA, cyclosporine; MMF, mycophenolate mofetil; MRCT, multicenter, randomized clinical trial; NA, not available; PGA, physician's global assessment; RCT, randomized clinical trial; RDPCT, randomized, double-blind, placebo-controlled clinical trial.
Data from Refs.[43–47]

study, mostly because of retinoid-related adverse events.[53]

A recent review of acitretin serves as an update to the 2009 AAD guidelines.[1,50] In short, acitretin as monotherapy usually reveals poor tolerability at doses required to achieve PASI 75. However, acitretin excels at treating the generalized, palmoplantar pustular, and hyperkeratotic variants of psoriasis.[54]

The side effects of acitretin are dose-limiting and may limit adherence. Most patients will experience some degree of mucocutaneous xerosis, which may become more tolerable as treatment continues. Dose-related hyperlipidemia occurs in 25% to 40% of acitretin users and may necessitate addition of a lipid-lowering medication.[50] Liver transaminase elevation also occurs but less frequently than with methotrexate. Acitretin is pregnancy category X, and women of childbearing potential should not conceive for 3 years after ceasing the drug, thus eliminating acitretin as a practical therapy for these patients. In addition, acitretin use has been associated with diminished night vision, rare diffuse skeletal hyperostosis, and pseudotumor cerebri.

Acitretin, like methotrexate, has been extensively investigated as a combination therapy. It is more effective when combined with ultraviolet phototherapy, and found to be safe when combined with biologic therapies.[50] Despite warning against its use with methotrexate, acitretin may be used in this combination in appropriate patients, with careful monitoring of the LFTs. It may also be used in sequential or rotational systemic therapy, although this approach is used far less frequently with the advent of the biologic therapies.

JANUS KINASE INHIBITORS

Tofacitinib is the first member of a novel class of medications, Janus kinase (JAK) inhibitors, to gain Food and Drug Administration (FDA) approval with an indication for rheumatoid arthritis. This drug is not currently approved for the treatment of moderate to severe psoriasis or psoriatic arthritis. JAK proteins are intracellular second messengers necessary for transmitting extracellular cytokine signals to the nucleus, and their inhibition attenuates these signals. Tofacitinib has relative specificity for JAK1 and JAK3, and preferentially blocks signaling through the common gamma chain-containing receptors for IL-2, IL-4, IL-7, IL-9, IL-15, and IL-21.[55] These immunomodulatory activities are hypothesized to be responsible for the efficacy of JAK inhibitors in rheumatoid arthritis and psoriasis.

There have been 3 major studies on tofacitinib in psoriasis, including 2 phase III multicenter trials with results posted to clinicaltrials.gov (**Table 5**). These multicenter, randomized, blinded, dose-response or placebo-controlled investigations show a significant improvement in skin symptoms with average week 12 PASI 75 response rates of approximately 40% at 5 mg twice a day and 64% at 10 mg twice a day dosing,[55,56] and week 24 PASI 75 response rates of 43.8% and 67.6%, respectively.[57,58] Importantly, they also demonstrated tofacitinib 10 mg twice a day was noninferior to etanercept 50 mg subcutaneously twice-weekly.[56]

Tofacitinib has several safety considerations, especially beyond the 5 mg twice daily dose. Lymphocytopenia, neutropenia, and anemia have all been reported, as well as increased LFTs, cholesterol, and serum creatinine.[55–57] Most of these effects have been transient and reversible on discontinuation, and only occurred in a small minority of patients.[58] Further, low-density lipoprotein (LDL) and high-density lipoprotein (HDL) cholesterol levels seem to increase in parallel with no change in LDL to HDL ratio. Herpes zoster occurs more frequently in patients receiving tofacitinib. Infections, some serious, and malignancies have also been reported with tofacitinib therapy; although they are not clearly related to the drug. There currently is an FDA boxed warning related to these adverse events. Because of these considerations, a complete blood count, lipid profile, renal function tests, and LFTs should be monitored regularly during therapy; significant and persistent perturbations should prompt dose adjustment or cessation of medication.

APREMILAST

Part of a novel class of immunomodulatory medications, apremilast, approved in the United States for the treatment of both psoriasis and psoriatic arthritis, inhibits phosphodiesterase 4 (PDE4), which degrades intracellular cyclic AMP and is particularly active in both cells of the immune system and keratinocytes.[59] Inhibition of PDE4 has been shown in vitro to decrease production of proinflammatory cytokines TNF-α, IL-2, IL-12, IL-23, and interferon-γ; to increase anti-inflammatory cytokines, including IL-10; and to reduce in vivo epidermal thickness.[60,61]

Robust phase II and III clinical trial data have been generated for apremilast in psoriatic patients with and without arthritis (**Table 6**). In psoriasis, phase III multicenter, randomized, placebo-controlled studies demonstrate PASI 75 achievement rates between 28.8% and 33.1% after 16 weeks of apremilast taken at a dose of 30 mg twice daily.[62,63]

Apremilast has demonstrated a good safety profile during its large clinical trials, with the most

Table 5
Clinical studies evaluating tofacitinib

Study, Year	Agents	Number of Subjects Evaluated	Study Type	Outcome Measure	Results	P	Comments
ClinicalTrials.gov[56] NCT01241591, April 2014	Tofacitinib vs etanercept vs placebo	1120 (712 received study drug)	MRDPCT	PASI 75	At 12 wk: tofacitinib 5 PASI 75 39.51%; tofacitinib 10 PASI 75 63.64%	Statistically better than placebo; noninferior to etanercept	BID dosing
Papp et al,[55] 2012	Tofacitinib vs placebo	197 (147 received study drug)	MRDPCT	PASI 75	At 12 wk: tofacitinib 2 PASI 75 25%; tofacitinib 5 PASI 75 40.8%; tofacitinib 15 PASI 75 66.7%	P<.001 or better vs placebo, all	BID dosing
A3921111, ClinicalTrials.gov[57] NCT01186744, Bissonnette, 2014	Tofacitinib 5 mg vs 10 mg twice daily (bid) for 24 wk	5 mg (n = 331) 10 mg (n = 335)	MRDCT	PASI 75	At 24 wk: tofacitinib 5 PASI 75 144/329 (43.8%); tofacitinib 10 PASI 75 225/333 (67.6%)	—	—

Abbreviations: MRDCT, multicenter, randomized, double-blind, clinical trial; MRDPCT, multicenter, randomized, double-blind, placebo-controlled clinical trial.
Data from Refs.[55–57]

Table 6
Clinical studies evaluating apremilast

Study, Year	Agent	Number of Subjects Evaluated	Study Type	Outcome Measure	Results	P	Comments
Paul et al,[62] 2014 (ESTEEM2, AAD 2014 poster)	Apremilast 30 mg bid vs placebo	413	MRDPCT	PASI 75	At 16 wk, apremilast 30 PASI 75 28.8%	P<.0001	Rare discontinuations due to diarrhea, nausea
Reich et al,[63] 2014 (ESTEEM1, AAD 2014 poster)	Apremilast 30 mg bid vs placebo	844	MRDPCT	PASI 75	At 16 wk, apremilast 30 PASI 75 33.1%	P<.0001	—
Kavanaugh et al,[59] 2014	Apremilast vs placebo	489 (324 received drug)	MRDPCT	PASI 75	At 24 wk apremilast 20 PASI 75 17.6%; apremilast 30 PASI 75 21%	P = .018, .004 for 20 and 30 mg bid vs placebo, respectively	Phase II trial also evaluating PsA
Papp et al,[60] 2012	Apremilast vs placebo	280	MRDPCT	PASI 75	At 16 wk apremilast 20 PASI 75 29%; apremilast 30 PASI 75 41%	P<.0001 vs placebo, both	10 mg bid apremilast not significantly better than placebo
Gottlieb et al,[61] 2008	Apremilast	17	Open-label single-arm treatment study	PASI 50	At 29 d, apremilast 20 mg daily PASI 50 17.6%	NA	—

Abbreviation: MRDPCT, multicenter, randomized, double-blind, placebo-controlled clinical trial; NA, not availabe; PsA, psoriatic arthritis.
Data from Refs.[59–63]

common side effects being nausea, vomiting, and diarrhea particularly in the early stages of therapy. Headaches, and upper respiratory or nasopharyngeal infection may also be noted. Discontinuation of therapy due to side effects has been a rare occurrence. In addition, no sustained and significant laboratory abnormalities are associated with apremilast treatment, which suggests there may be no need for laboratory monitoring beyond baseline evaluation and age-appropriate, routine surveillance. However, the mean weight loss in patients treated long-term with apremilast is approximately 2 kg. A weight decrease between 5% and 10% of baseline body weight occurred in 10% of apremilast-treated subjects compared with 3% of those treated with placebo. Additionally, the weight loss is not related to gastrointestinal adverse events. The mechanism of action of apremilast-related weight loss currently is unknown and is associated with no overt clinical consequences.[64] Although the package labeling also mentions a risk of depression and suicidal ideation associated with apremilast, the data supporting this risk in psoriasis patients are weak, with very low event rates and little difference between the groups receiving treatment or placebo in the phase III studies.[64]

MYCOPHENOLATE MOFETIL

A prodrug that had extensive use in transplant medicine before its introduction in dermatology, mycophenolate mofetil is metabolized to mycophenolic acid, an inhibitor of de novo purine synthesis in B and T cells. Mycophenolate mofetil typically is given starting at 1 to 2 g/d in divided doses, with titration up to 3 g/d, or higher, depending on side effects and the presence of normal laboratory results.

There have been limited high-quality clinical studies on mycophenolate mofetil in psoriasis (**Table 7**). Based on the open-label and comparison studies that have been published, mycophenolate mofetil is generally an inferior treatment compared with methotrexate or cyclosporine, although it may have some value in maintaining disease control obtained via cyclosporine.[46] As monotherapy, its PASI 75 achievement rate averages less than 20%, though its PASI 50 rate is reliably around 50%.[47,65,66]

Gastrointestinal symptoms, including nausea and diarrhea, are the most common and often dose-limiting side effects of mycophenolate mofetil therapy. Dose-dependent, reversible hematologic abnormalities occur with frequencies that mandate complete blood count monitoring. Electrolytes and LFTs should also be checked regularly. There are

reports, largely from the transplant literature, of hematologic malignancies, progressive multifocal leukoencephalopathy, and other serious infections in patients treated with mycophenolate mofetil.[67] Screening for these and other complications should be a routine part of follow-up visits, in addition to the recommended laboratory evaluations.

Mycophenolate mofetil is pregnancy category D, having been associated with a range of fetal anomalies. Women should have a negative pregnancy test before initiating therapy and avoid conception while being treated. There are numerous potential drug interactions with mycophenolate mofetil; narcotics, antibiotics, immunosuppressants, NSAIDS, thymidine kinase inhibitors, and levonorgestrel-containing oral contraceptives can all be significant. As in all pharmacologic interventions, verifying the absence of drug interactions is mandatory.

LEFLUNOMIDE

Leflunomide is a prodrug that has an active metabolite that inhibits pyrimidine synthesis. In a double-blind, multicenter, placebo-controlled study, the 24-week PASI 75 achievement rate for subjects receiving the drug at 20 mg taken daily was 17%, compared with 8% receiving placebo.[68] The baseline BSA of involvement and PASI scores for the enrolled subjects were low (3% and 9%, respectively), but there was significant improvement in the Dermatology Life Quality Index when compared with placebo. The most common side effects include diarrhea, nausea, upper respiratory tract infection, headache, hypertension, and alopecia. Like other antimetabolites, leflunomide is contraindicated in pregnancy. Monitoring for blood count and liver function is recommended at baseline and monthly.

FUMARIC ACID ESTERS

The mix of dimethyl fumarate and monomethyl fumarate salts, collectively termed fumarates or fumaric acid esters, has long been used in Europe as effective psoriasis therapy. These drugs are thought to act through antiproliferative effects on keratinocytes and preferential induction of apoptosis in activated T cells.[42] There are low-dose and high-dose preparations available in Europe that undergo dose escalation during therapy. Fumaric acid esters currently are not approved or available for psoriasis in the United States.

A randomized trial comparing fumaric acid esters to methotrexate in moderate to severe plaque psoriasis found comparable PASI responses between them.[42] In an unblinded study of 80 subjects

Table 7
Selected additional clinical studies evaluating mycophenolate mofetil

Study, Year	Agent	Number of Subjects Evaluated	Study Type	Outcome Measure	Results	P	Comments
Fallah Arani et al,[65] 2014	Enteric-coated mycophenolate sodium	8 (20 received drug)	Open label, noncontrolled	PASI improvement	At 24 wk, 2/8 subjects had PASI 75	NA	Enteric-coated preparation; 1440 mg maximum dose. Only 8/20 analyzed because of dropout due to psoriasis worsening or relapse
Zhou et al,[66] 2003	Mycophenolate mofetil	18	Open-label, noncontrolled	PASI improvement	At 12 wk, average PASI reduction was 47%	NA	2–3 g dose escalation

Abbreviation: NA, not available.

Data from Fallah Arani S, Waalboer Spuij R, Nijsten T, et al. Enteric-coated mycophenolate sodium in psoriasis vulgaris: an open pilot study. J Dermatolog Treat 2014;25(1):46–9; and Zhou Y, Rosenthal D, Dutz J, et al. Mycophenolate mofetil (CellCept) for psoriasis: a two-center, prospective, open-label clinical trial. J Cutan Med Surg 2003;7(3):193–7.

with severe, recalcitrant psoriasis addition of fumaric acid esters to their regimen improved disease control for 32%, and allowed dose reduction of other systemic agents without loss of disease control.[69] Side effects, including nausea, diarrhea, and flushing, occur in some patients, and often cause cessation of therapy. Leukopenia, eosinophilia, and transient LFT abnormalities have been documented, with the first 2 being significant enough to discontinue the drug.[70]

Overall, fumaric acid esters have a favorable safety profile and seem relatively effective in treating psoriasis, but larger randomized, double-blind controlled trials are needed to confirm these data. Approval in only a limited number of countries hinders the wider acceptance of fumaric acid esters for the treatment of psoriasis. However, larger studies are planned in North America.

HYDROXYUREA

Hydroxyurea is another antimetabolite that is thought to exert its effects via inhibition of DNA replication. Typically, hydroxyurea is prescribed at a dose of 500 mg taken 3 times daily. There have been a few open-label and retrospective studies demonstrating its efficacy, and 2 comparative studies with methotrexate (see Table 3). Overall, the data suggest hydroxyurea is inferior to methotrexate at achieving PASI 75 over a 3-month term.[40] However, hydroxyurea may be more effective when used for a longer duration (9–16 months).[41] Due to risk of bone marrow suppression, hydroxyurea has similar monitoring requirements to other antimetabolites and is contraindicated in pregnancy, nursing, or significant bone marrow suppression.

6-THIOGUANINE

6-Thioguanine is an antimetabolite that is the active form of azathioprine, and seems to be more effective than its parent drug in treating psoriasis.[1] It is thought to work by inhibition of purine synthesis. Two separate, open-label studies demonstrated 78% complete or almost-complete clearance and effective maintenance in 49% on varying doses of 6-thioguanine.[71,72] Pulse-dosing 2 to 3 times per week may decrease the risk of drug-associated myelosuppression. Monitoring for hepatotoxicity is also required, and nausea, headache, and fatigue are common.[73]

SULFASALAZINE

Sulfasalazine has been examined in a single double-blind, randomized, placebo-controlled study for moderate to severe psoriasis, during which 8 out of 25 subjects dropped out due to adverse effects, yet 7 out the remaining 17 subjects had 60% to 89% improvement.[74] More recently, a small comparative study demonstrated that 3 of 8 subjects on sulfasalazine alone had a 50% to 70% moderate PASI improvement, whereas 6 of 7 subjects in the methotrexate group had a very good response of 70% PASI improvement or better.[75] There were many dropouts, often due to side effects such as anorexia, headache, rash, and gastrointestinal symptoms. Sulfasalazine should be regularly monitored with a complete blood count and LFTs.

DISCUSSION

A summary of systemic, oral medications used in psoriasis is presented in Table 8, including useful parameters to help guide choice when selecting which agent to use. Practically, and assuming no contraindications, the following general principles may serve as a guide:

1. Methotrexate, begun at doses around 7.5 to 15 mg/wk and appropriate for long-term therapy at doses between 7.5 and 30 mg, has efficacy often revealed after 4 to 8 weeks of therapy. Full efficacy may require 3 to 6 months of therapy. Methotrexate also may serve as a bridge to biologic therapy while awaiting coverage decisions, or may be combined with biologic therapies indefinitely.
2. Cyclosporine, at 3 to 5 mg/kg/d, is a fast, short-term solution for severe incapacitating disease, flares, and erythrodermic psoriasis, but there must be a long-term exit strategy (biologic therapy, methotrexate, acitretin, ultraviolet phototherapy, or other).
3. Acitretin is a good choice in generalized, palmoplantar pustular or hyperkeratotic psoriasis but should be avoided in women of any childbearing potential. It is a viable long-term treatment in patients in whom immunosuppression is a concern, and may be combined with most any other modality.
4. Apremilast may be sufficient as a monotherapy in up to one-third of patients, with minimal laboratory testing and a good safety profile. It is a viable alternative to methotrexate or a biologic for some patients wary of side effects and self-injectable medications. Apremilast also treats psoriatic arthritis.
5. Mycophenolate mofetil is generally well tolerated but has poor efficacy as monotherapy. It is only suggested for use in patients who cannot tolerate first-line therapies or biologics,

Table 8
Summary of systemic, oral medications used in psoriasis

Agent	Dose Range	Expected % PASI 75	Onset of Effect	Monitoring	Common Side Effects	Comments
Methotrexate	7.5–25 mg/wk as a single dose	40	Few weeks to months	CMP, CBC, pregnancy	Nausea, fatigue, HA, LFT abnormalities	Folate 1–5 mg/d Folinic acid 15 mg/wk in 3 divided doses q 12 h, starting >6 h after methotrexate dose Avoid in alcohol abuse, hepatitis, pregnancy
Cyclosporine	3–5 mg/kg/d in 2 divided doses	60–70	Few weeks	CMP, CBC, magnesium, K, blood pressure	HA, HTN, increased creatinine, edema, nausea, hirsutism, gingival hyperplasia, tremor, infection parathesia	Fast-acting, good rescue medication Prolonged use associated with toxicity Safe in pregnancy
Acitretin	10–50 mg/d, increased as needed; maximum 75 mg/d; single dose with fatty meal	20–40	Few months	CMP, lipids, CBC, pregnancy	Xerosis (general + mucous membrane), alopecia, peeling, erythema, lipid abnormalities, LFT abnormalities	More effective for palmoplantar, pustular, or erythrodermic variants; more effective in combination with psoralen-UV-A or ultraviolet B phototherapy; used safely in combination with other oral agents, topicals, and biologics. Avoid in women of childbearing age, alcohol abuse, dyslipidemia Extremely long half-life
Apremilast	30 mg bid	30	Few weeks to months	Weight*	HA, nausea, diarrhea, URI	Pregnancy C, registry for exposure reporting *No sustained lab abnormalities identified in phase II/III studies

	Dosage		Onset of Action	Monitoring	Side Effects	Comments
Tofacitinib	5–10 mg bid	40–64	Several weeks	CBC, LFT, lipids	Infection, lymphopenia or neutropenia, LFT, lipid abnormalities herpes zoster	FDA approved for RA at 5 mg dose; safety concerns in RA at 10 mg Pregnancy C, registry for exposure reporting Avoid concomitant use with other immunosuppressive medications
Fumaric Acid Esters	Titrated up to maximum of 720 mg/d in 3 divided doses	40	Several weeks	CBC, LFT	Diarrhea, abdominal cramps, flushing, HA, eosinophilia, lymphopenia	Maximum dose requires tid administration Limited data Appears safe in pediatric population
Mycophenolate Mofetil	1–5 g/d in 2 divided doses	20	Few months	CMP, CBC, pregnancy	Nausea, diarrhea, CBC abnormalities, urinary symptoms	Significant number of partial responders and nonresponders Lack of long-term toxicity Pregnancy D
Hydroxyurea	500–1500 mg daily, as tolerated; alternately, 3–4.5 g/wk	40–50, yet poorly substantiated	Several months	CBC, pregnancy	gastrointestinal symptoms, rash, ulcers, alopecia	Poor quality data Pregnancy D
6-Thioguanine	120 mg twice per week, up to 160 mg thrice per week	50–80 yet poorly substantiated	Several months	CMP, CBC, pregnancy	Myelosuppression, liver toxicity	Poor quality data Pregnancy D
Sulfasalazine	1.5–4 g daily, as tolerated	<40	Several weeks	CBC, LFT, pregnancy	Anorexia, HA, nausea, vomiting, rash, oligospermia	Poor quality data Pregnancy B
Leflunomide	100 mg/d × 3 d loading dose, then 20 mg/d	17	Unclear	LFT, phosphate, CBC, pregnancy	Diarrhea, nausea, URI, HTN, HA, alopecia, rash	May benefit patients with significant PsA

Abbreviations: BP, blood pressure; CBC, complete blood count; CMP, comprehensive metabolic panel (electrolytes, renal, LFTs); HA, headache; HTN, hypertension; URI, upper respiratory tract infection.

Data from Nast A, Sporbeck B, Rosumeck S, et al. Which antipsoriatic drug has the fastest onset of action? Systematic review on the rapidity of the onset of action. J Invest Dermatol 2013;133(8):1963–70.

and may be an appropriate drug for use in combination with other modalities. Immunosuppression should be monitored.

6. Fumarates demonstrate efficacy on a par with methotrexate and may gain more worldwide approval in the coming decade. Three-times daily dosing may be a barrier to adherence.

7. More data on safety need to be reviewed for the higher (10 mg twice daily), more efficacious doses of tofacitinib. At the currently approved 5 mg twice-daily dose efficacy is relatively low, and cost remains high. Tofacitinib may gain acceptance as a small molecule, oral drug with significant efficacy, but laboratory evaluations and the close monitoring for infections will be required.

8. Leflunomide may offer some benefit as a secondary therapy in a limited number patients who also suffer from psoriatic arthritis.

9. Hydroxyurea, 6-thioguanine, and sulfasalazine remain last-line therapies, with lower efficacy and substandard safety profiles, compared with the other oral systemics.

SUMMARY

It has been 5 years since the last published guidelines from the AAD regarding the use of conventional systemic therapies in psoriasis.[1] During that time there has been great progress in drug development for the treatment of psoriasis, leading to 2 new classes of oral medications with significant clinical data, several new biologics, and a host of other compounds in very early clinical development that were excluded from this review. There have never been more options for treating moderate to severe psoriasis, and the quality of clinical data supporting conventional drugs, such as methotrexate, and newer drugs, such as apremilast and tofacitinib, continues to improve apace. How the newer medications fit into this increasingly complex therapeutic landscape will largely depend on their cost, availability, real-world efficacy, and long-term safety.

POTENTIAL CONFLICTS OF INTEREST

B.E. Strober. Speakers' Bureau: AbbVie (honoraria); Consultant: AbbVie, Amgen, Celgene, Dermira, Janssen, Leo, Eli Lilly, Maruho, Medac, Merck, Novartis, Pfizer, Stiefel/GlaxoSmithKline, UCB; Investigator: AbbVie, Amgen, Novartis, Lilly, Janssen, Merck, Xenoport; Grant Support to the University of Connecticut for Fellowship Program: AbbVie, Janssen; P. Foley. Consultant: Galderma, Leo/Peplin, Ascent, Clinuvel, Aspen, Janssen-Cilag, Eli Lilly, Australian Ultraviolet Services, Novartis, Wyeth/ Pfizer, Mayne Pharma, MedyTox, and Roche; Advisory boards/speakers' bureaus and/or as a clinical trial investigator: CSL, Galderma, 3M/iNova/Valeant, LEO/Peplin, Ascent, Clinuvel, GSK/Stiefel, Abbott/AbbVie, BiogenIdec, Janssen-Cilag, Merck Serono, Schering-Plough/MSD, Wyeth/Pfizer, Amgen, Novartis, Eli Lilly, Celgene, Roche, Aspen, Actelion, Sanofi Aventis, MedyTox, Shape, and BMS; Travel Grants: Galderma, LEO/Peplin, Biogen Idec, Merck Serono, Ascent, Abbott/Abbvie, Schering-Plough/MSD, Janssen Cilag, Wyeth/Pfizer, Novartis, and Roche.

REFERENCES

1. Menter A, Korman NJ, Elmets CA, et al. Guidelines of care for the management of psoriasis and psoriatic arthritis: section 4. Guidelines of care for the management and treatment of psoriasis with traditional systemic agents. J Am Acad Dermatol 2009; 61(3):451–85.

2. Mehta NN, Azfar RS, Shin DB, et al. Patients with severe psoriasis are at increased risk of cardiovascular mortality: cohort study using the general practice research database. Eur Heart J 2010;31(8):1000–6.

3. Miller IM, Ellervik C, Yazdanyar S, et al. Meta-analysis of psoriasis, cardiovascular disease, and associated risk factors. J Am Acad Dermatol 2013;69(6): 1014–24.

4. Hugh J, Van voorhees AS, Nijhawan RI, et al. From the Medical Board of the National Psoriasis Foundation: the risk of cardiovascular disease in individuals with psoriasis and the potential impact of current therapies. J Am Acad Dermatol 2014; 70(1):168–77.

5. Strober BE, Siu K, Menon K. Conventional systemic agents for psoriasis. A systematic review. J Rheumatol 2006;33(7):1442–6.

6. Smolen JS, Van der heijde D, Machold KP, et al. Proposal for a new nomenclature of disease-modifying antirheumatic drugs. Ann Rheum Dis 2014;73(1):3–5.

7. Chan ES, Cronstein BN. Molecular action of methotrexate in inflammatory diseases. Arthritis Res 2002;4(4):266–73.

8. Montesinos MC, Desai A, Delano D, et al. Adenosine A2A or A3 receptors are required for inhibition of inflammation by methotrexate and its analog MX-68. Arthritis Rheum 2003;48(1):240–7.

9. Dogra S, Krishna V, Kanwar AJ. Efficacy and safety of systemic methotrexate in two fixed doses of 10 mg or 25 mg orally once weekly in adult patients with severe plaque-type psoriasis: a prospective, randomized, double-blind, dose-ranging study. Clin Exp Dermatol 2012;37(7):729–34.

10. Chládek J, Martínková J, Simková M, et al. Pharmacokinetics of low doses of methotrexate in patients

with psoriasis over the early period of treatment. Eur J Clin Pharmacol 1998;53(6):437–44.

11. Pichlmeier U, Heuer K. Subcutaneous administration of methotrexate with a prefilled autoinjector pen results in a higher relative bioavailability compared with oral administration of methotrexate [abstract]. Arthritis Rheum 2013;65(Suppl 10):1355.

12. Schiff MH, Simon LS, Dave KJ, et al. Self-administered methotrexate using a medi-jet auto-injector improves bioavailability compared with oral methotrexate in adults with rheumatoid arthritis. Ann Rheum Dis 2013;72(Suppl 3):249.

13. Hamilton RA, Kremer JM. Why intramuscular methotrexate may be more efficacious than oral dosing in patients with rheumatoid arthritis. Br J Rheumatol 1997;36(1):86–90.

14. van Roon EN, van de Laar MA. Methotrexate bioavailability. Clin Exp Rheumatol 2010;28(5 Suppl 61):S27–32.

15. Braun J, Kästner P, Flaxenberg P, et al. Comparison of the clinical efficacy and safety of subcutaneous versus oral administration of methotrexate in patients with active rheumatoid arthritis: results of a six-month, multicenter, randomized, double-blind, controlled, phase IV trial. Arthritis Rheum 2008;58(1):73–81.

16. Islam MS, Haq SA, Islam MN, et al. Comparative efficacy of subcutaneous versus oral methotrexate in active rheumatoid arthritis. Mymensingh Med J 2013;22(3):483–8.

17. Hameed B, Jones H. Subcutaneous methotrexate is well tolerated and superior to oral methotrexate in the treatment of rheumatoid arthritis. Int J Rheum Dis 2010;13(4):e83–4.

18. Rutkowska-Sak L, Rell-Bakalarska M, Lisowska B. Oral vs. subcutaneous low-dose methotrexate treatment in reducing gastrointestinal side effects. Rheumatolgia 2009;47(4):207–11.

19. Whittle SL, Hughes RA. Folate supplementation and methotrexate treatment in rheumatoid arthritis: a review. Rheumatology (Oxford) 2004;43(3):267–71.

20. Morgan SL, Oster RA, Lee JY, et al. The effect of folic acid and folinic acid supplements on purine metabolism in methotrexate-treated rheumatoid arthritis. Arthritis Rheum 2004;50(10):3104–11.

21. Saurat JH, Stingl G, Dubertret L, et al. Efficacy and safety results from the randomized controlled comparative study of adalimumab vs. methotrexate vs. placebo in patients with psoriasis (CHAMPION). Br J Dermatol 2008;158(3):558–66.

22. Reich K, Langley RG, Papp KA, et al. A 52-week trial comparing briakinumab with methotrexate in patients with psoriasis. N Engl J Med 2011;365(17):1586–96.

23. Barker J, Hoffmann M, Wozel G, et al. Efficacy and safety of infliximab vs. methotrexate in patients with moderate-to-severe plaque psoriasis: results of an open-label, active-controlled, randomized trial (RESTORE1). Br J Dermatol 2011;165(5):1109–17.

24. Hébert HL, Ali FR, Bowes J, et al. Genetic susceptibility to psoriasis and psoriatic arthritis: implications for therapy. Br J Dermatol 2012;166(3):474–82.

25. Strober BE. Methotrexate-induced liver toxicity: replacing the liver biopsy. JAMA Dermatol 2014; 150(8):862–3. [Epub ahead of print].

26. Barker J, Horn EJ, Lebwohl M, et al. Assessment and management of methotrexate hepatotoxicity in psoriasis patients: report from a consensus conference to evaluate current practice and identify key questions toward optimizing methotrexate use in the clinic. J Eur Acad Dermatol Venereol 2011;25(7):758–64.

27. Van der voort EA, Koehler EM, Dowlatshahi EA, et al. Psoriasis is independently associated with nonalcoholic fatty liver disease in patients 55 years old or older: results from a population-based study. J Am Acad Dermatol 2014;70(3):517–24.

28. Rosenberg P, Urwitz H, Johannesson A, et al. Psoriasis patients with diabetes type 2 are at high risk of developing liver fibrosis during methotrexate treatment. J Hepatol 2007;46(6):1111–8.

29. Heydendael VM, Spuls PI, Opmeer BC, et al. Methotrexate versus cyclosporine in moderate-to-severe chronic plaque psoriasis. N Engl J Med 2003; 349(7):658–65.

30. Foley PA, Quirk C, Sullivan JR, et al. Combining etanercept with traditional agents in the treatment of psoriasis: a review of the clinical evidence. J Eur Acad Dermatol Venereol 2010;24(10):1135–43.

31. Salvarini C, Boiardi L, Macchioni P, et al. Multidisciplinary focus on cyclosporin A. J Rheumatol 2009; 36(Suppl 83):52–5.

32. Amor KT, Ryan C, Menter A. The use of cyclosporine in dermatology: part I. J Am Acad Dermatol 2010; 63(6):925–46.

33. Buchbinder R, Barber M, Heuzenroeder L, et al. Incidence of melanoma and other malignancies among rheumatoid arthritis patients treated with methotrexate. Arthritis Rheum 2008;59(6):794–9.

34. Griffiths CE, Dubertret L, Ellis CN, et al. Ciclosporin in psoriasis clinical practice: an International Consensus Statement. Br J Dermatol 2004; 150(Suppl 67):11–23.

35. Flytström I, Stenberg B, Svensson A, et al. Methotrexate vs. ciclosporin in psoriasis: effectiveness, quality of life and safety. A randomized controlled trial. Br J Dermatol 2008;158(1):116–21.

36. Ho SG, Yeung CK, Chan HH. Methotrexate versus traditional Chinese medicine in psoriasis: a randomized, placebo-controlled trial to determine efficacy, safety and quality of life. Clin Exp Dermatol 2010; 35(7):717–22.

37. Akhyani M, Chams-davatchi C, Hemami MR, et al. Efficacy and safety of mycophenolate mofetil vs. methotrexate for the treatment of chronic plaque psoriasis. J Eur Acad Dermatol Venereol 2010; 24(12):1447–51.

38. Radmanesh M, Rafiei B, Moosavi ZB, et al. Weekly vs. daily administration of oral methotrexate (MTX) for generalized plaque psoriasis: a randomized controlled clinical trial. Int J Dermatol 2011;50(10): 1291–3.

39. Baranauskaite A, Raffayová H, Kungurov NV, et al. Infliximab plus methotrexate is superior to methotrexate alone in the treatment of psoriatic arthritis in methotrexate-naive patients: the RESPOND study. Ann Rheum Dis 2012;71(4):541–8.

40. Ranjan N, Sharma NL, Shanker V, et al. Methotrexate versus hydroxycarbamide (hydroxyurea) as a weekly dose to treat moderate-to-severe chronic plaque psoriasis: a comparative study. J Dermatolog Treat 2007; 18(5):295–300.

41. Mahbub MS, Khondker L, Khan SI, et al. Comparative efficacy of hydroxyurea and methotrexate in treating psoriasis. Mymensingh Med J 2013;22(1): 116–30.

42. Fallah Arani S, Neumann H, Hop WC, et al. Fumarates vs. methotrexate in moderate to severe chronic plaque psoriasis: a multicentre prospective randomized controlled clinical trial. Br J Dermatol 2011; 164(4):855–61.

43. Ellis CN, Fradin MS, Messana JM, et al. Cyclosporine for plaque-type psoriasis. Results of a multidose, double-blind trial. N Engl J Med 1991;324(5): 277–84.

44. Reitamo S, Spuls P, Sassolas B, et al. Efficacy of sirolimus (rapamycin) administered concomitantly with a subtherapeutic dose of cyclosporin in the treatment of severe psoriasis: a randomized controlled trial. Br J Dermatol 2001;145(3):438–45.

45. Yoon HS, Youn JI. A comparison of two cyclosporine dosage regimens for the treatment of severe psoriasis. J Dermatolog Treat 2007;18(5):286–90.

46. Pedraz J, Daudén E, Delgado-jiménez Y, et al. Sequential study on the treatment of moderate-to-severe chronic plaque psoriasis with mycophenolate mofetil and cyclosporin. J Eur Acad Dermatol Venereol 2006;20(6):702–6.

47. Beissert S, Pauser S, Sticherling M, et al. A comparison of mycophenolate mofetil with ciclosporine for the treatment of chronic plaque-type psoriasis. Dermatology 2009;219(2):126–32.

48. Tauscher AE, Fleischer AB, Phelps KC, et al. Psoriasis and pregnancy. J Cutan Med Surg 2002;6(6):561–70.

49. Baroz B, Hackman R, Einarson T, et al. Pregnancy outcome after cyclosporine therapy during pregnancy: a meta-analysis. Transplantation 2001;71(8):1051–5.

50. Dogra S, Yadav S. Acitretin in psoriasis: an evolving scenario. Int J Dermatol 2014;53(5):525–38.

51. Gollnick H, Bauer R, Brindley C, et al. Acitretin versus etretinate in psoriasis. Clinical and pharmacokinetic results of a German multicenter study. J Am Acad Dermatol 1988;19(3):458–68.

52. Berbis P, Geiger JM, Vaisse C, et al. Benefit of progressively increasing doses during the initial treatment with acitretin in psoriasis. Dermatologica 1989;178(2):88–92.

53. Van de kerkhof PC, Cambazard F, Hutchinson PE, et al. The effect of addition of calcipotriol ointment (50 micrograms/g) to acitretin therapy in psoriasis. Br J Dermatol 1998;138(1):84–9.

54. Lassus A, Geiger JM. Acitretin and etretinate in the treatment of palmoplantar pustulosis: a double-blind comparative trial. Br J Dermatol 1988;119(6): 755–9.

55. Papp KA, Menter A, Strober B, et al. Efficacy and safety of tofacitinib, an oral Janus kinase inhibitor, in the treatment of psoriasis: a Phase 2b randomized placebo-controlled dose-ranging study. Br J Dermatol 2012;167(3):668–77.

56. A phase 3, multi site, randomized, double blind, placebo controlled study of the efficacy and safety comparing CP-690,550 and etanercept in subjects with moderate to severe chronic plaque psoriasis. ClinicalTrials.gov. Available at: http://clinicaltrials. gov/ct2/show/NCT01241591. Accessed May 10, 2014.

57. A study to evaluate the effects and safety of treatment, treatment withdrawal, followed by re-treatment with CP-690,550 in subjects with moderate to severe chronic plaque psoriasis. ClinicalTrials.gov. Available at: http://clinicaltrials.gov/ct2/show/NCT01186744. Accessed May 10, 2014.

58. Strober B, Buonanno M, Clark JD, et al. Effect of tofacitinib, a Janus kinase inhibitor, on haematological parameters during 12 weeks of psoriasis treatment. Br J Dermatol 2013;169(5):992–9.

59. Kavanaugh A, Mease PJ, Gomez-reino JJ, et al. Treatment of psoriatic arthritis in a phase 3 randomised, placebo-controlled trial with apremilast, an oral phosphodiesterase 4 inhibitor. Ann Rheum Dis 2014;73(6):1020–6.

60. Papp K, Cather JC, Rosoph L, et al. Efficacy of apremilast in the treatment of moderate to severe psoriasis: a randomised controlled trial. Lancet 2012;380(9843):738–46.

61. Gottlieb AB, Strober B, Krueger JG, et al. An open-label, single-arm pilot study in patients with severe plaque-type psoriasis treated with an oral anti-inflammatory agent, apremilast. Curr Med Res Opin 2008;24(5):1529–38.

62. Paul C, Cather J, Gooderham M, et al. Apremilast, an oral phosphodiesterase 4 inhibitor, in patients with moderate to severe psoriasis: 16-week results of a phase 3, randomized, controlled trial (ESTEEM 2). Poster presented at 72nd AAD Annual Meeting. Denver, CO. Available at: http://www.aad.org/Posters/Documents/AM2014/Poster/8412/8412. Accessed April 30, 2014.

63. Reich K, Papp K, Leonardi C, et al. Long-term safety and tolerability of apremilast, an oral phosphodiesterase 4 inhibitor, in patients with moderate to severe psoriasis: Results from a Phase III, Randomized, Controlled Trial (ESTEEM 1). Poster presented at 72nd AAD Annual Meeting. Denver, CO. Available at: http://www.aad.org/Posters/Documents/AM2014/Poster/8296/8296. Accessed April 30, 2014.

64. Otezla [Package Insert]. NJ: Celgene Corporation, Summit; 2014.

65. Fallah arani S, Waalboer Spuij R, Nijsten T, et al. Enteric-coated mycophenolate sodium in psoriasis vulgaris: an open pilot study. J Dermatolog Treat 2014;25(1):46–9.

66. Zhou Y, Rosenthal D, Dutz J, et al. Mycophenolate mofetil (CellCept) for psoriasis: a two-center, prospective, open-label clinical trial. J Cutan Med Surg 2003;7(3):193–7.

67. Kaltenborn A, Schrem H. Mycophenolate mofetil in liver transplantation: a review. Ann Transplant 2013;18:685–96.

68. Kaltwasser JP, Nash P, Gladman D, et al. Efficacy and safety of leflunomide in the treatment of psoriatic arthritis and psoriasis: a multinational, double-blind, randomized, placebo-controlled clinical trial. Arthritis Rheum 2004;50(6):1939–50.

69. Wain EM, Darling MI, Pleass RD, et al. Treatment of severe, recalcitrant, chronic plaque psoriasis with fumaric acid esters: a prospective study. Br J Dermatol 2010;162(2):427–34.

70. Heelan K, Markham T. Fumaric acid esters as a suitable first-line treatment for severe psoriasis: an Irish experience. Clin Exp Dermatol 2012;37(7):793–5.

71. Zackheim HS, Glogau RG, Fisher DA, et al. 6-Thioguanine treatment of psoriasis: experience in 81 patients. J Am Acad Dermatol 1994;30(3):452–8.

72. Zackheim HS, Maibach HI. Treatment of psoriasis with 6-thioguanine. Australas J Dermatol 1988; 29(3):163–7.

73. Silvis NG, Levine N. Pulse dosing of thioguanine in recalcitrant psoriasis. Arch Dermatol 1999;135(4):433–7.

74. Gupta AK, Ellis CN, Siegel MT, et al. Sulfasalazine improves psoriasis. A double-blind analysis. Arch Dermatol 1990;126(4):487–93.

75. El-Mofty M, El-Darouti M, Fawzy M, et al. Sulfasalazine and pentoxifylline in psoriasis: a possible safe alternative [serial online]. J Dermatolog Treat 2011;22(1):31–7. Available from: Academic Search Premier, Ipswich, MA. Accessed April 30, 2014.

Ten Years On
The Impact of Biologics on the Practice of Dermatology

Craig L. Leonardi, MD[a],*, Ricardo Romiti, MD[b],
Paul W. Tebbey, PhD[c]

KEYWORDS

- Psoriasis • Biologics • Monoclonal antibodies • Cytokines • Clinical trials • Efficacy • Safety
- Quality of life

KEY POINTS

- Evolving science has been translated into targeted and effective therapeutic tools that have enabled the dermatologist to control both the symptoms and underlying inflammation of psoriasis.
- The toolbox continues to expand with emerging knowledge on the pathophysiology of psoriasis, which will manifest in new therapeutic options that can better enhance patients' quality of life.
- The currently available biological therapies for psoriasis are etanercept, infliximab, adalimumab, and ustekinumab; each of these therapies displays differential properties based on their unique mechanisms of action, which target either tumor necrosis factor α or interleukin (IL)-12/23 cytokines, and each biologic has accumulated significant controlled clinical trial and long-term use data to support a positive benefit/risk profile in psoriasis.
- New, promising therapies are in development for psoriasis (brodalumab, ixekizumab, and secukinumab, which specifically target interleukin [IL]-17, and guselkumab and tildrakizumab, which specifically target IL-23); the IL-17 and IL-23 cytokines constitute part of the TH17 axis that is thought to be at the core of psoriasis pathogenesis.

THE POTENTIAL OF BIOLOGICAL THERAPIES FOR PSORIASIS

Psoriasis is a chronic, genetically defined, inflammatory condition that affects approximately 2% to 3% of the population worldwide. Men and women are affected equally, with the onset of disease usually before 40 years of age.[1] The disease manifests most notably with characteristic skin lesions, which are distinguished by red, scaly plaques most prevalent on the elbows, knees, and scalp, although any or all portions of the body surface may be affected. A proportion of patients with psoriasis (10%–30%) will also develop psoriatic arthritis (PsA).[1,2] In addition to its physical signs, psoriasis impacts health-related quality of life (HRQOL) to a degree that parallels other major

Conflict-of-interest Disclosures: C.L. Leonardi is a consultant for Abbott, Amgen, Centocor, and Pfizer. He has been an investigator for Abbott, Amgen, Celgene, Centocor, Genentech, Eli Lilly, Genzyme, Pfizer, Incyte, ScheringPlough, Novartis, Novo Nordisk, Vascular Biogenics and Wyeth. C.L. Leonardi is also a founding board member of IPC. R. Romiti is/has served as a consultant, investigator, or speaker for Abbott, Janssen-Cilag, Leo Pharma, Merck, Sharp and Dohme, and Wyeth-Pfizer. R. Romiti is an IPC councilor. P.W. Tebbey is/has served as a consultant or employee for the following: International Psoriasis Council, Abbvie, Baxter Healthcare, Incyte Corporation, Johnson and Johnson, and Wyeth.
[a] Saint Louis University School of Medicine, 1034 South Brentwood Boulevard, Suite 600, St Louis, MO 63117-1206, USA; [b] University of São Paulo, São Paulo, Brazil; [c] International Psoriasis Council, St Louis, MO, USA
* Corresponding author.
E-mail address: Craig.leonardi@centralderm.com

Dermatol Clin 33 (2015) 111–125
http://dx.doi.org/10.1016/j.det.2014.09.009

systemic diseases.[3] Moreover, psoriasis is associated with disease states that potentially increase morbidity and mortality and lower QOL.[4] Evidence continues to accumulate to support the association of psoriasis with established comorbidities that increase the risk of cardiovascular-related disease, including components of metabolic syndrome, such as hypertension, diabetes, dyslipidemia, and obesity.[5–8] Data to support increased mortality in the psoriatic population continues to be collected and reported.[9]

The advent of biological therapies in the past 10 years has been paralleled by advances toward elucidating the pathogenic mechanisms of psoriasis.[10,11] The selective targeting of cytokines (ie, tumor necrosis factor-α [TNF-α], interleukin [IL]-12 and IL-23) or cell surface receptors (ie, leukocyte function antigen [LFA]-1 and LFA-3) through monoclonal antibodies has delivered clinical validation that a dysregulated immune system is at the core of psoriasis disease pathogenesis.[11] Indeed, the monoclonal antibody-based biological therapies have delivered a variety of clinical tools with which the dermatologist can, for the most part, control both the symptoms of psoriasis as well as the underlying systemic inflammation and associated comorbidities.[12] Evidence, however, continues to accumulate to support that the full potential of these magic bullets has not been realized because patients continue to be considerably undertreated globally.[13–15] In a series of US surveys performed by the National Psoriasis Foundation from 2003 to 2011, the proportion of patients with moderate to severe psoriasis who remain untreated has plateaued at approximately 30%.[13] Moreover, more than 20% of patients with moderate to severe psoriasis continue to be treated with topical therapies alone and more than 50% of patients are dissatisfied with their treatment.[14] In Brazil, similar discrepancies exist between actual clinical practice and the recommendations included in the relevant guidelines, thus negatively influencing optimal patient care.[15] The reasons for these inconsistencies include low awareness of therapy availability; lack of understanding of therapy use or monitoring; concerns over adverse effects; lack of effectiveness; and the inability to secure appropriate national insurance coverage or payment for the recommended biological therapies. This finding begs the question as to whether the much-heralded new era for disease management from 2003 has actually been fulfilled.[16] Consequently, this review revisits the rationale for the development of biological therapies, inventories the available therapies of today in terms of the clinical trial and postmarketing data sets, and also evaluates the impact of these agents on dermatology practice as it relates to the management of patients with psoriasis.

PERSPECTIVES ON THE DEVELOPMENT OF BIOLOGICAL THERAPIES

Biopharmaceuticals are biopolymers of organic molecules that are manufactured in living systems, such as animal or plant cells. They are derived from a combination of understanding of the fundamental biology of disease and advances in the technological engineering of proteins that target specific elements of cell processes. The Nobel Prize winners Kohler and Milstein[17] first reported such technology in 1975. Their discovery permitted the mass production of monoclonal antibodies as a consequence of the fusion of antibody-producing spleen cells to immortal myeloma cell lines. The psoriasis biologics currently available are based primarily on this antibody platform technology in the development of therapeutic tools that are protein structures that bind to specific receptors or cytokines.[18] Biologic drugs exhibit great variability in design and structure, features that lead to divergence in function and therapeutic benefit. For example, etanercept is a receptor/antibody fusion protein; infliximab is a chimeric mouse/human monoclonal antibody; however, adalimumab and ustekinumab are both fully human monoclonal antibodies (Table 1).[19–22] Their function, as well as interaction with the human body, is based not only on the amino acid number and sequence but also on posttranslational modifications (eg, folding and glycosylation) that are added by virtue of their manufacture in living systems. The uniqueness of each biological agent manifests in differences in binding specificity, affinity, and tolerability, features that can impact the clinical outcome.[23] However, most biological candidates deliver therapeutic effectiveness because of their selective mechanisms of action, which is derived from a significant understanding of the role of specific cytokine or cellular targets involved in the pathogenesis of disease. Consequently, biological therapies delivered hope for a solution to chronic psoriasis management while circumventing the safety limitations of traditional agents, thus offering patients continuous relief.[24]

CURRENT BIOLOGICAL THERAPIES FOR PSORIASIS

Consistent with the uniqueness of each biological agent in terms of structure and function, the approved biological agents for psoriasis display

Table 1
Registration dates for biological therapies in psoriasis (FDA & EMA)

Nonproprietary Name	Proprietary Name	US FDA Regulatory Approval for Psoriasis[a]	EU EMA Regulatory Approval for Psoriasis[a]
Alefacept[b]	Amevive[b]	Jan 2003	Not registered
Efalizumab[b]	Raptiva[b]	Oct 2003	June 2004
Etanercept	Enbrel	May 2004	Sept 2004
Infliximab	Remicade	Sept 2006[c]	Oct 2005
Adalimumab	Humira	Jan 2008	Dec 2007
Ustekinumab	Stelara	Sept 2009	Jan 2009

Abbreviations: FDA, Food and Drug Administration; EMA, European Medicines Agency; EU, European Union.
 [a] Adults with moderate to severe chronic plaque psoriasis.
 [b] Withdrawn from the market (efalizumab in 2009, alefacept in 2011).
 [c] Adults with chronic, severe (ie, extensive and/or disabling) plaque psoriasis.

a wide clinical response in the pivotal trials that were conducted to support registration (**Table 2**).

T-Cell–Targeting Biological Therapies for Psoriasis

Although alefacept was the first biological therapy approved in the United States in January 2003 for the treatment of adult patients with moderate to severe chronic plaque psoriasis, it was later withdrawn from the market by the manufacturer in 2011 (see **Table 1**).[25] Alefacept is a recombinant dimeric fusion protein that consists of the extracellular CD2-binding portion of the human LFA-3 linked to the Fc (hinge, CH2 and CH3 domains) portion of human immunoglobulin G1 (IgG1). LFA-3 binds to the CD2 receptor located on memory-effector T lymphocytes, thus inhibiting these cells and thereby limiting the propagation of the inflammatory response.[26] Alefacept was dosed either intramuscularly (15 mg) or intravenously (IV, 7.5 mg) in a regimen of 12 weekly injections. Although the proportional response to

alefacept was fairly limited, a subset of patients (~20%) did achieve a high response with significant duration of 2.0 to 3.5 months and occasionally up to 1 year as defined by maintenance of psoriasis area and severity index (PASI)-75.[25,27] This responder cohort exhibited unique patterns of gene regulation in response to alefacept, characterized by the suppression of the genes for T-cell receptors as well as the CD2 and CD3 costimulatory molecules.[28] Thus, optimal response to alefacept (and indeed other biological therapies) may depend on the differential classification of responder patients based on pretreatment gene expression analysis.

Efalizumab is a recombinant humanized IgG1 monoclonal antibody that binds to human CD11a, a subunit of LFA-1, which is expressed on all leukocytes. Mechanistically, efalizumab inhibits the binding of LFA-1 to intercellular adhesion molecule-1, which inhibits T-cell activation, adhesion, and migration to sites of inflammation, including psoriatic skin. To support the registration of efalizumab in 2003 (see **Table 1**), 4 randomized

Table 2
Treatment response from pivotal trials in psoriasis

Nonproprietary Name	Proprietary Name	Dosage Form	Proportion Achieving PASI-75 at Primary End Point (%)
Etanercept	Enbrel	SQ, 25 mg	32, 32
Etanercept	Enbrel	SQ, 50 mg	46, 47
Infliximab	Remicade	IV, 3 mg/Kg	70
Infliximab	Remicade	IV, 5 mg/Kg	75, 80
Adalimumab	Humira	SQ, 40 mg	71, 78
Ustekinumab	Stelara	SQ, 45 mg	67, 67
Ustekinumab	Stelara	SQ, 90 mg	66, 76

Abbreviations: IV, intravenously; PASI, psoriasis area and severity index; SQ, subcutaneously.

controlled studies were performed in adults with chronic, stable, plaque psoriasis. Patients received doses of 1 mg/kg or 2 mg/kg or placebo administered once a week for 12 weeks. The proportion of patients who achieved a PASI-75 response ranged from 22% to 39% across the 4 clinical trials.[29] During the clinical program, the use of efalizumab was associated with various adverse events (AEs) that included serious infections, malignancy, immunosuppression, and, notably, thrombocytopenia, hemolytic anemia, as well as a characteristic worsening of psoriasis in some patients. With increasing temporal exposure to efalizumab, progressive multifocal leukoencephalopathy (PML) was observed in 3 patients who had exposure greater than 3 years. These events ultimately resulted in the voluntary withdrawal of efalizumab from the market in 2009.

Ustekinumab is the most recent biological therapy to join the armamentarium against psoriasis gaining registration in both the United States and the European Union in 2009 (see **Table 1**). Ustekinumab is a fully human monoclonal antibody that specifically binds to the p40 protein subunit, which is a component of the cytokines IL-12 and IL-23.[22] In so doing, ustekinumab inhibits human IL-12 and IL-23 from binding to its cognate receptor on natural killer (NK) and T cells, IL-12Rβ1/β2 for IL-12 and IL-12Rβ1/23R for IL-23. IL-12 and IL-23 are naturally occurring cytokines that are involved in inflammatory and immune responses, such as natural killer cell activation and CD4+ T-cell differentiation and activation. Overexpression of IL-12 and IL-23 has been documented in psoriasis lesions, and the levels of these cytokines may correlate with disease severity.[30,31] Two randomized controlled clinical trials that included more than 2000 subjects supported the registration of ustekinumab in psoriasis.[32,33] Subjects were randomized to placebo, 45 mg or 90 mg of ustekinumab and received subcutaneous doses at Weeks 0, 4, and 16. At the week 12 primary end point, the proportion of subjects who experienced an improvement in PASI-75 ranged from 66% to 76% (see **Table 2**).[22] Although subjects who weighed 100 kg or less responded similarly to either the 45- or 90-mg dose, those subjects who weighed greater than 100 kg experienced higher response rates with the 90-mg dose (68%–71% PASI-75) relative to the 45-mg dose (49%–54% PASI-75). Through the 52-week treatment regimen, 89% subjects who displayed a 75% improvement in their psoriasis retained the response with continued dosing.[22] The results demonstrate the validity of targeting IL-12/23 in psoriasis and also contribute additional insights as to the role of these cytokines in psoriasis pathophysiology. The most notable precautions related

to the use of ustekinumab were observed to include serious infections, malignancies, anaphylaxis, and reversible posterior leukoencephalopathy syndrome.[22] Emerging long-term data on the safety of ustekinumab are reviewed in subsequent paragraphs.

Tumor Necrosis Factor-α–Targeting Biological Therapies for Psoriasis

The TNF class of biologics (etanercept, infliximab, and adalimumab) appeared following the initial registration of both alefacept and efalizumab (see **Table 1**). Targeting TNF-α in psoriasis was based on the identification of elevated levels of the cytokine in psoriatic skin lesions and in the blood of patients with psoriasis.[34] Retrospectively, it can be asserted that anti–TNF-α therapies have shown remarkable efficacy in treating psoriatic skin lesions, enthesitis, dactylitis, as well as joint pain and, importantly, the capacity to inhibit radiographic progression of joint damage.[35] Etanercept, the first of the registered TNF biological agents, is a soluble form of the p75 TNF receptor, stabilized by the attachment of the human IgG1 Fc region, which competes with the natural cell-surface TNF receptor for the relevant ligand.[19] Etanercept mediates its function through the binding of either TNF-α or TNF-β (lymphotoxin alpha) thereby inactivating the targeted cytokines. This effect dampens systemic inflammation through altered neutrophil migration as well as dendritic cell and T-cell maturation.[35] Today, etanercept is typically provided to patients as a single-use prefilled syringe or as a single-use autoinjector for subcutaneous administration.[19] The US Food and Drug Administration (FDA)–approved initial dosage for etanercept in psoriasis of 50 mg twice weekly for 12 weeks is higher than that in the other FDA-approved indications for etanercept (25 mg twice weekly for 12 weeks). In contrast, the European Medicines Agency–approved dose of etanercept is consistent with the other indications at 25 mg twice weekly for 12 weeks.[35] Maintenance doses of 50 mg weekly are recommended similarly in the United States and the European Union. The pivotal trials evaluated etanercept in 2 well-controlled clinical trials that included more than 1200 patients. At the primary end points, the proportion of patients achieving a PASI-75 was 46% (study 1) and 47% (study 2) for patients receiving 50 mg twice weekly (see **Table 2**). For those patients who received 25 mg twice weekly, the proportion of PASI-75 responders was 32% in each study.[19] Responses with etanercept were evaluated through 24 weeks wherein improvement continued up to 59% PASI-75 responders for those patients on 50 mg twice weekly and 44% PASI-75 responders for those on 25 mg twice weekly.[36] However, loss of response was observed in patients who experienced a decrease in dose from 50 mg to 25 mg at week 12, with only 70 out of 91 (77%) maintaining a PASI-75 response at week 24.[19] The most serious precautions relevant to etanercept are typical of the TNF class as a whole and include infections (including tuberculosis), malignancies (including lymphoma), anaphylaxis, pancytopenia, aplastic anemia, demyelinating disease, and the development of lupuslike syndrome or autoimmune hepatitis. In addition, it has been reported that mostly mild injection site reactions can occur in approximately 37% of patients.[12,19]

Infliximab is a chimeric monoclonal antibody with specificity for both soluble and membrane-bound forms of TNF-α and, in that regard, has a more restricted specificity versus etancercept.[19,20] Infliximab potentially inhibits a variety of functions, including induction of proinflammatory cytokines (eg, IL-1, IL-6), enhancement of leukocyte migration and expression of adhesion molecules by endothelial cells and leukocytes, activation of neutrophil and eosinophil functional activity, induction of acute phase reactants, and tissue degrading enzymes produced by synoviocytes and/or chondrocytes. Because infliximab can bind to cell-associated TNF-α that has already bound to its cognate receptor, it also induces apoptosis resulting in cell lysis, which is thought to be one of the mechanisms of action of this therapy.[37] Infliximab was studied in 2 phase 3 trials that included 1213 patients with moderate to severe psoriasis. Patients were dosed by IV infusion with either 3 mg/kg or 5 mg/kg at weeks 0, 2, and 6, followed by a maintenance dosing regimen at every 8 weeks. At the week 10 primary end point, the proportion of patients who achieved a PASI-75 response was 70% for the 3-mg/kg dose versus 75% to 80% for the 5-mg/kg dose (see **Table 2**).[20,38,39] The infliximab trials also demonstrated a reduction in response over time, similar to the other biological therapies, with only 61% of those that demonstrated a PASI-75 improvement at week 10 being maintained at week 52.[38] Nevertheless, it is recognized that few dermatologists have infusion centers or use IV-administered infliximab relative to other biologics that are subcutaneously injected.[40] The most serious precautions related to infliximab therapy include serious infections (including tuberculosis), invasive fungal infections, malignancies (including lymphoma), hepatitis B virus reactivation, hypersensitivity, cytopenia, hepatotoxicity, heart failure, demyelinating disease, and lupuslike syndrome.[20] Because infliximab is IV administered,

infusion-related reactions are a concern for approximately 16% of patients, although these tend to be mostly mild, with less than 1% considered serious, and can be managed with appropriate medications and infusion rate adjustments.[12]

Adalimumab is a fully human monoclonal antibody with specificity for TNF-α, thus blocking the interaction of TNF-α with the cell-surface TNF receptors.[41] Like infliximab, adalimumab binds to both soluble and receptor-bound TNF, which can result in cell lysis in the presence of complement.[21] The safety and efficacy of adalimumab was evaluated in 2 randomized and controlled trials that included 1696 subjects with moderate to severe chronic plaque psoriasis.[41,42] Patients received subcutaneously injected adalimumab at an initial dose of 80 mg at week 0 followed by 40-mg doses every other week thereafter. The proportion of patients who achieved a PASI-75 from baseline to week 16, the primary end point of the trials, was 71% and 78% for studies 1 and 2, respectively (see **Table 2**). The proportion of subjects who maintained a PASI-75 response from week 33 through week 52 was 79% of those who reached PASI-75 at week 16. Like most fixed-dose drugs, a lesser response was observed in heavy patients (>125 kg). Interestingly, 43% of the week 16 PASI-75 responders maintained a PASI-75 response at week 52 even with placebo treatment from week 33 onward, possibly indicating an impact on the natural history of disease in a subset of patients.[41] The most serious precautions related to the use of adalimumab are similar to the other TNF-biologic class members, etanercept and infliximab. Consequently, they include serious infections, invasive fungal infections, malignancies, anaphylaxis or serious allergic reactions, hepatitis B virus reactivation, pancytopenia, heart failure, lupuslike syndrome, and demyelinating disease.[21] The most common adverse reactions related to the use of adalimumab are infections (eg, upper respiratory, sinusitis), injection site reactions, headache, and rash.[21]

A fourth potential member of the TNF class remains in development for psoriasis. Certolizumab pegol (CZP) is a pegylated anti-TNF agent that is composed of a TNF-α–targeting Fab' portion of an antibody that has been pegylated to preserve stability of the therapy.[43] CZP has been studied in a controlled phase 2 trial of 176 patients with moderate to severe psoriasis. Patients received either placebo or 400 mg CZP at week 0 followed by placebo or CZP (200 or 400 mg) every other week dosed subcutaneously through week 10. At the week 12 primary end point for the study, 75% and 83% of patients in the 200-mg and 400-mg groups, respectively, achieved PASI-75 versus only 7% of those who received placebo. Serious AEs (SAEs) occurred in 3%, 5%, and 2% of CZP 200-mg, CZP 400-mg, and placebo patients, respectively.

THE LONG-TERM EXPERIENCE WITH BIOLOGICAL THERAPIES FOR PSORIASIS

To determine if biological therapies are appropriate as maintenance treatments for psoriasis, studies over longer-term time horizons are required. To this end, many of the currently approved biological therapies have and continue to be evaluated in postapproval follow-up studies. As a consequence of regulatory approval, manufacturers of new biological agents are required to perform continuous studies of their therapies either in controlled trials or, more typically, in registries. Thus, data are beginning to emerge on the use and utility of biological therapies in the real-life clinical setting over multiple years.[44–46] One such example is the Psoriasis Longitudinal Assessment and Registry (PSOLAR), an 8-year international study sponsored by Janssen Scientific Affairs, LLC to prospectively enroll a targeted 12,000 patients who are receiving or who are candidates for systemic therapies. Although data on therapy use from PSOLAR are currently in press, the design and demographics of the patients enrolled have been reported.[40] Additionally, several national registries have been designed for ongoing evaluation and long-term follow-up related to the use of biological therapies. The British Association of Dermatologists has developed a Biologic Interventions Register, which collects primarily long-term safety data on biologics and conventional systemic therapies.[47] In addition, many studies of long-term use tend to focus on evaluating only the safety profiles of biological treatments for psoriasis. In one such recent study, a cohort of 173 patients with psoriasis (409 patient-years of follow-up) on biologics was prospectively followed for 5 years between February 2005 and April 2010.[48] In this cohort, only the safety of the biological therapies was evaluated and deemed favorable with a low incidence of therapy-related SAEs.

Long-term Safety Studies

Ustekinumab has now been evaluated for 5 years in 800 patients (517 of whom completed the study) demonstrating a stable clinical response and safety profile that are conducive to the chronic management of psoriasis. Patients were initially randomized to either placebo or ustekinumab (45 mg or 90 mg) at weeks 0 and 4 and every 12 weeks thereafter. However, partial responders were permitted to adjust their dosing interval to every 8 weeks. The clinical response was generally maintained through week 244 with a PASI-75 achieved in 63.4% and 72.0% patients receiving the 45-mg and 90-mg doses, respectively.[49] Concomitant with such clinical responses, improvements in HRQOL as measured by the Dermatology Life Quality Index (DLQI) were also consistently maintained through the 5-year trial evaluation period. Moreover, immunogenicity rates remained low through year 5, with antibodies to ustekinumab detected in only 5.2% of patients. The extended trial was calculated to span 3104 patient-years of follow-up, with rates of overall AEs, SAEs, serious infections, malignancies, and major adverse cardiovascular events that were generally consistent over time and comparable between doses. Notably, the cumulative rates of overall AEs, AEs leading to discontinuation, SAEs, infections, malignancies, and major adverse cardiac event (MACE) were generally comparable between patients receiving ustekinumab 45 and 90 mg, suggesting no dose effect. There were 32 serious infections reported in 30 patients, 14 reports of nonmelanoma skin cancers, and 15 reports of other malignancies. Also, there were 10 cases of MACE (8 in the 45-mg group and 2 in the 90-mg group) that occurred in patients with at least 3 established cardiovascular risk factors. Thus, through 5 years of continuous treatment, ustekinumab maintained a stable effectiveness and safety profile in patients with psoriasis that was consistent with the observations seen in the shorter-term pivotal trials used for product registration.[49] These results help dermatologists determine the likelihood of treatment success in patients with psoriasis who may be candidates for biological therapies, such as ustekinumab. Thus, the results confirm that ustekinumab is an effective and well-tolerated therapeutic regimen that is appropriate for long-term management of patients with moderate to severe psoriasis.

Collectively, the use of TNF biologics has been found to reduce the risk for myocardial infarction (MI) in patients with psoriasis.[50] Wu and colleagues[50] performed a retrospective cohort study spanning 6 years between 2004 and 2010 to investigate the impact of anti-TNF therapy on MI. The cohort included patients who had received diagnoses of psoriasis or PsA. The study population of Kaiser Permanente Southern California health system included a total of 8845 patients composed of 1673 patients who received a TNF-inhibitor for at least 2 months (TNF-inhibitor cohort), 2097 who were TNF-inhibitor naive and received other systemic agents or phototherapy (oral/phototherapy cohort), and 5075 who were not treated with TNF-inhibitors, other systemic therapies, or phototherapy (topical cohort). The collective cohort was observed for a median of 4.3 years translating into 42,424 patient-years of follow-up. The entire cohort experienced 221 episodes (2.5%) of incident MI, for an overall rate of 5.21 per 1000 patient-years. The incident rates of MI for the TNF-inhibitor, oral/phototherapy, and topical cohorts were 3.05, 3.85, and 6.73 per 1000 patient-years, respectively ($P<.001$). After adjusting for MI risk factors, the TNF-inhibitor cohort had a 50% lower hazard of MI compared with the topical cohort (adjusted hazard ratio, 0.50; 95% confidence interval). Future and more comprehensive research in this area is still needed to better define the potential of TNF therapy in reducing the risk of major adverse cardiovascular events in patients with systemic inflammatory conditions.

Etanercept has been studied in open-label extensions of controlled trials for up to 4 years.[51] In the 108 patients that completed the treatment regimen, the incidence of SAEs (infections, malignancies, or cardiovascular events) did not increase over time. The numbers of AEs per 100 patient-years of treatment were measured at 96.9 for infections and 0.9 for serious infections, the latter of which included bronchitis, cellulitis, fasciitis, diverticulitis, enteritis, and viral meningitis. The most common infections in the study were nasopharyngitis (26.1 events per 100 patient-years) and upper respiratory tract infections (14.9 events per 100 patient-years). There were no reports of opportunistic infections or tuberculosis reactivation. The rate for malignancies was found to be similar to that in the general population, and the rate did not increase with continued exposure to etanercept. Nineteen malignancies were reported through the study, with 6 nonmelanoma skin cancers and 5 nonskin malignancies being reported as serious. However, no cases of malignant melanoma or lymphoma were reported. Several cardiovascular events were reported in the study, but these did not correlate with etanercept dose of time on therapy. The adjusted event rates were 2.8 per 100 patient-years for cardiovascular events and 1.7 per 100 patient-years for serious cardiovascular events, the latter of which included 2 MIs and 1 congestive heart failure that were considered possibly related to etanercept use. Consequently, these studies support the long-term safety for the use of etanercept in patients with chronic plaque psoriasis.

Infliximab has been studied for more than 5 years in specific populations with psoriasis.[51] This controlled trial that included 54 Japanese patients observed the safety of infliximab for 78 weeks. SAEs were reported in 6 patients and consisted of infections (herpes zoster) and malignancies (adenoma). The most common AEs reported were nasopharyngitis (50%), back pain (16%), tinea pedis (12%), arthralgia (12%), headache (10%), and abnormal liver function tests in 10% of patients. This study supports the safety of infliximab in the psoriasis population over the long-term and demonstrates that infliximab is generally well tolerated for periods of up to 78 weeks.[52]

Beyond the 52-week pivotal trials in psoriasis, adalimumab has been studied in patients with psoriasis continuously treated for more than 3 years.[46] The study consists of an open-label extension to the REVEAL controlled clinical trial in which patients received doses of either 40 mg every other week for those that indicated a PASI-75 response or 40 mg weekly for those patients who failed to achieve PASI-50 relative to their enrollment baseline scores. The data indicated that the AE profile for adalimumab as a result of this 3-year open-label extension was consistent with that observed in the initial controlled portion of the REVEAL trial.[46] Indeed the rate of AEs declined through the study period with 245 events per 100 patient-years as compared with the 399 events per 100 patient-years observed in the original REVEAL trial. Similarly, the rate of patient discontinuation on therapy declined with increasing exposure to adalimumab. There were no reported cases of tuberculosis, lupuslike syndrome, or demyelinating disorders in the extension study. Additionally, the rates of infections, malignancies, and cardiovascular events were similar between the long-term extension study and the controlled REVEAL trial. The data, therefore, support the stable safety profile of long-term adalimumab use in patients with moderate to severe psoriasis.

THE IMPACT OF BIOLOGICAL THERAPIES ON THE QUALITY OF LIFE OF PATIENTS WITH PSORIASIS

Psoriasis is a lifelong disorder with a major impact on patients' QOL. Patients with psoriasis often report feelings of embarrassment, helplessness, and depression.[53] Although physical measures give a partial indication of the degree of psychosocial impairment experienced by patients, they are not adequate in accurately depicting the extent of morbidity in all cases. Optimal therapy can only be achieved by taking the patients' perception of illness into account. Even objectively mild disease needs to be aggressively treated if its impact on QOL is judged to be severe by patients.[54] Several instruments have been developed over the years for evaluating patients' QOL, including different generic, dermatology-specific, and psoriasis-specific self-administered psychometric instruments. DLQI is the most widely used QOL measure among these instruments in psoriasis-related clinical trials.[55]

In 1990, Finlay and colleagues[56] demonstrated that psoriasis was more detrimental to life quality than angina or hypertension. Rapp and colleagues[3] showed that patients with psoriasis reported reduction in physical functioning and mental functioning comparable to that seen in cancer, arthritis, hypertension, heart disease, diabetes, and depression. By means of a non–skin-validated instrument (Psychological General Well-Being Index) that permits comparison with other medical conditions, Bhutani and colleagues[57] further showed that patients with untreated psoriasis have as much impairment in psychological well-being as patients with other major medical diseases, including breast cancer, coronary artery disease, congestive heart failure, and diabetes.

Different studies have indicated that the most important factor related to QOL was extent of skin involvement with psoriasis.[58] Decrements in QOL-related to psoriasis were also associated with patients seeking care from multiple physicians for their psoriasis. This observation likely reflects that patients who are affected by psoriasis are often dissatisfied with their treatment.[59]

Immediate and substantial intervention is warranted so as to improve psychosocial morbidity and HRQOL. Different studies have reported higher levels of satisfaction when biologics are used compared with other treatment options, including both systemic and phototherapy treatments.[60,61] More recently, a cross-sectional study of 1182 patients with moderate to severe psoriasis in the Dermatology Clinical Effectiveness Research Network in the United States showed highest overall satisfaction scores for patients receiving biological monotherapies, biologic-methotrexate combinations, or phototherapy (83.3); scores were lowest for those receiving topical therapies only or acitretin (66.7). In adjusted models, compared with patients receiving methotrexate monotherapy, those receiving adalimumab, etanercept, ustekinumab, phototherapy, or adalimumab with methotrexate had significantly higher median overall satisfaction scores by 7.2 to 8.3 points, whereas those receiving topical therapies only had significantly lower overall satisfaction by 8.9 points.[62] The positive effect of TNF-α antagonist, etanercept, as well as of the anti–IL-12/23 antagonist on improvement of HRQOL has been evaluated in different studies and in a meta-analysis of clinical trials in psoriasis.[63]

A review of the clinical trials with infliximab on the correlation between skin clearance and changes of HRQOL in psoriasis demonstrated a clear correlation between the absence of skin symptoms and maximum improvement in HRQOL. For example, data from the phase III multicenter European and Canadian EXPRESS study evaluating the impact of long-term infliximab maintenance therapy for moderate to severe psoriasis demonstrated that at week 24, 70% of patients with a PASI of 0 also had a DLQI of 0, whereas only a small percentage of patients with a PASI greater than 5 achieved this goal. Furthermore, the loss of PASI-75 or PASI-90 responses in some patients between week 24 and week 50 was paralleled by a loss in the percentage of patients reporting a DLQI of 0.[38]

Analyses of the correlation between PASI responses and improvements in HRQOL in patients with psoriasis treated with adalimumab showed similar results.[64] These findings supported the concept that only if patients achieved high levels of PASI reduction (PASI-75), was this associated with achievement of DLQI scores of 0 or 1 (no effect on overall HRQOL). Concerning etanercept therapy, improvements in HRQOL have been shown to be similar to other studies using anti–TNF antagonists. Data analyses from 528 patients with rheumatoid arthritis (RA), 205 patients with PsA, and 583 patients with psoriasis treated with etanercept evidenced improvement in HRQOL across all indications. Although there were differences in the magnitude of change between the 3 diseases, the ability of patients with RA, PsA, and psoriasis to achieve HRQOL improvements were consistently similar.[65] Tyring and colleagues[66] further assessed the effect of etanercept on fatigue and symptoms of depression, both of which are common in the psoriasis population and are thought to be associated with increased levels of TNF. In a placebo-controlled study evaluating 618 patients with moderate to severe psoriasis, these investigators demonstrated significant and clinically meaningful improvements in fatigue and symptoms of depression in the etanercept-treated group of patients.

Effects of ustekinumab on symptoms, such as anxiety and depression, as well as on skin-related QOL in patients with psoriasis have also been thoroughly evaluated in different populations. A phase III trial evaluating 1230 American, Canadian, and European patients with moderate to severe psoriasis evidenced, at baseline, 40.3% and 26.7% of patients reported symptoms of anxiety and depression, respectively, and 54.6% reported DLQI scores greater than 10. Greater improvements at week 12 in mean Hospital Anxiety and

Depression Scale-Anxiety (13.9%), Hospital Anxiety and Depression Scale-Depression (29.3%), and DLQI (76.2%) scores were reported in ustekinumab groups compared with placebo (P<.001 each).[67] Studies with Korean/Taiwanese patients also evidenced that individual DLQI domains in the ustekinumab-treated group were significantly improved compared with placebo. For ustekinumab-randomized patients, HRQOL improvements were sustained through week 28. Placebo patients who crossed over to ustekinumab experienced similar improvements compared with those randomized to ustekinumab.[68]

Various biologic therapies have also been strictly associated with improvement in mental status in patients with PsA, particularly in those patients who also had improvements in their disease activity.[69] In a recent study, drug survival was used as a marker for treatment success. A prospective registry was used to collect data, which was analyzed using Kaplan-Meier estimates. Happy drug survival was calculated and split for happy (DLQI ≤5) versus unhappy (DLQI>5) at baseline and month 3, 6, 9, and 12. One-year drug survival for ustekinumab, adalimumab, and etanercept was 85%, 74%, and 68%, respectively. At baseline, the majority (n = 115, 73%) was considered unhappy and the minority happy (n = 42, 27%) (ratio happy/unhappy = 1:2.7). The percentage of happy on-drug patients increased to 79% after 1 year of biological therapy.[70]

THE FUTURE OF TARGETED THERAPIES FOR PSORIASIS

Despite the progress made to date in using targeted therapies for psoriasis, none of the currently available therapies can be considered completely effective and safe for all patients. In addition, because of the diversity of phenotypic expression of psoriasis and the wide spectrum of comorbidities, the quest remains for therapies that display longer-term efficacy, elimination of relapse after drug withdrawal, enhanced safety, and lower cost. The advances to date have illuminated knowledge on the pathogenesis of psoriasis to such a degree that now biological therapies are in development specifically to target the TH17 axis of inflammation, which is regarded as the master switch in the propagation of the psoriasis march.[71–73] The evidence supporting a central role for IL-17A as an important effector cytokine in the pathogenesis of psoriasis derives from its overexpression in psoriatic plaques and by virtue of its production by TH17 cells, likely in response to activation by IL-23, a proinflammatory cytokine

playing an essential role in the maintenance of psoriatic lesions.[74] Thus, the selective targeting of IL-17A represents a potential therapeutic strategy that could address a broad spectrum of patients' needs, which continue to persist despite the availability of our current multiple systemic and biological agents.

Secukinumab is a fully human, anti–IL-17A IgG1, monoclonal antibody, which is in development for moderate to severe plaque psoriasis and to date has completed a phase II controlled trial. Almost 150 patients were randomized to placebo or one of 4 subcutaneously administered secukinumab regimens: 1 × 25 mg, 3 × 25 mg, 3 × 75 mg or 3 × 150 mg at weeks 0, 4, and 8. After 12 weeks of treatment with secukinumab, PASI-75 response rates were 82% and 57% for the 150-mg and 75-mg doses, respectively. Similar to the currently approved biological therapies for psoriasis, the PASI-75 responses gradually declined during the follow-up period.[71] The PASI-90 response rate was significantly higher in the 150-mg dose group at 52% at week 12, and this remained higher during the follow-up period. In addition, a weight-based dose dependency was observed, as patients weighing less than 90 kg displayed better responses versus patients in the greater-than-90 kg group. The overall incidence of AEs was higher in the 150-mg group (89%), compared with the other secukinumab dose cohorts (73%–76%), which were similar in incidence to the placebo group. The most frequently reported AEs across all cohorts were worsening of psoriasis, nasopharyngitis, and upper respiratory tract infection. Overall, secukinumab was considered to be well tolerated; its monthly use in doses of either 3 × 75 mg or 3 × 150 mg was found to be statistically efficacious in moderate to severe psoriasis, as measured by the primary outcome of PASI-75 response at 12 weeks.

Secukinumab phase 3 data were released in 2013 at the twenty-second annual European Academy of Dermatology and Venereology congress held in Istanbul, Turkey.[75] At the week 12 primary end point for the controlled part of the FIXTURE phase 3 trial, 67.0% and 77.1% of patients achieved PASI-75 for the 150-mg and 300-mg doses, respectively, that were administered subcutaneously at weeks 0, 1, 2, 3, 4, and 8 (Table 3). The incidence of AEs was reported to be similar between the secukinumab and etanercept control group. Rare SAEs of special interest were noted, including candida infections (2.6% and 4.7% for the 150-mg and 300-mg dose groups, respectively). However, overall secukinumab demonstrated a positive benefit/risk profile consisting of rapid onset with high and sustained effectiveness

Table 3
Treatment response in PsO from drugs in development

Nonproprietary Name	Proprietary Name	FDA Status for Psoriasis	Proportion Achieving PASI-75 at Primary End Point (%)
Certolizumab-pegol	Cimzia	Phase 2	75–83[a]
Guselkumab	—	Phase 2	43.9–81.0[a]
Tildrakizumab	—	Phase 3	35–76.2[a]
Secukinumab[b]	—	Phase 3	67–77.1[c]
Ixekizumab	—	Phase 3	77–83[a]
Brodalumab	—	Phase 3	60.3–83.3[c]

Abbreviations: PsO, psoriasis; PASI, psoriasis area and severity index.
[a] Phase 2 results.
[b] Submitted for registration to FDA.
[c] Phase 3 results.

in patients with psoriasis, thus supporting the submission of the biologics license application (BLA) application to the US FDA for registration.

Brodalumab is a human, anti–IL-17 receptor antagonist monoclonal antibody that binds with high affinity to the human IL-17 receptor, thus blocking the action of IL-17A as well as IL-17E and F. Brodalumab has been evaluated in a phase 2 clinical trial that included 198 patients and is currently being assessed in larger phase 3 trials.[72] The phase 2 trial used subcutaneously administered doses of 70, 140, and 210 mg brodalumab injected at weeks 0, 1, 2, 4, 6, 8, and 10. In addition, a dose of 280 mg, administered at weeks 0, 4, and 8, was also included. At the week 12 primary end point, 33% (70 mg), 77% (140 mg), and 82% (210 mg) and 67% (280 mg with 3 doses) achieved PASI-75, respectively. This finding was statistically significant for all doses versus the placebo. Moreover, 18% (70 mg), 72% (140 mg), 75% (210 mg), and 57% (280 mg with 3 doses) of patients achieved PASI-90. This trial also reported PASI-100 rates of 10% (70 mg), 38% (140 mg), 62% (210 mg), and 29% (280 mg with 3 doses), respectively.[72] The results in patients who experienced the higher doses indicate a dose response effect relative to the 70-mg group. But the data also indicated a higher rate of AEs in the brodalumab groups, with 2 cases of grade 3 asymptomatic neutropenia noted. The most commonly reported AEs in the combined brodalumab groups were nasopharyngitis, upper respiratory tract infection, and injection-site erythema.

Recently, phase 3 results were released for brodalumab in patients with moderate to severe plaque psoriasis.[76] In the AMAGINE-1 study, patients were randomized to receive 210 mg of brodalumab, 140 mg of brodalumab, or placebo every 2 weeks by subcutaneous injection. The results at

the primary end point of 12 weeks demonstrated that 83.3% of patients in the 210-mg group and 60.3% of patients in the 140-mg group achieved PASI-75 responses (see **Table 3**), which were significantly elevated versus placebo (2.7%). Moreover, 70.3% of patients in the 210-mg group and 42.5% of patients in the 140-mg group achieved PASI-90 responses compared with placebo (0.9%). PASI-100 responses were observed in 41.9% of patients in the 210-mg group and 23.3% of patients in the 140-mg group relative to placebo (0.5%). The most common AEs occurring in the controlled portion of the trial for the brodalumab group (ie, more than 5% of participants) were nasopharyngitis, upper respiratory tract infection, and headache. SAEs occurred at a rate of 1.8% in the 210-mg group, 2.7% in the 140-mg group, and 1.4% in the placebo group.

Ixekizumab is a humanized anti–IL-17A monoclonal antibody that similarly has to date been evaluated in a 142-patient, phase 2 clinical trial for moderate to severe chronic plaque psoriasis.[73] The trial consisted of 4 dose groups of 10, 25, 75, and 150 mg compared with placebo and administered at weeks 0, 2, 4, 8, 12, and 16. At the primary end point of 12 weeks, the 25-, 75-, and 150-mg dose groups yielded a statistically significant proportion of patients who reached PASI-75 (see **Table 3**). There were no statistical differences for the 10-mg group. The percentage of patients with a PASI-90 was 71.4% (150 mg), 58.6% (75 mg), and 50.0% (25 mg). PASI-100 was achieved in the 150-mg group (39.3%) and the 75-mg group (37.9%). The results were reported to be observable as early as week 1 and were sustained through the 20-week trial. Additionally, significant improvements were also reported in nail and scalp psoriasis for the 75- and 150-mg dose groups. Joint pain was relieved to a statistical degree in those that received 150 mg ixekizumab. No SAEs or major cardiovascular events were observed. The most common AEs were nasopharyngitis, upper respiratory infection, injection site reaction, and headache.[73]

The TH17 axis also includes therapies that selectively target IL-23 because IL-23 is a major regulator of TH17 T cells. Guselkumab is an IL-23–specific monoclonal antibody (mAb) that has demonstrated clinical and molecular response in a small phase 1, first-in-human study in patients with moderate to severe psoriasis. Twenty-four patients received a single subcutaneous dose of 10, 30, 100, or 300 mg of guselkumab or placebo with the primary end point for the trial at week 12.[77] The results demonstrated that neutralization of IL-23 improved the clinical manifestations of psoriasis (see **Table 3**). At week 12, elevated PASI-75 responses were observed in those patients who receive 10 mg (50%), 30 and 100 mg (60%), and 300 mg (100%) of guselkumab, respectively, as compared with 0% of placebo-treated patients. It was noted that these improvements in PASI score were maintained through the week-24 course of the trial for those patients that received guselkumab. From a safety perspective, the proportion of patients experiencing an AE was comparable between the combined guselkumab (13 of 20 [65.0%]) and placebo (2 of 4 [50.0%]) groups through week 24.

Tildrakizumab is a humanized anti–IL-23–specific monoclonal antibody that has been studied in phase 2 clinical trials. Tildrakizumab specifically binds to the p19 subunit of IL-23 but does not bind to the p40 subunit that is a component of both the IL-23 and IL-12 cytokines.[78] In the controlled phase 2b trial that was performed in 355 adult patients with psoriasis, tildrakizumab was dosed at 5, 25, 100, or 200 mg by subcutaneous injection at weeks 0 and 4 and every 12 weeks thereafter through the yearlong study. The proportion of patients, who improved their psoriasis at the week 16 end point, as measured by PASI-75, was 35.0, 65.5, 67.1 and 76.2 in the dose groups of 5, 25, 100, and 200 mg, respectively. In contrast, only 4.9% of placebo patients achieved a PASI-75 improvement.[78] No dose-dependent increase in AEs was observed across treatment groups. However, 4 SAEs were reported in the 16-week placebo-controlled portion of the trial consisting of bacterial arthritis (reported as possibly related to the 25-mg dose tildrakizumab); death (unlikely related to the 100-mg dose); ovarian cyst (unlikely related to the 200-mg dose); and lymphedema (possibly related to the 200-mg dose of tildrakizumab).

Taken together, the outcomes of these clinical studies targeting the IL-23/TH17 axis have indicated that the inhibition of IL17A and IL-23 has significant potential as a new therapeutic strategy for psoriasis. Each of the IL-17 and IL-23 targeting agents have displayed high efficacy, a rapid onset of action, and relatively sustained effectiveness through the trials. Therefore, the results validate the pivotal role played by IL-17 and IL-23 and, inferentially, TH17 T cells in the pathogenesis of psoriasis. However, the confirmation of these patterns of benefit to risk in larger and more comprehensive phase III trials will be important to support the IL-17 and IL-23 classes of biologics as a realistic supplement to the psoriasis biological family of therapies.

THE PAST, PRESENT, AND FUTURE OF BIOLOGICAL THERAPIES FOR PSORIASIS

The new era of biologics in psoriasis was heralded in 2003 with the introduction of alefacept and efalizumab (see **Table 1**), and with it came an unprecedented period for drug development for patients with psoriasis. The parallel focus on cell biology and immunology has led to a comprehension of psoriasis pathogenesis that has and continues to manifest in the development of specific targeted therapies that provide a never-ending sequence of therapeutic options available to the dermatologist and their patients. As a consequence, dermatologists have evolved as basic and clinical scientists as well as clinicians. We have become more sophisticated in our approach to clinical trial development and in the interpretation of complex clinical data. In addition, we have come to better realize the true and significant impact that a life with psoriasis has on each and every patients' QOL both day to day and in the long-term with respect to an assortment of associated comorbidities. Without question, the highlight of this watershed period in dermatology has been that many of our patients have benefited from impressive, well-tolerated clinical responses that have been maintained for many years.

Retrospectively, the first generation of biological therapies for psoriasis (alefacept and efalizumab) was suboptimal, possibly because of their cell surface receptor costimulatory molecule targets but more likely because their clinical profile and administration challenges impeded broad and sustained use. Alefacept displayed limited efficacy in most patients achieved only through many weeks of persistent treatment before learning whether the drug was indeed consistently effective in any given patient. It was indeed unfortunate that the small percentage of patients who attained up to 1 year of remission were not studied further using pharmacogenomics, which would have allowed alefacept to remain available to a small group of targeted patients. Efalizumab, although an enhancement relative to alefacept, only produced a modest improvement by current standards in most patients. Again, like alefacept, a small subset of patients, particularly those with severe palmar plantar disease, cleared completely with efalizumab despite having failed all prior systemic and TNF-α agents. Unfortunately, a minority of patients with efalizumab experienced a series of treatment-related side effects consisting of flare/rebound on abrupt discontinuation; new onset of PsA; and ultimately, in 3 patients, the PML that resulted in its market withdrawal.

Despite these setbacks, the dermatology community persevered in the development of enhanced biological therapies, which resulted in the reward of the second biological generation that focused on the targeting of TNF-α and included the therapies etanercept, infliximab, and adalimumab. Although these biologics were already approved for the treatment of the arthritides and inflammatory bowel diseases, they nevertheless offered dermatology dramatically increased efficacy and a highly favorable benefit/risk reward. In addition, they expanded dermatology's scope of psoriasis to include the early detection and treatment of PsA. For many dermatologists, this was their first opportunity to learn about the spectrum of PsA as well as to institute rational steps toward treating the disease. But, as a consequence of their introduction into dermatology, it was apparent that differences in efficacy existed between the agents in their capacity to clear skin, with adalimumab and infliximab being considered high-performance skin-clearing therapies but also fostering new questions about the immunobiology of psoriasis.

The third generation of biologic drugs involved the serendipitous discovery of the importance of IL-12/23 blockade. Ustekinumab was the first drug to successfully exploit this pathway. Initially touted as an IL-12 antagonist, the meaningful therapeutic impact was subsequently revealed to be its targeting of IL-23 through the binding of the p40 subunit that was found to be shared by both of the IL-12 and IL-23 cytokines. This IL-12/23 class of biologics displays highly effective and long-lasting effects on psoriasis, which facilitated intermittent dosing at 3-month intervals during the maintenance phase of therapy. However, although ustekinumab has been recently approved for use in PsA, it does not seem to be as potent as the TNF-α antagonist class of therapies for this indication. Additionally, a meta-analysis review of ustekinumab's safety during early stages of clinical trials revealed a pattern of MACE potentially associated with the treatment class.[79]

The IL-12/23 class of biologics stimulated biological investigation, which led to the identification of the TH17 axis that today is considered to be central to the propagation of psoriasis. Consequently, there are now multiple agents in various stages of development that target the TH17 axis, including secukinumab and ixekizumab (IL-17A antagonists), brodalumab (IL-17 receptor targeting mAb), as well as tildrakizumab and guselkumab (IL-23–specific mAbs). As with the prior generations of biological entrants, this class of therapies is destined to once again expand the treatment armamentarium for dermatologists as well as deliver knowledge to better illuminate our understanding of this complex inflammatory condition.

REFERENCES

1. Griffiths CE, Christophers E, Barker JN, et al. A classification of psoriasis vulgaris according to phenotype. Br J Dermatol 2007;156:258–62.
2. Menter A, Griffiths CE. Current and future management of psoriasis. Lancet 2007;370:272–84.
3. Rapp SR, Feldman SR, Exum ML, et al. Psoriasis causes as much disability as other major medical diseases. J Am Acad Dermatol 1999;41:401–7.
4. Menter A, Griffiths CE, Tebbey PW, et al. Exploring the association between cardiovascular and other disease-related risk factors in the psoriasis population: the need for increased understanding across the medical community. J Eur Acad Dermatol Venereol 2010;24:1371–7.
5. Mehta NN, Yu Y, Pinnelas R, et al. Attributable risk estimate of severe psoriasis on major cardiovascular events. Am J Med 2011;124(8):775.e1–6.
6. Neimann AL, Shin DB, Wang X, et al. Prevalence of cardiovascular risk factors in patients with psoriasis. J Am Acad Dermatol 2006;55:829–35.
7. Sterry W, Strober BE, Menter A. Obesity in psoriasis: the metabolic, clinical and therapeutic implications. Report of an interdisciplinary conference and review. Br J Dermatol 2007;157:649–55.
8. Kaye JA, Li L, Jick SS. Incidence of risk factors for myocardial infarction and other vascular diseases in patients with psoriasis. Br J Dermatol 2008;159: 895–902.
9. Ogdie A, Haynes K, Troxel AB, et al. Risk of mortality in patients with psoriatic arthritis, rheumatoid arthritis and psoriasis: a longitudinal cohort study. Ann Rheum Dis 2014;73(1):149–53.
10. Griffiths CE, Barker JN. Pathogenesis and clinical features of psoriasis. Lancet 2007;370:263–71.
11. Nestle FO, Kaplan DH, Barker JN. Psoriasis. N Engl J Med 2009;361:496–509.
12. Menter A, Gottlieb A, Feldman SR, et al. Guidelines of care for the management of psoriasis and psoriatic arthritis: section 1. Overview of

psoriasis and guidelines of care for the treatment of psoriasis with biologics. J Am Acad Dermatol 2008;58:826–50.

13. Horn EJ, Fox KM, Patel V, et al. Are patients with psoriasis undertreated? Results of National Psoriasis Foundation survey. J Am Acad Dermatol 2007;57(6): 957–62.

14. Armstrong AW, Robertson AD, Wu J, et al. Undertreatment, treatment trends, and treatment dissatisfaction among patients with psoriasis and psoriatic arthritis in the United States: findings from the National Psoriasis Foundation surveys, 2003-2011. JAMA Dermatol 2013;149(10): 1180–5.

15. Silveira MS, do N, de Camargo IA, et al. Adherence to guidelines in the use of biological agents to treat psoriasis in Brazil. BMJ Open 2014;4: e004179.

16. Kanitakis J, Butnaru AC, Claudy A. Novel biological immunotherapies for psoriasis. Expert Opin Investig Drugs 2003;12(7):1111–21.

17. Kohler G, Milstein C. Continuous cultures of fused cells secreting antibody of predefined specificity. Nature 1975;256:495–7.

18. Strober BE, Armour K, Romiti R, et al. Biopharmaceuticals and biosimilars in psoriasis: what the dermatologist needs to know. J Am Acad Dermatol 2012;66(2):317–22.

19. Enbrel (etanercept) [package insert]. Thousand Oaks, CA: Immunex Corp; 2013.

20. Remicade (infliximab) [package insert]. Horsham, PA: Janssen Biotech, Inc; 2013.

21. Humira (adalimumab) [package insert]. North Chicago, IL: AbbVie Inc; 2013.

22. Stelara (ustekinumab) [package insert]. Horsham, PA: Janssen Biotech, Inc; 2012.

23. Furst DE, Wallis R, Broder M, et al. Tumor necrosis factor antagonists: different kinetics and/or mechanisms of action may explain differences in the risk for developing granulomatous infection. Semin Arthritis Rheum 2006;36:159–67.

24. Pariser DM. The age of biologics: we've never seen anything like this. Manag Care 2003;12(Suppl 5):1.

25. Amevive (alefacept) [package insert]. Deerfield, IL: Astellas Pharma US, Inc; 2011.

26. Ellis C, Krueger GG. Treatment of chronic plaque psoriasis by selective targeting of memory effector T lymphocytes. N Engl J Med 2001;345: 248–55.

27. Gordon KB, Langley RG. Remittive effects of intramuscular alefacept in psoriasis. J Drugs Dermatol 2003;2(6):624–8.

28. Haider AS, Lowes MA, Gardner H, et al. Novel insight into the agonistic mechanism of alefacept in vivo: differentially expressed genes may serve as biomarkers of response in psoriasis patients. J Immunol 2007;178(11):7442–9.

29. Raptiva (efalizumab) [package insert]. South San Francisco, CA: Genentech, Inc; 2009.

30. Yawalkar N, Karlen S, Hunger R, et al. Expression of interleukin-12 is increased in psoriatic skin. J Invest Dermatol 1998;111(6):1053–7.

31. Lowes MA, Kikuchi T, Fuentes-Duculan J, et al. Psoriasis vulgaris lesions contain discrete populations of Th1 and TH17 T cells. J Invest Dermatol 2008; 128(5):1207–11.

32. Leonardi CL, Kimball AB, Papp KA, et al. Efficacy and safety of ustekinumab, a human interleukin-12/23 monoclonal antibody, in patients with psoriasis: 76-week results from a randomised, double-blind, placebo-controlled trial (PHOENIX 1). Lancet 2008; 371:1665–74.

33. Papp KA, Langley RG, Lebwohl M, et al. Efficacy and safety of ustekinumab, a human interleukin-12/23 monoclonal antibody, in patients with psoriasis: 52-week results from a randomised, double-blind, placebo-controlled trial (PHOENIX 2). Lancet 2008; 371:1675–84.

34. Villanova F, Di Meglio P, Nestle FO. Biomarkers in psoriasis and psoriatic arthritis. Ann Rheum Dis 2013;72(Suppl 2):ii104–10.

35. Reich K, Burden AD, Eaton JN, et al. Efficacy of biologics in the treatment of moderate to severe psoriasis: a network meta-analysis of randomized controlled trials. Br J Dermatol 2012;166(1):179–88.

36. Leonardi CL, Powers JL, Matheson RT, et al, Etanercept Psoriasis Study Group. Etanercept as monotherapy in patients with psoriasis. N Engl J Med 2003;349(21):2014–22.

37. Malaviya R, Sun Y, Tan JK, et al. Induction of lesional and circulating leukocyte apoptosis by infliximab in a patient with moderate to severe psoriasis. J Drugs Dermatol 2006;5(9):890–3.

38. Reich K, Nestle FO, Papp K, et al. Infliximab induction and maintenance therapy for moderate-to-severe psoriasis: a phase III, multicentre, double-blind trial. Lancet 2005;366(9494):1367–74.

39. Menter A, Feldman SR, Weinstein GD, et al. A randomized comparison of continuous vs. intermittent infliximab maintenance regimens over 1 year in the treatment of moderate-to-severe plaque psoriasis. J Am Acad Dermatol 2007;56(1): 31.e1–15.

40. Kimball A, Leonardi C, Stahle M, et al. Demography, baseline disease characteristics, and treatment history of patients with psoriasis enrolled in a multicenter, prospective, disease-based registry (PSOLAR). Br J Dermatol 2014. http://dx.doi.org/10.1111/bjd.13013.

41. Gordon KB, Langley RG, Leonardi C, et al. Clinical response to adalimumab treatment in patients with moderate to severe psoriasis: double-blind, randomized controlled trial and open-label extension study. J Am Acad Dermatol 2006;55(4):598–606.

42. Menter A, Tyring SK, Gordon K, et al. Adalimumab therapy for moderate to severe psoriasis: a randomized, controlled phase III trial. J Am Acad Dermatol 2008;58(1):106–15.

43. Reich K, Ortonne JP, Gottlieb AB, et al. Successful treatment of moderate to severe plaque psoriasis with the PEGylated Fab' certolizumab pegol: results of a phase II randomized, placebo-controlled trial with a re-treatment extension. Br J Dermatol 2012; 167(1):180–90.

44. Romero-Mate A, Garcia-Donoso C, Cordoba-Guijarro S. Efficacy and safety of etanercept on psoriasis/psoriatic arthritis: an updated review. Am J Clin Dermatol 2007;8:143–55.

45. Papousatki M, Talamonti M, Giunta A, et al. The impact of methodological approaches for presenting long-term clinical data on estimates of efficacy in psoriasis illustrated by three-year treatment data on infliximab. Dermatology 2010; 221(Suppl 1):43–7.

46. Gordon K, Papp K, Poulin Y, et al. Long-term efficacy and safety of adalimumab in patients with moderate to severe psoriasis treated continuously over 3 years; results from an open-label extension study for patients from REVEAL. J Am Acad Dermatol 2011;66:241–51.

47. Burden AD, Warren RB, Kleyn CE, et al. The British Association of Dermatologists' Biologic Interventions Register (BADBIR) design, methodology, and objectives. Br J Dermatol 2012;166:545–54.

48. van Lümig PP, Driessen RJ, Berends MA, et al. Safety of treatment with biologics for psoriasis in daily practice: 5-year data. J Eur Acad Dermatol Venereol 2012;26(3):283–91.

49. Kimball AB, Papp KA, Wasfi Y, et al. Long-term efficacy of ustekinumab in patients with moderate to severe psoriasis treated for up to 5 years in the PHOENIX 1 study. J Eur Acad Dermatol Venereol 2013;27(12):1535–45.

50. Wu JJ, Poon KY, Channual JC, et al. Association between tumor necrosis factor inhibitor therapy and myocardial infarction risk in patients with psoriasis. Arch Dermatol 2012;148(11):1244–50.

51. Papp KA, Poulin Y, Bissonette R, et al. Assessment of the long-term safety and effectiveness of etanercept for the treatment of psoriasis in an adult population. J Am Acad Dermatol 2012;66:e33–45.

52. Torii H, Nakagawa H. Infliximab monotherapy in Japanese patients with moderate to severe plaque psoriasis and psoriatic arthritis. A randomized, double- blind, placebo controlled multicenter trial. J Dermatol Sci 2010;59:40–9.

53. Mease PJ, Menter MA. Quality-of-life issues in psoriasis and psoriatic arthritis: outcome and psoriatic arthritis: outcome measures and therapies from a dermatological perspective. J Am Acad Dermatol 2006;54(4):685–704.

54. Choi J, Koo JY. Quality of life issues in psoriasis. J Am Acad Dermatol 2003;49(Suppl 2):S57–61.

55. Basra MK, Hussain S. Application of the dermatology life quality index in clinical trials of biologics for psoriasis. Chin J Integr Med 2012;18(3):179–85.

56. Finlay AY, Khan GK, Luscombe DK, et al. Validation of sickness impact profile and psoriasis disability index in psoriasis. Br J Dermatol 1990;123:751–6.

57. Bhutani T, Patel T, Koo B, et al. A prospective, interventional assessment of psoriasis quality of life using a nonskin-specific validated instrument that allows comparison with other major medical conditions. J Am Acad Dermatol 2013;69:e79–88.

58. Zachariae R, Zachariae H, Blomqvist K, et al. Quality of life in 6497 Nordic patients with psoriasis. Br J Dermatol 2002;146:1006–16.

59. Stern RS, Nijsten T, Feldman SR, et al. Psoriasis is common, carries a substantial burden even when not extensive, and is associated with widespread treatment dissatisfaction. J Investig Dermatol Symp Proc 2004;9:136–9.

60. Mahler R, Jackson C, Ijacu H. The burden of psoriasis and barriers to satisfactory care: results from a Canadian patient survey. J Cutan Med Surg 2009; 13(6):283–93.

61. Panigalli S, Coccarielli D, Germi L, et al. Non-randomized pilot study on the evaluation of the quality of life and psychosocial stress before and after systemic therapy in patients affected by moderate to severe psoriasis. J Biol Regul Homeost Agents 2009;23(2):111–7.

62. Callis Duffin K, Yeung H, Takeshita J, et al. Patient satisfaction with treatments for moderate-to-severe plaque psoriasis in clinical practice. Br J Dermatol 2014;170(3):672–80.

63. Katugampola RP, Lewis VJ, Finlay AY. The Dermatology Life Quality Index: assessing the efficacy of biological therapies for psoriasis. Br J Dermatol 2007;156:945–50.

64. Revicki DA, Willian MK, Menter A, et al. Relationship between clinical response to therapy and health-related quality of life outcomes in patients with moderate to severe plaque psoriasis. Dermatology 2008; 216(3):260–70.

65. Strand V, Sharp V, Koenig AS, et al. Comparison of health-related quality of life in rheumatoid arthritis, psoriatic arthritis and psoriasis and effects of etanercept treatment. Ann Rheum Dis 2012;71(7): 1143–50.

66. Tyring S, Gottlieb A, Papp K, et al. Etanercept and clinical outcomes, fatigue, and depression in psoriasis: double-blind placebo-controlled randomized phase III trial. Lancet 2006;367:29–35.

67. Langley RG, Feldman SR, Han C, et al. Ustekinumab significantly improves symptoms of anxiety, depression, and skin-related quality of life in patients with moderate-to-severe psoriasis: results

from a randomized, double-blind, placebo-controlled phase III trial. J Am Acad Dermatol 2010;63(3):457–65.

68. Tsai TF, Song M, Shen YK, et al, PEARL Investigators. Ustekinumab improves health-related quality of life in Korean and Taiwanese patients with moderate to severe psoriasis: results from the PEARL trial. J Drugs Dermatol 2012;11(8):943–9.

69. Saad AA, Ashcroft DM, Watson KD, et al. Improvements in quality of life and functional status in patients with psoriatic arthritis receiving anti-tumor necrosis factor therapies. Arthritis Care Res 2010; 62(3):345–53.

70. van den Reek JM, Zweegers J, Kievit W, et al. 'Happy' drug survival of adalimumab, etanercept and ustekinumab in psoriasis in daily practice care - results from the BioCAPTURE network. Br J Dermatol 2014. [Epub ahead of print].

71. Papp KA, Langley RG, Sigurgeirsson B, et al. Efficacy and safety of secukinumab in the treatment of moderate to severe plaque psoriasis: a randomized, double-blind, placebo-controlled phase II dose-ranging study. Br J Dermatol 2013;168:412–21.

72. Papp KA, Leonardi C, Menter A, et al. Brodalumab, an anti-interleukin-17-receptor antibody for psoriasis. N Engl J Med 2012;366(13):1181–9.

73. Leonardi C, Matheson R, Zachariae C, et al. Anti-interleukin-17 monoclonal antibody ixekizumab in chronic plaque psoriasis. N Engl J Med 2012; 366(13):1190–9.

74. Harper EG, Guo C, Rizzo H, et al. TH17 cytokines stimulate CCL20 expression in keratinocytes in vitro and in vivo: implications for psoriasis pathogenesis. J Invest Dermatol 2009;129:2175–83.

75. Langley R, Reich K, Griffiths C, et al. Secukinumab compared with placebo and etanercept: a head-to-head comparison of two biologics in a phase 3 study of moderate-to-severe plaque psoriasis (FIXTURE) [poster]. Presented at the 22nd European Academy of Dermatology and Venereology Congress. Istanbul, Turkey, October 26, 2013.

76. Amgen and AstraZeneca (THOUSAND OAKS, Calif. and LONDON, UK.) Positive results from phase 3 study Of brodalumab (AMG 827) in patients with moderate-to-severe plaque psoriasis study evaluating novel investigational IL-17 receptor antibody meets all primary and secondary endpoints, 2014/ PRNewswire/Press Release.

77. Sofen H, Smith S, Matheson RT, et al. Guselkumab (an IL-23–specific mAb) demonstrates clinical and molecular response in patients with moderate-to-severe psoriasis. J Allergy Clin Immunol 2014;133:1032–40.

78. Leonardi CL, Gordon KB. New and emerging therapies in psoriasis. Semin Cutan Med Surg 2014; 33(2 Suppl 2):S37–41.

79. Ryan C, Leonardi CL, Krueger JG, et al. Association between biologic therapies for chronic plaque psoriasis and cardiovascular events: a meta-analysis of randomized controlled trials. JAMA 2011;306(8): 864–71.

Psoriatic Arthritis for the Dermatologist

Suzanne J. Tintle, MD, MPH*, Alice B. Gottlieb, MD, PhD

KEYWORDS

• Psoriatic arthritis • Synovitis • Dactylitis • Enthesitis • Joint • Osteoclastogenesis • Interleukin-17

KEY POINTS

• Psoriatic arthritis (PsA) is underdiagnosed and undertreated, and dermatologists are in a unique position to recognize symptoms of the disease early and initiate disease-modifying therapy before significant effects on patients' quality of life and functional capacity occur.
• All patients with psoriasis require screening for PsA.
• Characteristics of PsA include enthesitis, dactylitis, spondylitis and sacroiliitis, stiffness after inactivity, and involvement of the distal interphalangeal joints and nails.
• Joint damage begins early in the course of the disease, and a tumor necrosis factor α inhibitor is required to halt progression of synovitis, bone resorption, formation of osteophytes, enthesitis, and dactylitis.
• Apremilast and tofacitinib are promising new orally administered medications for PsA.
• The interleukin (IL)-17 inhibitors and IL-23p19 inhibitors have been developed in response to improved understanding of the immunopathogenesis of PsA and osteoclastogenesis; these targeted therapies have shown excellent efficacy in PsA in early investigational studies.

OVERVIEW: NATURE OF THE PROBLEM

Psoriatic arthritis (PsA) is an underdiagnosed, undertreated, chronic, progressive spondyloarthropathy occurring in 11% to 42% of patients with cutaneous psoriasis.[1–5] Similar to psoriasis, PsA affects men and women equally, and usually develops between the ages of 30 and 50 years, although it can develop in childhood.[2] Patients with PsA have significantly impaired physical functioning and quality of life (QOL), with high rates of anxiety, depression, and poor self-image.[5] The disease is characterized by flares and remissions; but only about 18% of patients will experience sustained periods of remission, lasting on average 2.5 years.[6] Many patients with PsA are undertreated or are not treated systematically.[1] For instance, in Lebwohl and colleagues'[1] 2014 multinational study, approximately 15% of patients with PsA had not seen a health care provider in the past year, and almost 60% were not being treated for their joint disease.

Our understanding of the immune dysregulation that triggers psoriatic pathophysiology has greatly improved over the past 20 years and has driven the development of targeted therapies for psoriasis and PsA. Innate and adaptive immune

Disclosures: S.J. Tintle has no relevant disclosures; A.B. Gottlieb currently serves as a consultant and on advisory boards for Amgen Inc; Astellas, Akros, Centocor (Janssen), Inc; Celgene Corp, Bristol Myers Squibb Co, Beiersdorf, Inc, Abbott Labs (Abbvie), TEVA, Actelion, UCB, Novo Nordisk, Novartis, Dermipsor Ltd, Incyte, Pfizer, Canfite, Lilly, Coronado, Vertex, Karyopharm, CSL Behring Biotherapies for Life, Glaxo Smith Kline, Xenoport, Catabasis, Sanofi Aventis, and DUSA. A.B. Gottlieb receives research/educational grants paid to Tufts Medical Center from Centocor (Janssen), Amgen, Abbott (Abbvie), Novartis, Celgene, Pfizer, Lilly, Coronado, Levia, and Merck.
Department of Dermatology, Tufts Medical Center, 800 Washington Street, Box #114, Boston, MA 02111, USA
* Corresponding author.
E-mail address: suzanne.tintle@gmail.com

Dermatol Clin 33 (2015) 127–148
http://dx.doi.org/10.1016/j.det.2014.09.010
0733-8635/15/$ – see front matter © 2015 Elsevier Inc. All rights reserved.

responses are abnormally activated in PsA, and, in genetically susceptible patients, may acquire the ability to attack peripheral joints and other sites following an environmental trigger or inciting event (eg, mechanical stress and trauma including microtrauma).[7] PsA is highly heritable: In a 2009 study, 7.6% of first-degree relatives of patients with PsA also had PsA (17.7% of first-degree relatives had psoriasis).[8] Genome-wide studies have identified important risk loci for the disease; the psoriasis susceptibility 1 locus (PSORS1) was among the first identified and mapped to the major histocompatibility complex class I region.[9,10] The presence of the HLA-Cw*0602 allele accounts for an estimated one-third to one-half of genetic susceptibility to psoriasis, whereas the human leukocyte antigen (HLA)-B27, HLA-B38, and HLA-B39 alleles are more highly associated with PsA (specifically, HLA-B27 is linked to spinal involvement, and HLA-B38 and HLA-B39 to peripheral polyarthritis).[9,11] A strong genetic association of PsA with variants of the interleukin (IL)-23 receptor (IL-23R) and the IL-23p40 subunit has also been demonstrated, implicating the central pathophysiologic function of the IL-23/IL-17 axis in triggering the joint inflammation and downstream effects seen in the disease.[12]

PsA is characterized by inflammation of the tendons, ligaments, synovia, and bone, with the development of focal bone erosions mediated by osteoclasts at the bone-pannus junction. Histopathologically, PsA displays an influx of Th17 cells, a thin layer of synovial epidermal hyperplasia, and increased levels of proinflammatory, osteoclastogenic cytokines.[13] This cytokine milieu includes elevated levels of tumor necrosis factor (TNF)-α, IL-1B, IL-17, IL-12, IL-23, interferon-γ (IFN-γ), and receptor activator of NF-kappa B ligand (RANKL), together acting as potent inducers of the proliferation and activation of synovial and epidermal fibroblasts.[14] Long-term inflammation at this site leads to bone erosions alongside new bone formation in the form of syndesmophytes, enthesophytes, and ankylosis (peripheral bony fusion). IL-23 is a crucial upstream mediator of this process. Comprising a specific p19 subunit and a p40 subunit which it shares with IL-12, IL-23 is a mucosal defense factor derived from resident lymphoid or epidermal cells in the skin that acts synergistically with IL-6 and transforming growth factor β1 to promote rapid Th17 development, potentiating IL-17 and IL-22 release.[15] Mouse models of spondyloarthropathy have shown that early features of bone remodeling (early enthesitis, arthritis, and bone formation) are ameliorated by the addition of anti–IL-23 antibodies.[16,17] Following induction by IL-23, IL-17

and IL-22 stimulate proliferation of synovial fibroblasts and subsequent joint inflammation,[9] and STAT-3 (signal transducer and activator of transcription 3) dependent osteoblast-mediated bone remodeling.[17] In addition to induction of enthesitis and synovial hyperplasia, IL-17 and IL-23 are associated with changes in the RANKL-RANK axis, which further increases osteoclast formation and promotes bone remodeling in PsA.[18,19] Further knowledge regarding how simultaneous bone formation and bone resorption in PsA occurs, and how the osteoclast-osteoblast homeostasis becomes dysregulated in the psoriatic joint, is required and will further guide therapeutic development. IL-33, which may abrogate the effects of TNF-α on the RANKL pathway, and drugs inhibiting IL-1 and Bruton tyrosine kinase, both of which are costimulatory signals for osteoclastogenesis, are additional targets being studied that may have potential in PsA treatment.[20]

Juvenile psoriatic arthritis (JPsA) has traditionally been considered a subset of juvenile idiopathic arthritis (JIA), representing about 7% of all JIA cases. JPsA epidemiologically, pathologically, and clinically manifests similarly to adult PsA. As in adults, cutaneous psoriasis may not be present and joint symptoms may significantly precede cutaneous disease.[21] Treatment options for JPsA are discussed within each medication section that follows.

PATIENT EVALUATION

Patients with PsA typically present with an inflammatory arthritis, have a personal or family history of psoriasis, and are seronegative for rheumatoid factor. The clinical spectrum of PsA includes 5 major components, although not all are necessary for diagnosis: peripheral arthritis; axial disease/spondylitis; skin disease; dactylitis; and enthesitis.[22] Approximately 50% to 60% of patients have peripheral arthritis only, 6% have spondylitis only, and 35% to 40% have both peripheral arthritis and spondylitis.[23] Pain and stiffness are usually worse with rest and improved with activity, and patients may complain of morning stiffness (often >30 minutes in duration).[4] Joint symptoms typically improve with activity but can present, regardless of activity level, as inflamed, warm, tender, and swollen, with limited range of motion.[24] Dystrophy of the fingernails and/or toenails (eg, onycholysis, pitting, oil spots, hyperkeratosis, leukonychia, and/or nail plate crumbling) is strikingly common in PsA: up to 87% of PsA patients will present with this component of disease.[4] Risk factors for the development of PsA include: scalp involvement, increased extent of body surface area psoriasis plaque involvement, increased duration of psoriasis, presence of nail disease, intergluteal/perianal involvement, and increased body mass index.[25–27] In patients with psoriasis, skin symptoms are present for an average of 12 years before joint symptoms.[28] Thus, dermatologists are in a unique position to recognize and diagnose PsA early in the course of disease and initiate disease-modifying therapy before musculoskeletal destruction progresses to irreversible damage. All patients with psoriasis should be screened for PsA.

Each of the peripheral and axial joints should be assessed for stiffness, tenderness, and swelling, with careful attention particularly to the hands and feet, which are frequently involved. Enthesitis, disease at the site of insertion of tendon, ligament, or joint capsule fibers into the bone, may be the sole manifestation of PsA and is seen most commonly at the insertion sites of the plantar fascia, the Achilles tendon, as "tennis elbow," and at attachment sites of ligaments to the ribs, spine, and pelvis.[2] Dactylitis, the combination of inflammation of the soft tissue, tendons, and/or ligaments and synovial lining of the joint, resulting in a "sausage digit" appearance of the affected digit, occurs in about one-fifth of patients with PsA.[29] The distal interphalangeal joints (DIPs) are commonly affected in PsA, involved in about 41% of patients, and are frequently accompanied by psoriasis nail changes.[29,30] The knee is the most commonly affected joint in PsA monoarthritis, and the spine is most often affected at the lumbosacral transition and the neck.[31] Involvement of sacroiliac joints (sacroiliitis) typically presents as asymmetric back pain and stiffness in the morning.[31]

The American College of Rheumatology (ACR) 68 tender joint and 66 swollen joint assessment, developed for rheumatoid arthritis (RA), may be used as a guideline in PsA, although it is mostly used for outcome studies. This evaluation includes the DIPs and the feet, and has shown minimal intraobserver and interobserver variation in PsA studies.[32] The temporomandibular, sternoclavicular, acromioclavicular, shoulder, elbow, wrist (including the carpometacarpal and intercarpal joints as one unit), metacarpophalangeal (MCP), proximal interphalangeal (PIP), DIP, hip, knee, talotibial, midtarsal (including subtalar), metatarsophalangeal, and interphalangeal joints of the toes are each evaluated.[32] As it may be difficult to distinguish between PIP and DIP joint inflammation of the toes, inflammation of the PIP or DIP of the toe is counted as one unit.[32] Consideration of cutaneous disease is as important in the evaluation and choice of medication in PsA patients. A full body skin examination to evaluate the severity of current psoriasis, optimally with determination of body surface area of involvement with use of the Psoriasis Area and Severity Index (PASI), should be performed in all patients.

Radiographic evaluation to examine osteitis, bone erosions, and new bone formation is typically performed by rheumatologists to aid in the differential diagnosis of PsA, although results affect the dermatologist's choice of therapy, as only the TNF-α inhibitors and ustekinumab have been found to delay radiographic disease progression.[33] Additional radiographic findings in PsA are joint erosion, joint narrowing, new bone growth (including spur formation, spondylitis, "flail" or ankylotic deformities of the digits, and syndesmophytes), and/or profound phalangeal osteolysis ("pencil-in-cup" deformity). Ultrasonographic examination may also be performed by rheumatologists to further evaluate enthesitis, which can be difficult to assess on both clinical examination and conventional radiography.[34]

Diagnosis of PsA should be based on the modified CASPAR (ClASsification criteria for Psoriatic Arthritis) criteria (Table 1), in which a patient with musculoskeletal symptoms (arthritis, enthesitis, and/or spondylitis) meets at least 3 points from the criteria shown in Table 1. The CASPAR criteria have a high specificity and sensitivity for diagnosing PsA.[35]

Patients should be advised of certain environmental factors that have been implicated in the pathogenesis of both psoriasis and PsA, and

Table 1
Classification criteria for psoriatic arthritis (CASPAR)

Criterion	Point Value
Current psoriasis	2
Personal history of psoriasis (unless current psoriasis is present)	1
Family history of psoriasis (unless current psoriasis is present or there is a personal history of psoriasis)	1
Dactylitis (current or personal history)	1
Juxta-articular new bone formation	1
Rheumatoid factor negativity	1
Nail dystrophy (onycholysis, pitting, and/or hyperkeratosis)	1

A total score of at least 3 points must be established.
Adapted from Taylor W, Gladman D, Helliwell P, et al. Classification criteria for psoriatic arthritis: development of new criteria from a large international study. Arthritis Rheumatism 2006;54(8):2665–73; with permission.

may lead to flare of the latter. Mainly physical trauma/injury and emotional stress have been shown to drive inflammatory pathways in both psoriasis and PsA.[36–39] Both increased body mass index and smoking are risk factors for PsA and are associated with increased severity of PsA; thus, increases in body weight in addition to increased or new smoking may be expected to flare disease.[40,41]

Following clinical evaluation of the joints and skin, patient QOL and loss of function attributable to PsA should be assessed. Patients with hand and/or foot involvement can have severely impaired ability to perform activities of daily living. All patients should be educated as to the nature of their condition and to the effect of stress on their disease. Rates of depression and anxiety are high (prevalence rates range from 19.2% to 62%) in patients with all types and severities of psoriatic disease.[42,43] Furthermore, patients with PsA have been found to have a worse QOL than patients with psoriasis alone, and the presence of joint pain is associated with higher rates of depression.[43,44] In a 2014 study of 306 patients with PsA, the prevalence of depression and anxiety were approximately 22.2% and 36.6%, respectively.[42] There are variable results on the association of PsA treatment with a decrease in prevalence of anxiety and/or depression in PsA patients.[45,46] Depression and anxiety symptoms may be less likely to improve with psoriatic disease treatment in patients with PsA compared with patients with psoriasis alone, which highlights the value of identifying PsA patients with symptoms of psychiatric illness and applying a multidisciplinary approach.

All patients should be evaluated for the presence of comorbidities associated with psoriasis and PsA (diabetes, obesity, metabolic syndrome, nonalcoholic fatty liver disease [NAFLD], coronary artery disease, cerebral artery disease, depression) that may affect overall health and selection of treatment. In evaluating the patient's medical history, particular attention should also be given to the presence of liver disease including a history of hepatitis B or hepatitis C, impaired renal function, congestive heart disease, a personal or family history of demyelinating disease, anemia and other cytopenias, personal history of malignancy, history of tuberculosis and other chronic, serious infections. In patients with liver enzyme levels greater than 3 times the upper limit of normal, an ultrasonogram of the liver should be performed to evaluate for NAFLD and other causes of liver disease, which may preclude the patient from receiving certain medications. Laboratory evaluation of erythrocyte sedimentation rate and

C-reactive protein (CRP), which are elevated in about 50% of PsA patients, may be used for prognostic reasoning and to monitor disease activity, but are nonspecific for PsA and generally do not contribute to choice of medical therapy nor to determination of disease severity.[24,47]

MANAGEMENT GOALS

Improving joint pain and soreness, mobility, patient QOL, and emotional health are major goals for PsA patients, ideally through management by both a dermatologist and rheumatologist. Treatment of cutaneous disease alone is insufficient and has little effect on joint symptoms of PsA.[30] Treatment algorithms for PsA have been suggested by the European League Against Rheumatism (EULAR) (most recently, in 2013)[48] and by the Group for Research and Assessment of Psoriasis and Psoriatic Arthritis (GRAPPA), most recently in 2009.[49] The authors recommend that patients with severe disease, examples of whom are given in **Box 1**, receive treatment with a biological agent as first-line therapy. Although PsA should not be defined by the number of joints involved alone but in combination with patient QOL and functional status, in general, patients with 2 or more swollen joints and 2 or more tender/painful joints, or with sacroiliitis or spondylitis in 1 or more joint have at least moderate PsA and may be candidates for a TNF-α inhibitor, ustekinumab, apremilast, or combination therapy.[28]

Axial involvement of PsA presents a unique treatment challenge. Data on adequacy of available medications has been adapted from ankylosing spondylitis (AS) studies, and have not been adequately studied in PsA.[50] However, each of the available TNF-α inhibitors has shown significant improvements in axial spondyloarthropathy in AS; response rates were similar,

---

Box 1
PsA patient groups requiring initiation of a biological agent

Presence of 3 or more swollen and tender joints causing functional disability

Axial joint involvement

Moderate-to-severe cutaneous psoriasis (high Psoriasis and Area Severity Index [PASI] score and joint disease with a severely affected quality of life)

Presence of enthesitis or dactylitis unresponsive to nonsteroidal anti-inflammatories, intra-articular corticosteroids, and/or disease-modifying antirheumatics

averaging at about 60%.[51–55] Ustekinumab also has promise for effectiveness in treating axial disease: A 2014 open-label trial on the use of ustekinumab in 24 patients with AS found an improvement in BASDAI (Bath Ankylosing Spondylitis Disease Activity Index) of at least 50% in 55% of patients.[56,57]

In addition to improving patient QOL, mobility, and functional capability, dermatologists need to encourage patient medication compliance, even in the absence of symptoms, to prevent disease flares.

PHARMACOLOGIC TREATMENT OPTIONS

PsA therapy has historically relied on the nonsteroidal anti-inflammatory drugs (NSAIDs) and disease-modifying antirheumatic drugs (DMARDs), but these agents are not ideal because of long-term potential toxicity.[58] The TNF-α inhibitors and ustekinumab are the mainstay for moderate-to-severe PsA in preventing disease progression and slowing joint damage.[59,60] However, given practical and financial restraints, patients are often placed on methotrexate (MTX) or another DMARD before initiation of a biologic.[51,53–55,61]

Mild PsA (simple enthesopathy alone, or involvement of one joint that does not affect QOL or functioning) may be treated with NSAIDs, which reduce inflammation through nonselective inhibition of cyclo-oxygenase enzymes COX1 and COX2, thereby preventing formation of proinflammatory prostaglandins and leukotrienes, and/or with intra-articular glucocorticoid injections. Enteric-coated aspirin, naproxen, ibuprofen, diclofenac, or ketoprofen are used for peripheral arthropathy, and indomethacin or tolmetin are often chosen for axial disease.[49] NSAIDs are associated with a high rate of adverse events: Endoscopic studies indicate that gastric or duodenal ulcers develop in 15% to 30% of patients who regularly take NSAIDs,[62] and the medications attenuate the efficacy of certain antihypertensive agents.[63] Rarely, NSAIDs may lead to flaring or exacerbation of psoriasis.[49]

Rheumatologists often perform intra-articular injections of glucocorticoids for PsA that is either mild or limited to only 1 or 2 joints. Repetitive intra-articular glucocorticoid injection is safe and has good efficacy in the short term: McCarty[64] reported that 88% of patients receiving intra-articular glucocorticoid injection in the small joints of the hands and/or wrists achieved relative remission with symptomatic control lasting an average of 22 months. Doses of glucocorticoid used in PsA are based on the standards for RA. Repetitive glucocorticoid injections may be

particularly valuable as a nonsystemic treatment of pauciarticular-onset JIA.[65] Systemic corticosteroids are seldom used by dermatologists for the treatment of PsA, given the risk of potentially severe cutaneous disease flare, particularly pustular psoriasis. In patients with little or no psoriasis, some rheumatologists use low-dose prednisone (5–10 mg) for long-term treatment of mild PsA.

Disease-Modifying Antirheumatic Drugs

MTX is the most commonly used oral drug for PsA in clinical practice. It competitively inhibits the enzyme dihydrofolate reductase, necessary for synthesis of nucleic acids; significant lymphoid tissue proliferation also occurs with MTX treatment. Of note, MTX is more efficacious in joint disease than in skin disease, and may be one of the better options for a patient with PsA without cutaneous psoriasis or with severe PsA and only mild skin symptoms.[66] Two randomized, placebo-controlled studies of MTX (15 mg/wk) in PsA found significant improvements in global assessment ratings with treatment, although tender and swollen joint counts and composite measures of PsA (PsARC, ACR20, and DAS28) did not improve in either study at 3 or 6 months.[67,68] MTX has demonstrated good retention rates (approximately 65% at 2 years).[69]

Oral MTX has an advantage in that it is only given once a week, at doses ranging from 7.5 to 25 mg weekly as a single dose or divided into 3 doses within a 24-hour period. Recommendations for testing before initiating treatment are the same as that in psoriasis or other diseases: Before MTX initiation, a complete blood count with differential, chemistry panel, hepatitis panel, tuberculosis testing, and a pregnancy test should be performed.[70] A low-level test dose may be given to evaluate for bone marrow suppression in susceptible patients.[70]

Once an adequate dose is reached, patient response can take 4 to 6 weeks.[71] Folic acid, which can prevent elevations in liver enzymes, is usually prescribed once weekly to 6 days a week (there are no randomized controlled trials to determine the optimal dose).[72] Slow tapering of MTX in patients who do not respond after 6 to 8 weeks of therapy is recommended to prevent potentially severe flares of both skin and joint disease.[2]

Common toxicities of MTX are nausea, anorexia, stomatitis, and fatigue (typically at the time of administration), effects that can be minimized by splitting the dose throughout the day of administration and administering the drug with food.[2] The most serious potential side effects of

MTX include liver toxicity, interstitial lung disease, and bone marrow suppression.[2] Complete blood counts and chemistry panels with liver function enzymes and albumin should be monitored once every 2 to 4 weeks during the first few months of treatment (and when treatment doses are increased), then once every 1 to 3 months. Monitoring guidelines for hepatotoxicity are given in **Box 2**. In psoriasis patients, the risk of hepatic fibrosis has been most common in patients with additional risk factors for liver disease (obesity, diabetes, and alcohol use).[73]

MTX is Food and Drug Administration (FDA) pregnancy category X and is contraindicated in women trying to conceive. Its use in pediatric PsA patients has primarily been evaluated in JIA, and low-dose weekly MTX has been highly effective, safe, and well tolerated in this pediatric population; primary side effects are similar to those seen in adults, and adult liver biopsy guidelines may be followed.[74] According to the ACR 2011 recommendations, a course of MTX is recommended for children with high disease activity and features of poor prognosis, or if they have failed intra-articular glucocorticoid injections.[74]

Leflunomide, an inhibitor of de novo pyrimidine synthesis, is approved for use in RA, and is less frequently used and not FDA-approved in the treatment of psoriasis and PsA. However, leflunomide has shown efficacy equivalent to that of MTX in randomized, double-blind, placebo-controlled studies in PsA: In a 2013 multicenter European study of 514 patients treated with leflunomide for PsA, PsARC response was achieved by 86% of the patients at week 24, and significant improvement was seen in tender and swollen joint counts, dactylitis, nail lesions, skin lesions, and patient self-assessment.[75] Other studies have found significantly lower response rates: A 2004 randomized controlled study of patients with PsA in the United States found that 59% of patients were receiving leflunomide according to the PsARC.[76] Diarrhea and increased serum aminotransferase levels are adverse effects of the drug that are well described in RA trials.[75] Leflunomide can be considered for patients who fail MTX treatment or in whom an oral medication is required. It is given in a loading dose of 100 mg/d for 3 days followed by 20 mg/d thereafter, and is associated with gastrointestinal upset, weight loss, headache, dizziness, elevated liver enzymes, leukopenia, and an increased risk of infections. The drug is teratogenic and its use has not been studied in the pediatric PsA population, although it is effective in pediatric RA.

Similar to leflunomide, sulfasalazine is not FDA-approved for the treatment of either psoriasis or PsA, but several double-blind, placebo-controlled studies of the drug in both psoriasis and PsA have shown that it is moderately effective (dosages escalated over time as tolerated from 1.5 to 4.0 g daily).[77] It is thought to exert

---

Box 2
Monitoring for hepatotoxicity in patients receiving methotrexate

Patients at low risk for liver disease

Monitor LFTs monthly for the first 6 months of treatment, then once every 1 to 3 months thereafter

- Elevations of LFTs less than twice the upper limit of normal: repeat testing in 2 to 4 weeks
- Elevations greater than twice the upper limit of normal, repeat testing in 2 to 4 weeks and decrease the dose of methotrexate

First biopsy at 3.5 to 4 g total cumulative dose; subsequent biopsies to be considered at additional 1.5 g of drug

- Biopsy for a persistent elevations of LFTs during a 12-month period, or if there is a decline in serum albumin level in a patient with normal nutritional status

Patients at high risk for liver disease

Baseline biopsy, then subsequent biopsies every 6 months or with after additional 1 to 1.5 g of drug

Risk factors for liver disease

Personal history of diabetes mellitus, obesity, persistent abnormal LFT results, history of or current excessive alcohol consumption, history of chronic liver disease including hepatitis B or C, family history of inheritable liver disease, history of significant exposure to hepatotoxic drugs or chemicals, lack of folate supplementation, hyperlipidemia

Abbreviation: LFT, liver function test.

Adapted from Kalb RE, Strober B, Weinstein G, et al. Methotrexate and psoriasis: 2009 National Psoriasis Foundation Consensus Conference. J Am Acad Dermatol 2009;60(5):824–37; with permission.

anti-inflammatory effects through inhibition of the 5-lipoxygenase pathway. Adverse effects associated with sulfasalazine include gastrointestinal disturbances, arthralgias, reversible oligospermia, leukopenia, and agranulocytosis.[78] Sulfasalazine is FDA pregnancy category B and has been used rarely, but safely and efficaciously, in the pediatric population.[79] Before instituting therapy with sulfasalazine, it is important to ascertain that the patient does not have an allergic history to sulfa drugs.[50]

Cyclosporine A (CsA) is a rapidly acting immunosuppressive agent FDA-approved for severe, recalcitrant psoriasis. The drug binds to cyclophilin, subsequently inhibiting calcineurin and its downstream proinflammatory signal pathways that lead to T-cell activation. In PsA, CsA is used in low doses (typically 2.5–5 mg/kg/d). In a 2001 open-label study of patients with PsA, CsA was significantly better than both sulfasalazine alone and "usual care" (prednisone, NSAIDs, and analgesics) in decreasing pain and cutaneous lesions. In reducing tender and swollen joint counts, CsA was similarly effective as sulfasalazine and significantly more effective than usual care.[80]

CsA is particularly useful in crisis management of psoriasis; comparative studies have found greater efficacy of CsA in comparison with MTX in psoriasis, including in patients with PsA.[80,81] However, owing to its side effects of nephrotoxicity and hypertension, use of CsA should not exceed 12 months to prevent irreversible renal damage. Before initiation of the drug, 2 blood pressure readings, 2 serum creatinine measurements, a complete blood count, a complete chemistry panel with magnesium, and a lipid panel are performed, and monitoring is recommended every other week after initiation of treatment, then once every 1 to 3 months.[78] Additional side effects of CsA include hypomagnesemia, hyperkalemia, hyperlipidemia, drug-to-drug interactions, hypertrichosis, and lymphoproliferative disease.[78] The FDA has classified CsA as category C; it should be used during pregnancy only if the potential benefit outweighs the potential risk to the fetus. CsA use in JPsA has been reported only rarely, although its use in children with other dermatologic and rheumatologic conditions suggests that the side effect profile is similar to that seen in adults.[82]

Tumor Necrosis Factor α Inhibitors

TNF-α plays a pivotal role in the chronic inflammation underlying PsA and psoriasis, and the TNF-α inhibitors have revolutionized therapy for PsA. TNF-α inhibitors etanercept, infliximab, and adalimumab are remarkably effective in psoriasis and have become first-line for patients with moderate-to-severe PsA.[83] Of note, the TNF-α inhibitors etanercept, infliximab, adalimumab, and golimumab are efficacious in improving enthesitis and dactylitis, and can markedly inhibit radiographic progression of disease.[59] Recommended dosages of the TNF-α inhibitors and their respective PsA and psoriasis response rates are given in **Table 2**.[84–97] Importantly, although TNF-α inhibitors have great benefits for many patients with psoriasis, their efficacy is not universal and the magnitude and durability of their effect is variable.[7]

There are limited data on the use of TNF-α inhibitors in the pediatric population, but etanercept is approved for the treatment of DMARD-resistant polyarticular JIA, and glucocorticoids, NSAIDs, or other analgesics may be continued during therapy.[98] Recommended (off-label) dosages are 0.8 mg/kg (maximum: 50 mg/dose) once weekly or 0.4 mg/kg (maximum: 25 mg/dose) twice weekly.[98,99] Infliximab is approved for children aged 4 years and older at doses of 3 mg/kg (weeks 0, 2, and 6), then 3 to 6 mg/kg/dose every 8 weeks thereafter. Infliximab has been used in children with JIA in combination with MTX.[100,101] Similarly, data on adalimumab use in JIA is sparse, but the drug has been recommended for severe cases for children of at least 4 years in doses of 20 mg subcutaneously every other week (patient weight 15 kg to <30 kg), and 40 mg subcutaneously every other week for children weighing 30 kg and greater.[102,103]

Newer anti–TNF-α agents include golimumab and certolizumab pegol, both of which are FDA-approved for the treatment of PsA. Neither is yet approved for psoriasis, although improvement of skin lesions has been observed in clinical trials on PsA.[104]

Interestingly, certolizumab pegol lacks the Fc portion of the TNF-α antibody, and hypothetically may be less likely to induce antibody-related complement activation, apoptosis, or cellular toxicity.[104] In a double-blind phase III trial on certolizumab pegol use in 368 patients with PsA (the RAPID-PsA trial), 20% of patients with PsA who had previously experienced inadequate responses to another TNF-α inhibitor demonstrated responses similar to those of the overall study population.[84] ACR20 response was achieved in 58.0% and 51.9% of the 2 treatment arms (200 mg certolizumab once every 2 weeks or 400 mg once every 4 weeks) at week 12, independent of prior TNF-α inhibitor exposure.[104] PsARC improved in 78% of treated patients, and

Table 2
Currently available biological agents for psoriatic arthritis (PsA)

Biologic[a]	Recommended Dose in PsA	% Achieving ACR20	% Achieving PASI-75	Beneficial Effect on Radiographic Damage	Adverse Effects
Etanercept: Anti-TNF agent; recombinant fusion protein of p75 unit of TNF receptor and Fc portion of human IgG1	25 or 50 mg SubQ twice weekly	59% (week 24)	26% of PsA patients (week 24) 49% of Ps patients (week 12)	Yes	Pruritus Headache Immunosuppression Injection-site reaction
Adalimumab: Anti-TNF agent; Fully human monoclonal antibody	40 mg SubQ every 2 wk	58% (week 24)	59% of PsA patients (week 24) 76% of Ps patients (week 160)	Yes	Immunosuppression
Infliximab: Anti-TNF agent; chimeric mouse/human antibody	Initial: 5 mg/kg IV infusion at weeks 0, 2, and 6; Maintenance: 5 mg/kg IV infusion every 8 wk	65% (week 16)	65% of PsA patients 80% of Ps patients (week 10)	Yes	Lupus-like symptoms Serum sickness/delayed reactions Infusion reactions Elevated liver enzymes
Golimumab: Anti-TNF agent; fully human monoclonal antibody	50 mg SubQ every 4 wk	51% (week 256)	62.8%–69.9% of PsA patients (week 256) 60.8%–72.2% of Ps patients (week 256)	Yes	Headache Nasopharyngitis Increased risk of nonmelanoma skin cancers[7] Immunosuppression

Drug/Class	Dosing			Immunosuppression	Side Effects
Certolizumab pegol: Anti-TNF agent; pegylated fully human monoclonal antibody	Initial: 400 mg SubQ, at weeks 0, 2 and 4; Maintenance: 200 mg every 2 wk	58.0% (week 12)	62.2% of PsA patients (week 24) 75%-83% of Ps patients (week 12)	Yes	Headache, Nasopharyngitis, Diarrhea, URI, Immunosuppression, Elevated liver enzymes
Ustekinumab: Anti-IL12/23p40	45 or 90 mg SubQ every 12 wk	42% receiving 45 mg (week 16) 49.5% receiving 90 mg (week 16)	62% of PsA patients (week 16) 74% of Ps patients (week 12)	Yes	Increased risk of infection, Headache, Upper respiratory infection, Immunosuppression
Apremilast: Anti-phosphodiesterase-4	20 or 30 mg orally every day	40% (week 16) (30 mg BID group)	21% of PsA patients (week 16) 24% of Ps patients (30 mg BID)	Unknown	Nausea, Diarrhea, URI, Immunosuppression

Abbreviations: ACR20, at least a 20% improvement in American College of Rheumatology criteria; BID, twice daily; FDA, Food and Drug Administration; Ig, immunoglobulin; IL, interleukin; IV, intravenously; JAK, Janus kinases; PASI-75, improvement of at least 75% in Psoriasis and Area Severity Index; Ps, psoriasis; PsA, psoriatic arthritis; SubQ, subcutaneously; TNF, tumor necrosis factor; URI, upper respiratory infections.

[a] Food and Drug Administration (FDA)-approved dose.

sustained improvements were observed in psoriatic skin involvement, enthesitis, dactylitis, and nail disease.[84] Both dosage intervals of certolizumab pegol also resulted in rapid improvements in dermatologic-specific, PsA-specific, and generic health-related QOL outcome measures[104]: At week 24, clinically meaningful and statistically significant differences in fatigue, pain, QOL, and Dermatology Life Quality Index (DLQI) measures were observed in both certolizumab pegol treatment arms, irrespective of prior TNF-inhibitor exposure.[104]

Head-to-head comparison studies of the TNF-α inhibitors have not been performed. Some investigators have suggested combination therapy (see later discussion) or switching from one biologic to another to improve clinical efficacy in PsA, although this has not been supported by clinical evidence.[105,106] A 2012 meta-analysis performed an indirect comparison of PsARC and patient-reported outcomes for the available anti-TNF agents at that time (adalimumab, etanercept, golimumab, and infliximab).[107] Data from 20 publications representing 7 PsA clinical trials were analyzed; the investigators and did not find any statistically significant differences between the TNF-α inhibitors,[107] as the data compiled in **Table 2** also suggest.

TNF-α inhibitors do have significant limitations; namely, a substantial number of patients may lose efficacy over time, likely related to development of antibodies against the biologic.[28,59] Additional major prohibiting factors to the use TNF-α inhibitors include their expense and the inconvenience of intravenous or subcutaneous administration.[108]

TNF-α inhibitors are contraindicated in patients with serious infections, those with a history of demyelinating diseases, those with New York Heart Association (NYHA) class I or II heart failure and an ejection fraction of less than 50%, and in patients with NYHA class III or class IV heart failure.[2] Likewise, adverse effects of TNF-α inhibitors include an increased risk of bacterial, viral, invasive fungal, and mycobacterial infections (all patients require annual tuberculosis testing), the development of or worsening peripheral or central demyelinating disease, lymphomas and other malignancies, reactivation of hepatitis B, and exacerbation of congestive heart failure.[2] A small number of cases of new-onset psoriasis in patients have been reported.[105] The TNF-α inhibitors are pregnancy category B. Live vaccines are contraindicated in patients receiving the drugs.[2] The risk of malignancy may be higher in children, and these agents are used very cautiously in JPsA.[109]

Ustekinumab

Ustekinumab is the only available fully human G1κ monoclonal antibody that binds to the p40 subunit of IL-12 and IL-23; it was approved in the United States in 2013 for the treatment of PsA. Single-nucleotide polymorphisms in the IL-23 receptor and IL-12 genes have been found to increase susceptibility to PsA.[110] IL-23 potently promotes IL-17 and Th17 activation, and enhances osteoclastogenesis and bone resorption in mouse models.[111] Inhibition of IL-12 has been shown to dramatically reduce pathogenic IL-12–induced synovial tissue levels of TNF-α and IFN-γ.[112]

In PsA, ustekinumab at a dose of 45 mg (if <100 kg; 90 mg if >100 kg) subcutaneously at weeks 0, 4, 12, then every 12 weeks thereafter leads to significant improvements in enthesitis, dactylitis, physical functioning, radiographic progression of disease, and patient QOL.[33,113,114] Its long half-life allows for ongoing efficacy with a dosing interval of 12 weeks, giving it the longest dosing interval of all currently available medications for PsA.[7] Of note, ustekinumab also has shown good efficacy in PsA patients who have previously received NSAIDs, DMARDs, and TNF-α inhibitors.[59,85,115] Of consideration is the fact that in some markets the 90-mg dose is twice as expensive as the 45-mg dose. Ustekinumab fills an unmet need in PsA therapy; it is an option for nonresponders to TNF-α inhibitors and for patients in whom the TNF inhibitors are contraindicated, whether for prior adverse effects or comorbid conditions.

Most adverse effects associated with ustekinumab are mild and include nasopharyngitis, upper respiratory infections (URI), and headache.[33] No opportunistic infections (including tuberculosis), malignancies, or deaths occurred in either of the large phase III PSUMMIT-1 or -2 trials. Although there has been particular concern regarding cardiovascular risks associated with anti–IL-12/23 agents, leading to the withdrawal of briakinumab from the market,[116] a large 2013 postmarketing study reported that ustekinumab use for up to 5 years in patients with psoriasis did not lead to an increased risk of major adverse cardiovascular events (MACE).[117] Similarly, the Psoriasis Longitudinal Assessment and Registry (PSOLAR) study found comparably low rates of MACE with ustekinumab (0.21 events per patient-years of observation) as seen with adalimumab and etanercept.[118]

Ustekinumab is FDA pregnancy category B. A theoretic increased risk for infection with *Mycobacterium* and *Salmonella* has been suggested, given reports of increased susceptibility to these infections of patients with IL-12 receptor deficiency.[78]

Apremilast

Apremilast, a phosphodiesterase-4 inhibitor, is a recently FDA-approved, orally administered small molecule that has shown substantial efficacy in PsA and many other inflammatory arthritides. In the PALACE trials, apremilast (30 mg twice daily) led to an average ACR20 achievement at week 52 in 43%, 28%, and 32% of PsA patients who were biologic-naïve, biologic-experienced, and DMARD-naïve, respectively.[86] Reductions in enthesitis and dactylitis, and improvements in QOL and physical functioning, were also statistically significant at week 52.[49]

Apremilast is unique to the PsA market. It acts at an intracellular level, indirectly blocking TNF-α and other proinflammatory cytokines via inhibition of the cyclic adenosine monophosphate pathway.[111] Adverse effects of apremilast include diarrhea and nausea, the incidence of which decreases with length of treatment time, URI, and headache (see **Table 2**).[119] Effects of apremilast on radiographic progression of PsA and studies on its long-term efficacy are under way.

Emerging Therapies for Psoriatic Arthritis

IL-17 and other Th-17 cytokines play a crucial role in PsA pathogenesis,[120,121] and therapies targeting this pathway (including IL-17A and the IL-17 receptor), secukinumab, brodalumab, and ixekizumab, are under investigation for the treatment of PsA. The IL-17 cytokine family consists of 6 cytokines (interleukins 17A to 17F) and 5 receptors (interleukins 17RA to 17RE),[122] and overproduction of interleukins 17A, 17F, and 17A/F induces expression of proinflammatory cytokines with pathologic consequences, including the proliferation of keratinocytes in psoriasis.[122] Levels of IL-17 are elevated in the lesional skin, serum, and synovial fluid of patients with psoriasis and PsA,[121,123] and correlate with disease severity in psoriasis.[124] In animal models of inflammatory arthritis, IL-17 neutralization reduces arthritis severity by diminishing joint inflammation and inhibiting structural damage.[125]

Each of the IL-17 agents currently under investigation is administered subcutaneously at varying intervals (**Table 3**).[122,126–131] Secukinumab is a fully human monoclonal immunoglobulin G1 (IgG1) monoclonal antibody that selectively binds to and neutralizes IL-17A, with demonstrated success in trials for moderate-to-severe plaque psoriasis, PsA, RA, and AS. In a phase II randomized clinical trial in 42 patients with active PsA,

ACR20 was reached by 43% of patients receiving secukinumab at week 24 (see **Table 3**).[126] Patient-reported outcomes of health-related disability and QOL also showed improvements,[126] and further study of the drug in larger patient populations is under way. Adverse events in the study were comparable with those observed in patients receiving placebo.[126] Further study of secukinumab in larger patient populations is needed, as the drug has shown remarkable efficacy in cutaneous psoriasis in phase III studies. In a head-to-head comparison study of secukinumab to etanercept in plaque psoriasis, secukinumab (in both 150-mg and 300-mg doses) showed improved efficacy to etanercept throughout the 52-week study period.[132]

Ixekizumab (given as 150 or 300 mg once every 2 weeks) has also demonstrated good efficacy in PsA. In a trial of 142 patients with psoriasis with or without PsA, among patients with PsA, significant reductions in joint pain from baseline (assessed by the joint-pain visual analog scale) and improvements in DLQI were observed in the ixekizumab group.[127] At week 12, a striking 82% of patients receiving the drug achieved PASI-75.[127] Significant differences occurred as early as 1 week and were maintained during 20 weeks of follow-up. The drug has just completed phase II studies in RA with good efficacy in patients who were biologic-naïve and in patients who were deemed inadequate responders to TNF-α inhibitors.[121] The most frequently reported adverse events of ixekizumab trials in plaque psoriasis were nasopharyngitis, URI, injection-site reaction, and headache; no serious adverse events were reported. Phase III trials of ixekizumab in plaque psoriasis are under way, including a comparator study of the drug with etanercept.

Brodalumab is also a fully human monoclonal antibody, but binds to IL-17RA, the shared common receptor subunit for signaling through interleukins IL-17A, -17F, and -17A/F, all of which play a role in inflammatory signaling in psoriasis and PsA.[125] Brodalumab treatment has resulted in dramatic improvements in phase II trials on psoriasis (see **Table 3**), and trials on its efficacy in PsA are ongoing.[122] Adverse effects and contraindications of these medications are similar to those seen with the TNF-α-inhibitors; risk of mild infections is increased, and reported severe adverse events have been rare.

Anti–IL-23p19 agents (tildrakizumab and guselkumab) and the IL-22 inhibitor fezakizumab are also in development and will likely become additional options in therapy for PsA, although current results are only available from studies in moderate-to-severe chronic plaque psoriasis. Tildrakizumab is a monoclonal antibody administered

Table 3
Biological agents in development (phase III investigation) for potential use in psoriatic arthritis

	Route of Administration	Efficacy	Adverse Effects
Brodalumab: Anti–IL-17 receptor fully human monoclonal antibody[a]	SubQ	Ps: PASI-75 achieved by 86.3% (210 mg every 2 wk) and 76.0% (280 mg every 4 wk) (week 12) ACR20: Not yet available	Nasopharyngitis URI Injection-site erythema Neutropenia
Ixekizumab: Anti–IL-17; fully human monoclonal antibody	SubQ	PASI-75 in 82% (week 12) ACR20: Not yet available	Nasopharyngitis URI Injection-site reaction Headache
Secukinumab: Anti–IL-17; fully human monoclonal antibody	SubQ	PASI-75 in 82% (week 12) ACR20 in 43% (week 24)	Nasopharyngitis URI Headache
Tildrakizumab: Anti-23p19; fully human monoclonal antibody	SubQ	PASI-75 in 74% (week 16) ACR20: Not yet available	Unknown
Abatacept: Anti–CTLA-4; fusion protein (CTLA-4 and IgG1), inhibits T-cell costimulation	IV	ACR20 in 48% (10 mg/kg) (week 24)	Dizziness Headache Hypertension Increased risk of infections
Tofacitinib: JAK Inhibitor	Oral	PASI-75 in 66.7% (week 12) ACR20: Not yet available	URI Nasopharyngitis Headache

Abbreviations: ACR20, at least a 20% improvement in American College of Rheumatology criteria; CTLA-4, cytotoxic T lymphocyte antigen 4; FDA, Food and Drug Administration; Ig, immunoglobulin; IV, intravenously; JAK, Janus kinases; PASI-75, improvement of at least 75% in Psoriasis and Area Severity Index; Ps, psoriasis; PsA, psoriatic arthritis; SubQ, subcutaneously; URI, upper respiratory infections.
[a] Food and Drug Administration (FDA)-approved dose.

subcutaneously and given in doses of 100 mg or 200 mg once every 2 weeks. In a phase II randomized controlled trial in which 339 patients with moderate-to-severe chronic plaque psoriasis were given 100 or 200 mg of tildrakizumab, 66% and 74% of patients achieved PASI-75, respectively.[133] Incidence of adverse events was uniform across treatment groups. In phase I study in patients with moderate-to-severe psoriasis, 100% of patients treated with 300 mg guselkumab subcutaneously achieved a 75% improvement in PASI scores from baseline at week 12, improvements which were largely maintained through week 24.[134] Data on fezakizumab are still limited.

A fully human CTLA-4–IgG1 fusion protein, abatacept, selectively blocks T-cell costimulation and activation through CD80 or CD86, and although not yet approved for PsA is used successfully in treatment of RA. Administered intravenously, abatacept demonstrated ACR20 achievement rates of up to 48% in a 2011 study of 170 PsA patients who received the drug at doses of 10 mg/kg administered in 3 initial doses at 2-week intervals and then every 4 weeks for 6 months (see **Table 3**).[128]

Of note, all patients in that 2011 study had a history of an inadequate response to a nonbiological DMARD (usually MTX), a biological agent (usually a TNF inhibitor), or both.[128] Modest improvements in skin disease were seen.[128] Improvements in JIA at the same dose (10 mg/kg) have also been observed.[128,135] Risks of abatacept include an increased risk of infections and malignancies; all patients should be screened for tuberculosis and hepatitis B before treatment initiation, and live vaccines should be avoided during therapy. Infusion-related events include dizziness, headache, and hypertension. The drug is pregnancy category C (risk to the fetus unknown or unclear).

Lastly, tofacitinib, an oral Janus kinase (JAK) inhibitor that is FDA-approved for the treatment of RA, has shown good efficacy in psoriasis[129] and is undergoing evaluation in PsA. Inhibitors of the JAK family of nonreceptor tyrosine kinases, which are stimulated by various cytokines, have been shown to ameliorate inflammation in murine models of inflammatory arthritides.[136] No studies to date have evaluated bone homeostasis in patients treated with JAK inhibitors, but given the prominent role of inflammatory cytokines on osteoclastogenesis, it is plausible that an indirect effect of JAK inhibition will be a lower state of bone resorption.[137] In support of the potential bone-protective effects of JAK inhibitors, van der Heijde and colleagues[138] presented data showing that the oral JAK inhibitor tofacitinib was associated with decreased radiographic progression in RA patients after 1 year of therapy.

NONPHARMACOLOGIC TREATMENT OF PSORIATIC ARTHRITIS

All patients should be instructed on joint protection, encouraged to exercise, lose weight, reduce stress, and, if needed, can be referred for physical therapy, occupational therapy, and/or for orthotics. Despite historical recommendation of physical therapy for PsA symptoms,[31] there are no randomized controlled therapies to assess the benefit of physical therapy in PsA.

COMBINATION THERAPIES

For PsA patients in whom monotherapy does not lead to adequate, sustained response of disease, combination therapies are considered. In many patients with PsA, a single systemic agent will not be sufficient for disease control. The presence of PsA itself in patients with concomitant moderate-to-severe psoriasis is considered by some investigators an indication for the use of combination therapy,[139] and experts suggest that combination therapies of systemic agents may be underused.[66]

Loss of efficacy is commonly observed with long-term treatment of PsA with both major classes of drugs currently used most commonly, the DMARDs and TNF-α inhibitors. Long-term monotherapy, particularly with DMARDs, may also require significant dose escalation, increasing toxicity risks. With combination therapy, lower dosages of individual agents can be used, limiting toxicity and improving overall efficacy.[66] The potentially increased risk of adverse effects when using 2 immunosuppressive agents is a crucial consideration.[70,140] These patients require frequent surveillance.

Various combinations of therapies have been used in PsA, although randomized controlled studies on their use versus monotherapy are sparse and mostly compare older medications. A 2008 study found that combination NSAID plus MTX in standard doses for 6 months resulted in significantly greater reductions of swollen and tender joint counts compared with sequential therapy with NSAIDs followed by MTX in PsA patients.[141] However, there were no significant differences in

other clinical measures, including the pain assessment scale, patient's global assessment, or physician's global assessment.[141] Thus, a clinical benefit of combination NSAID-MTX therapy for PsA has not been established.

A second randomized, placebo-controlled trial evaluating MTX in combination with CsA in 72 PsA patients with an incomplete response to MTX monotherapy showed improvements in swollen joint counts, PASI, synovitis (detected by ultrasonography), radiographic (change in Larsen score of radiographs of +7.4 vs +1.7, respectively), and CRP levels in patients receiving combination therapy versus MTX monotherapy, although the results were not statistically significant.[142] CsA is required only in the most severe cases, usually in patients with both skin and joint involvement, and, as in monotherapy, the drug should not be used for longer than 12 months given its nephrotoxicity and other adverse effects.[70] Combination therapy for MTX with sulfasalazine is used less frequently, but has been reported.[66]

The biological agents have greatly expanded the options for combination therapy. Current recommendations for PsA treatment position combination therapy with a DMARD plus TNF-α inhibitor or a DMARD plus a non-TNF inhibitor second agent as treatment for moderate-to-severe PsA in patients with inadequate response to conventional courses of both DMARD monotherapy and TNF-α inhibitor monotherapy. MTX in combination with a TNF-α inhibitor has been shown to be more effective in PsA than MTX monotherapy: The 2012 RESPOND study of 115 MTX-naïve patients with PsA found an ACR20 response at week 16 of 86% in patients receiving combination infliximab-MTX therapy, versus only 67% in the MTX-alone arm.[143] Improvements in CRP levels, DAS28 response and remission rates, dactylitis, fatigue, and morning stiffness duration were also significantly greater in the group receiving combination infliximab-MTX, as were improvements in skin disease, as measured by PASI-75. More patients in the combination therapy arm (46%) experienced adverse events compared with the MTX monotherapy arm (24%).

Combination of MTX with each of the TNF-α inhibitors etanercept and adalimumab has been shown to result in greater patient responses than combination with MTX alone in patients with psoriasis; however, studies in patients with PsA have shown only modest improvement in outcomes with etanercept or adalimumab plus MTX.[144–146] The few studies on TNF-α inhibitors in combination with CsA in PsA have found results consistent with combination MTX and TNF-α inhibitor therapy, with slightly greater improvements in cutaneous disease in those on the CsA combination compared with those on the MTX combination.[147] Clinical trials to date have not shown superiority of combination DMARD plus TNF-α inhibitor use to TNF-α inhibitor therapy alone, thus, further study is needed.

Evidence of ustekinumab used in combination with other systemic agents is encouraging: in PSUMMIT-1 and PSUMMIT-2, about 50% of patients in each trial were receiving concomitant MTX.[85,115] In PSUMMIT-1, at week 24, 43.5% of patients receiving concomitant MTX achieved ACR20, compared with 42.4% of patients overall.[85] Although the data suggested that addition of MTX did not add additional benefit to ustekinumab use, tests of significance were not performed, as the study was not powered to detect differences among these groups.[85] Inhibition of radiographic progression was observed for ustekinumab (both doses) versus placebo, regardless of MTX use at baseline.[33] Combination therapy has also been reported in pediatric patients. In a study of 60 patients with JIA, infliximab plus MTX was superior to 2 DMARDs in combination and strikingly superior to MTX alone: ACR75 was achieved in 100% (19 of 19) of patients receiving a TNF-α inhibitor, 65% (13 of 20) on combination TNF-α inhibitors and MTX, and 50% (10 of 20) on MTX.[79]

SURGICAL TREATMENT OPTIONS

There are limited data on the epidemiology and efficacy of surgery in patients with PsA. One study of 440 patients with PsA revealed that 31 (7%) had undergone musculoskeletal surgery.[148] Surgical interventions used include synovectomy, arthroplasty, and reconstructive surgery.[149] In that study, the probability for surgery increased with disease duration, increased actively inflamed joints, and radiographic evidence of damage. Joint replacements (usually hip, knee, or hand surgeries) have been performed when PsA leads to damage that limits movement and impairs function. Most commonly, silicone arthroplasty of the MCP joints is performed, given the high prevalence of hand involvement with severe loss of function. There is a paucity of evidence for surgery-associated risks in PsA patients; the study referenced above reported 1 infection in 71 procedures.[148] One study suggested that while initial results for total hip replacement were good, there appeared to be excess bone proliferation with a decrease in mobility, and experts have noted the frequent appearance of fibrosis around prostheses, particularly in small joint arthroplasty.[150]

TREATMENT RESISTANCE AND DISEASE RECURRENCE/COMPLICATIONS
Treatment Resistance

Treatment resistance is a major problem in PsA. In patients with inadequate responses to monotherapy, combination therapy (see earlier discussion) may be considered. To prevent flare of disease, initiation of a biologic may be performed without a washout period of any conventional DMARD.[49] If patients develop resistance or loss of efficacy to a biological agent, switching to a second biologic (at present, either a second TNF-α inhibitor or ustekinumab) is recommended, although evidence of improved efficacy with biologic switching has not yet been proved.[151] At the same time, an inadequate response to one TNF inhibitor does not predict resistance to other agents in the class, although inefficacy and discontinuation rates increase with successive switches.[106] New biologics can also be given at the next scheduled dosage date without a washout period, unless the discontinuation of the first biologic is due to an adverse effect.[49] Apremilast and emerging therapies (eg, secukinumab, brodalumab, ixekizumab, abatacept, tildrakizumab, guselkumab, tofacitinib, and tocilizumab) will become increasingly important for the treatment of patients who do not respond to TNF-α inhibitors and/or ustekinumab (even with long periods of treatment, eg, 3–6 months).

In general, continuous rather than intermittent therapy for PsA is thought to provide greater efficacy.[152,153] In clinical trials in which drugs leading to a response are discontinued then reinitiated, or primary responding drugs are introduced after cessation, up to 20% of patients have failed to regain a PASI-75 response after reintroduction of the drug.[154] There are limited data on the benefit of sequential use of TNF-α inhibitors in PsA, and there are no randomized controlled trials of switching between the drugs in PsA. A retrospective review of more than 27,000 patients in the United States with PsA, RA, psoriasis, or AS who received etanercept, adalimumab, or infliximab, identified 53% of patients as having discontinued treatment over 1 to 3 years of follow-up.[106] Within 360 days of discontinuing the initial TNF inhibitor, 53.4% restarted the same drug, about 17% of patients switched to a second TNF-α inhibitor, and about 5.3% switched from the initial TNF-α agent to a non-TNF biological therapy.[106] Although a majority (61% to 66%) of patients restarted therapy within 3 months after initial discontinuation, the study confirmed that long gaps in the treatment of psoriasis, PsA, and RA are common (differences across the disease entities were insignificant).[106]

Interestingly a significantly higher proportion of etanercept patients restarted etanercept within 3 months of discontinuation, compared with patients taking adalimumab or infliximab.[106]

Also in 2014, Jani and colleagues[154] published results of a United Kingdom survey of 548 PsA patients, 94 of whom were switched at least once from a TNF-α inhibitor to a second or third PsA therapy. Of these, 72% were on a concomitant DMARD (84% of which comprised MTX).[57] Twelve weeks after initiation of a TNF-α inhibitor, 74% had an adequate response, and of the remainder, the main reason for cessation of the initial biologic was lack of inefficacy of initial response, followed by inefficacy over time.[154] Of all patients on TNF-α inhibitors, 17% switched to a second TNF-α inhibitor, and 3% switched to a different biologic (either rituximab, tocilizumab, or ustekinumab).[154] Sixty percent of patients were recorded to have an adequate response to a second-line or third-line agent, and 18% were awaiting assessment of disease activity at the time of the survey.[154]

Further studies are warranted in PsA on treatment resistance, sequential therapy, combination therapy in PsA, efficacy rates after switching agents, and discerning associations between switching behavior and clinical response to therapy.

Complications

Of importance, the increased cardiovascular risk associated with psoriasis appears further enhanced in PsA, likely reflecting the overall burden of systemic inflammation contributing to atherogenic processes.[155] The 2008 American Journal of Cardiology Editor's Consensus on Psoriasis and Coronary Artery Disease recommended that all patients with moderate-to-severe psoriasis be informed of a potential increased risk for coronary artery disease,[156] and these guidelines may be followed for all patients with PsA as well. The panel also recommended ascertaining the family history of the patient, assessing the patient's blood pressure, and performing screening lipid profiles and fasting blood glucose testing.[156] A 2008 consensus statement from the National Psoriasis Foundation also addressed recommendations for the assessment of psoriasis comorbidities[157]: In addition to supporting the standard recommendations for identifying and reducing cardiovascular risk (smoking cessation, weight loss, and physical activity), the consensus panel recommended interventions to recognize and control depression, moderate alcohol intake, and maintain vigilance for signs of lymphoma, cutaneous malignancies, and solid tumors (age-appropriate screening,

annual skin examinations on patients on immunosuppressants or with a history of psoralen/ultraviolet A treatment, vigilance for plaques that appear atypical for psoriasis). Lastly, aggressive treatment and symptom management of PsA is essential in that it may improve cardiovascular risk factors in patients. In a 2013 retrospective cohort study of 210 PsA patients with metabolic syndrome treated with etanercept, adalimumab, or methotrexate for 24 months, patients who received drugs proven to halt PsA disease progression (etanercept and adalimumab) showed a significant improvement of metabolic syndrome components (including waist circumference, triglycerides, high-density lipoprotein cholesterol, and fasting glucose) when compared with patients receiving MTX.[158]

Other comorbidities specific to PsA include various manifestations of ocular inflammation, similar to the risk seen with other seronegative spondyloarthropathies. Eye inflammation (presenting as uveitis, episcleritis, blepharitis, or keratoconjunctivitis sicca) has been reported in about 10% of patients with PsA at some time during the course of disease.[159] The most common type of uveitis that complicates PsA is chronic anterior uveitis.[159] Patients with uveitis should be referred promptly to an ophthalmologist.[160]

SUMMARY

PsA is a chronic, progressive, systemic inflammatory disease that is often painful, debilitating, and difficult to treat. It is one of the most common and most significant comorbidities of psoriasis; patients with PsA have a diminished health-related QOL, and productivity and functionality similar to those of patients with other serious, chronic diseases, including cancer, diabetes, and heart disease. Increased understanding of the immunopathogenesis of psoriasis has led to the development of multiple biological drugs targeting specific molecules that are essential for the development of joint and soft-tissue inflammation, osteoclastogenesis, and psoriatic plaque lesions. As new insights into osteoimmunology are acquired and applied to what is known about joint disease, the study of osteoblast and osteoclast homeostasis will likely become a pivotal area of focus in PsA.

The TNF-α inhibitors, ustekinumab, apremilast, and several agents in the pipeline hold promise in achieving adequate efficacy in PsA symptomatology in addition to slowing radiographic progression by inhibiting the dysregulated osteoclastogenesis and bone resorption that characterize the disease. Ongoing studies and registries will help to provide long-term data, particularly data on adverse events that investigational trials are not powered to detect. It will also be imperative to determine biomarkers for disease to determine patient-specific PsA therapies, as there remain significant fractions of patients who are unresponsive to each class of medication. Biomarkers are also needed to determine which patients with psoriasis will develop PsA and for prediction of which patients are most likely to develop severe disease with radiographic progression.

Dermatologists frequently are the first providers to encounter patients with PsA and those who are at risk of developing the disease. It is essential for the provider to be familiar with the presenting signs and symptoms of PsA as well as the currently available and quickly growing number of therapeutic options for the disease. Long-term goals of therapy in PsA are to maintain health-related QOL, limit progression of structural damage, and control cutaneous and joint symptoms such as pruritus, swelling, pain, and functional disability. Collaboration of dermatologists with rheumatologists in managing patients who have psoriasis and PsA is likely to yield more optimal control of psoriatic dermal and joint symptoms, and improve long-term patient outcomes. Although further clinical comparative studies on the efficacy of available therapeutic options, their influence on QOL, and rates of patient adherence are needed, great strides have been made in the past decade in the management of this debilitating disease.

REFERENCES

1. Lebwohl MG, Bachelez H, Barker J, et al. Patient perspectives in the management of psoriasis: results from the population-based multinational assessment of psoriasis and psoriatic arthritis survey. J Am Acad Dermatol 2014;70(5):871–81.e1-30.
2. Gottlieb A, Korman NJ, Gordon KB, et al. Guidelines of care for the management of psoriasis and psoriatic arthritis: section 2. Psoriatic arthritis: overview and guidelines of care for treatment with an emphasis on the biologics. J Am Acad Dermatol 2008;58(5):851–64.
3. Gelfand JM, Gladman DD, Mease PJ, et al. Epidemiology of psoriatic arthritis in the population of the United States. J Am Acad Dermatol 2005; 53(4):573.
4. Gladman DD, Antoni C, Mease P, et al. Psoriatic arthritis: epidemiology, clinical features, course, and outcome. Ann Rheum Dis 2005;64(Suppl 2): ii14–7.
5. Mease PJ, Menter MA. Quality-of-life issues in psoriasis and psoriatic arthritis: outcome measures and therapies from a dermatological perspective. J Am Acad Dermatol 2006;54(4):685–704.
6. Gladman DD, Hing EN, Schentag CT, et al. Remission in psoriatic arthritis. J Rheumatol 2001;28(5): 1045–8.
7. Weitz JE, Ritchlin CT. Ustekinumab: targeting the IL-17 pathway to improve outcomes in psoriatic arthritis. Expert Opin Biol Ther 2014;14(4):515–26.
8. Chandran V, Schentag CT, Brockbank JE, et al. Familial aggregation of psoriatic arthritis. Ann Rheum Dis 2009;68(5):664–7.
9. Nograles KE, Brasington RD, Bowcock AM. New insights into the pathogenesis and genetics of psoriatic arthritis. Nat Clin Pract Rheumatol 2009;5(2):83–91.
10. Gladman DD, Cheung C, Ng CM, et al. HLA-C locus alleles in patients with psoriatic arthritis (PsA). Hum Immunol 1999;60(3):259–61.
11. Liu Y, Helms C, Liao W, et al. A genome-wide association study of psoriasis and psoriatic arthritis identifies new disease loci. PLoS Genet 2008; 4(3):e1000041.
12. Frleta M, Siebert S, McInnes IB. The interleukin-17 pathway in psoriasis and psoriatic arthritis: disease pathogenesis and possibilities of treatment. Curr Rheumatol Rep 2014;16(4):414.
13. Anandarajah AP, Ritchlin CT. The diagnosis and treatment of early psoriatic arthritis. Nat Rev Rheumatol 2009;5(11):634–41.
14. Ritchlin CT. Pathogenesis of psoriatic arthritis. Curr Opin Rheumatol 2005;17(4):406–12.
15. Weaver CT, Elson CO, Fouser LA, et al. The Th17 pathway and inflammatory diseases of the intestines, lungs, and skin. Annu Rev Pathol 2013;8: 477–512.
16. Lories RJ, McInnes IB. Primed for inflammation: enthesis-resident T cells. Nat Med 2012;18(7): 1018–9.
17. Sherlock JP, Joyce-Shaikh B, Turner SP, et al. IL-23 induces spondyloarthropathy by acting on ROR-gammat+ CD3+CD4-CD8- entheseal resident T cells. Nat Med 2012;18(7):1069–76.
18. Raychaudhuri SP, Raychaudhuri SK, Genovese MC. IL-17 receptor and its functional significance in psoriatic arthritis. Mol Cell Biochem 2012;359(1–2): 419–29.
19. Adamopoulos IE, Suzuki E, Chao CC, et al. IL-17A gene transfer induces bone loss and epidermal hyperplasia associated with psoriatic arthritis. Ann Rheum Dis 2014. [Epub ahead of print].
20. Rahimi H, Ritchlin CT. Altered bone biology in psoriatic arthritis. Curr Rheumatol Rep 2012;14(4): 349–57.
21. Nigrovic PA. Juvenile psoriatic arthritis: bathwater or baby? J Rheumatol 2009;36(9):1861–3.
22. Daly M, Alikhan A, Armstrong AW. Combination systemic therapies in psoriatic arthritis. J Dermatolog Treat 2011;22(5):276–84.

23. Kristensen LE, Gulfe A, Saxne T, et al. Efficacy and tolerability of anti-tumour necrosis factor therapy in psoriatic arthritis patients: results from the South Swedish Arthritis Treatment Group register. Ann Rheum Dis 2008;67(3):364–9.

24. Garg A, Gladman D. Recognizing psoriatic arthritis in the dermatology clinic. J Am Acad Dermatol 2010;63(5):733–48 [quiz: 749–50].

25. Thumboo J, Uramoto K, Shbeeb MI, et al. Risk factors for the development of psoriatic arthritis: a population based nested case control study. J Rheumatol 2002;29(4):757–62.

26. Scarpa R, Cosentini E, Manguso F, et al. Clinical and genetic aspects of psoriatic arthritis "sine psoriasis". J Rheumatol 2003;30(12):2638–40.

27. Wilson FC, Icen M, Crowson CS, et al. Incidence and clinical predictors of psoriatic arthritis in patients with psoriasis: a population-based study. Arthritis Rheum 2009;61(2):233–9.

28. Gottlieb AB, Kircik L, Eisen D, et al. Use of etanercept for psoriatic arthritis in the dermatology clinic: the Experience diagnosing, understanding care, and treatment with etanercept (EDUCATE) study. J Dermatolog Treat 2006;17(6):343–52.

29. Reich K, Kruger K, Mossner R, et al. Epidemiology and clinical pattern of psoriatic arthritis in Germany: a prospective interdisciplinary epidemiological study of 1511 patients with plaque-type psoriasis. Br J Dermatol 2009;160(5):1040–7.

30. Brockbank J, Gladman D. Diagnosis and management of psoriatic arthritis. Drugs 2002;62(17): 2447–57.

31. Wollina U, Unger L, Heinig B, et al. Psoriatic arthritis. Dermatol Ther 2010;23(2):123–36.

32. Gladman DD, Farewell V, Buskila D, et al. Reliability of measurements of active and damaged joints in psoriatic arthritis. J Rheumatol 1990;17(1):62–4.

33. Kavanaugh A, Ritchlin C, Rahman P, et al. Ustekinumab, an anti-IL-12/23 p40 monoclonal antibody, inhibits radiographic progression in patients with active psoriatic arthritis: results of an integrated analysis of radiographic data from the phase 3, multicentre, randomised, double-blind, placebo-controlled PSUMMIT-1 and PSUMMIT-2 trials. Ann Rheum Dis 2014;73(6):1000–6.

34. Anandarajah A. Imaging in psoriatic arthritis. Clin Rev Allergy Immunol 2013;44(2):157–65.

35. Taylor W, Gladman D, Helliwell P, et al. Classification criteria for psoriatic arthritis: development of new criteria from a large international study. Arthritis Rheum 2006;54(8):2665–73.

36. Ritchlin C, Haas-Smith SA, Hicks D, et al. Patterns of cytokine production in psoriatic synovium. J Rheumatol 1998;25(8):1544–52.

37. Thorleifsdottir RH, Sigurdardottir SL, Sigurgeirsson B, et al. Improvement of psoriasis after tonsillectomy is associated with a decrease in the frequency of circulating T cells that recognize streptococcal determinants and homologous skin determinants. J Immunol 2012;188(10):5160–5.

38. Grice EA, Segre JA. The skin microbiome. Nat Rev Microbiol 2011;9(4):244–53.

39. Pattison E, Harrison BJ, Griffiths CE, et al. Environmental risk factors for the development of psoriatic arthritis: results from a case-control study. Ann Rheum Dis 2008;67(5):672–6.

40. Eder L, Shanmugarajah S, Thavaneswaran A, et al. The association between smoking and the development of psoriatic arthritis among psoriasis patients. Ann Rheum Dis 2012;71(2):219–24.

41. Soltani-Arabshahi R, Wong B, Feng BJ, et al. Obesity in early adulthood as a risk factor for psoriatic arthritis. Arch Dermatol 2010;146(7):721–6.

42. McDonough E, Ayearst R, Eder L, et al. Depression and anxiety in psoriatic disease: prevalence and associated factors. J Rheumatol 2014;41(5):887–96.

43. Rosen CF, Mussani F, Chandran V, et al. Patients with psoriatic arthritis have worse quality of life than those with psoriasis alone. Rheumatology (Oxford) 2012;51(3):571–6.

44. Harvima RJ, Viinamaki H, Harvima IT, et al. Association of psychic stress with clinical severity and symptoms of psoriatic patients. Acta Derm Venereol 1996;76(6):467–71.

45. Freire M, Rodriguez J, Moller I, et al. Prevalence of symptoms of anxiety and depression in patients with psoriatic arthritis attending rheumatology clinics. Reumatol Clin 2011;7(1):20–6 [in Spanish].

46. Tyring S, Gottlieb A, Papp K, et al. Etanercept and clinical outcomes, fatigue, and depression in psoriasis: double-blind placebo-controlled randomised phase III trial. Lancet 2006;367(9504):29–35.

47. Punzi L, Podswiadek M, Oliviero F, et al. Laboratory findings in psoriatic arthritis. Reumatismo 2007; 59(Suppl 1):52–5.

48. Gossec L, Smolen JS, Gaujoux-Viala C, et al. European League Against Rheumatism recommendations for the management of psoriatic arthritis with pharmacological therapies. Ann Rheum Dis 2012; 71(1):4–12.

49. Ritchlin CT, Kavanaugh A, Gladman DD, et al. Treatment recommendations for psoriatic arthritis. Ann Rheum Dis 2009;68(9):1387–94.

50. Clegg DO, Reda DJ, Abdellatif M. Comparison of sulfasalazine and placebo for the treatment of axial and peripheral articular manifestations of the seronegative spondylarthropathies: a Department of Veterans Affairs cooperative study. Arthritis Rheum 1999;42(11):2325–9.

51. Brandt J, Haibel H, Cornely D, et al. Successful treatment of active ankylosing spondylitis with the anti-tumor necrosis factor alpha monoclonal antibody infliximab. Arthritis Rheum 2000;43(6): 1346–52.

52. Baraliakos X, Brandt J, Listing J, et al. Outcome of patients with active ankylosing spondylitis after two years of therapy with etanercept: clinical and magnetic resonance imaging data. Arthritis Rheum 2005;53(6):856–63.

53. van der Heijde D, Kivitz A, Schiff MH, et al. Efficacy and safety of adalimumab in patients with ankylosing spondylitis: results of a multicenter, randomized, double-blind, placebo-controlled trial. Arthritis Rheum 2006;54(7):2136–46.

54. Inman RD, Davis JC Jr, Heijde D, et al. Efficacy and safety of golimumab in patients with ankylosing spondylitis: results of a randomized, double-blind, placebo-controlled, phase III trial. Arthritis Rheum 2008;58(11):3402–12.

55. Landewe R, Braun J, Deodhar A, et al. Efficacy of certolizumab pegol on signs and symptoms of axial spondyloarthritis including ankylosing spondylitis: 24-week results of a double-blind randomised placebo-controlled Phase 3 study. Ann Rheum Dis 2014;73(1):39–47.

56. Poddubnyy D, Hermann KG, Callhoff J, et al. Ustekinumab for the treatment of patients with active ankylosing spondylitis: results of a 28-week, prospective, open-label, proof-of-concept study (TOPAS). Ann Rheum Dis 2014;73:817–23.

57. Nash P. Therapies for axial disease in psoriatic arthritis. A systematic review. J Rheumatol 2006; 33(7):1431–4.

58. Gottlieb AB. Psoriasis: emerging therapeutic strategies. Nat Rev Drug Discov 2005;4(1):19–34.

59. Gottlieb A, Narang K. Ustekinumab in the treatment of psoriatic arthritis: latest findings and clinical potential. Ther Adv Musculoskelet Dis 2013; 5(5):277–85.

60. Ritchlin CM, IK A, Puig L, et al. Maintenance of efficacy and safety of ustekinumab in patients with active psoriatic arthritis despite prior conventional nonbiologic and anti-TNF biologic therapy: 1 year results of a phase 3, multicenter, double-blind, placebo-controlled trial. American College of Rheumatology/ARHP Annual Meeting. San Diego, October 26–30, 2013.

61. Baraliakos X, Davis J, Tsuji W, et al. Magnetic resonance imaging examinations of the spine in patients with ankylosing spondylitis before and after therapy with the tumor necrosis factor alpha receptor fusion protein etanercept. Arthritis Rheum 2005; 52(4):1216–23.

62. Laine L. Nonsteroidal anti-inflammatory drug gastropathy. Gastrointest Endosc Clin N Am 1996; 6(3):489–504.

63. Gislason GH, Rasmussen JN, Abildstrom SZ, et al. Increased mortality and cardiovascular morbidity associated with use of nonsteroidal anti-inflammatory drugs in chronic heart failure. Arch Intern Med 2009;169(2):141–9.

64. McCarty DJ. Treatment of rheumatoid joint inflammation with triamcinolone hexacetonide. Arthritis Rheum 1972;15(2):157–73.

65. Papadopoulou C, Kostik M, Gonzalez-Fernandez MI, et al. Delineating the role of multiple intraarticular corticosteroid injections in the management of juvenile idiopathic arthritis in the biologic era. Arthritis Care Res 2013;65(7):1112–20.

66. Lebwohl M, Ali S. Treatment of psoriasis. Part 2. Systemic therapies. J Am Acad Dermatol 2001; 45(5):649–61 [quiz: 662–4].

67. Kingsley GH, Kowalczyk A, Taylor H, et al. A randomized placebo-controlled trial of methotrexate in psoriatic arthritis. Rheumatology (Oxford) 2012;51(8):1368–77.

68. Willkens RF, Williams HJ, Ward JR, et al. Randomized, double-blind, placebo controlled trial of low-dose pulse methotrexate in psoriatic arthritis. Arthritis Rheum 1984;27(4):376–81.

69. Lie E, van der Heijde D, Uhlig T, et al. Effectiveness and retention rates of methotrexate in psoriatic arthritis in comparison with methotrexate-treated patients with rheumatoid arthritis. Ann Rheum Dis 2010;69(4):671–6.

70. Menter A, Korman NJ, Elmets CA, et al. Guidelines of care for the management of psoriasis and psoriatic arthritis. Section 3. Guidelines of care for the management and treatment of psoriasis with topical therapies. J Am Acad Dermatol 2009; 60(4):643–59.

71. Hamilton RA, Kremer JM. Why intramuscular methotrexate may be more efficacious than oral dosing in patients with rheumatoid arthritis. Br J Rheumatol 1997;36(1):86–90.

72. van Ede AE, Laan RF, Rood MJ, et al. Effect of folic or folinic acid supplementation on the toxicity and efficacy of methotrexate in rheumatoid arthritis: a forty-eight week, multicenter, randomized, double-blind, placebo-controlled study. Arthritis Rheum 2001;44(7):1515–24.

73. Rosenberg P, Urwitz H, Johannesson A, et al. Psoriasis patients with diabetes type 2 are at high risk of developing liver fibrosis during methotrexate treatment. J Hepatol 2007;46(6):1111–8.

74. Schmeling H, Foeldvari I, Horneff G. A39: efficacy and safety of methotrexate in oligoarticular persistent juvenile idiopathic arthritis. Arthritis Rheumatol 2014;66(Suppl 11):S59.

75. Behrens F, Finkenwirth C, Pavelka K, et al. Leflunomide in psoriatic arthritis: results from a large European prospective observational study. Arthritis Care Res 2013;65(3):464–70.

76. Kaltwasser JP, Nash P, Gladman D, et al. Efficacy and safety of leflunomide in the treatment of psoriatic arthritis and psoriasis: a multinational, double-blind, randomized, placebo-controlled clinical trial. Arthritis Rheum 2004;50(6):1939–50.

77. Mease PJ, Armstrong AW. Managing patients with psoriatic disease: the diagnosis and pharmacologic treatment of psoriatic arthritis in patients with psoriasis. Drugs 2014;74(4):423–41.

78. Menter A, Korman NJ, Elmets CA, et al. Guidelines of care for the management of psoriasis and psoriatic arthritis: section 4. Guidelines of care for the management and treatment of psoriasis with traditional systemic agents. J Am Acad Dermatol 2009; 61(3):451–85.

79. Tynjala P, Vahasalo P, Tarkiainen M, et al. Aggressive combination drug therapy in very early polyarticular juvenile idiopathic arthritis (ACUTE-JIA): a multicentre randomised open-label clinical trial. Ann Rheum Dis 2011;70(9):1605–12.

80. Salvarani C, Macchioni P, Olivieri I, et al. A comparison of cyclosporine, sulfasalazine, and symptomatic therapy in the treatment of psoriatic arthritis. J Rheumatol 2001;28(10):2274–82.

81. Flytstrom I, Stenberg B, Svensson A, et al. Methotrexate vs. ciclosporin in psoriasis: effectiveness, quality of life and safety. A randomized controlled trial. Br J Dermatol 2008;158(1):116–21.

82. Dadlani C, Orlow SJ. Treatment of children and adolescents with methotrexate, cyclosporine, and etanercept: review of the dermatologic and rheumatologic literature. J Am Acad Dermatol 2005; 52(2):316–40.

83. Menter A, Korman NJ, Elmets CA, et al. Guidelines of care for the management of psoriasis and psoriatic arthritis: section 6. Guidelines of care for the treatment of psoriasis and psoriatic arthritis: case-based presentations and evidence-based conclusions. J Am Acad Dermatol 2011;65(1): 137–74.

84. Mease PJ, Fleischmann R, Deodhar AA, et al. Effect of certolizumab pegol on signs and symptoms in patients with psoriatic arthritis: 24-week results of a Phase 3 double-blind randomised placebo-controlled study (RAPID-PsA). Ann Rheum Dis 2014;73(1):48–55.

85. McInnes IB, Kavanaugh A, Gottlieb AB, et al. Efficacy and safety of ustekinumab in patients with active psoriatic arthritis: 1 year results of the phase 3, multicentre, double-blind, placebo-controlled PSUMMIT 1 trial. Lancet 2013;382(9894):780–9.

86. Kavanaugh A, Mease PJ, Gomez-Reino JJ, et al. Treatment of psoriatic arthritis in a phase 3 randomised, placebo-controlled trial with apremilast, an oral phosphodiesterase 4 inhibitor. Ann Rheum Dis 2014;73:1020–6.

87. Mease PJ, Kivitz AJ, Burch FX, et al. Etanercept treatment of psoriatic arthritis: safety, efficacy, and effect on disease progression. Arthritis Rheum 2004;50(7):2264–72.

88. Gottlieb AB, Matheson RT, Lowe N, et al. A randomized trial of etanercept as monotherapy for psoriasis. Arch Dermatol 2003;139(12):1627–32 [discussion: 1632].

89. Salvarani C, Pipitone N, Catanoso M, et al. Adalimumab in psoriatic arthritis. J Rheumatol Suppl 2012;89:77–81.

90. Gordon KB, Langley RG, Leonardi C, et al. Clinical response to adalimumab treatment in patients with moderate to severe psoriasis: double-blind, randomized controlled trial and open-label extension study. J Am Acad Dermatol 2006;55(4):598–606.

91. Antoni CE, Kavanaugh A, Kirkham B, et al. Sustained benefits of infliximab therapy for dermatologic and articular manifestations of psoriatic arthritis: results from the infliximab multinational psoriatic arthritis controlled trial (IMPACT). Arthritis Rheum 2005;52(4):1227–36.

92. Reich K, Nestle FO, Papp K, et al. Infliximab induction and maintenance therapy for moderate-to-severe psoriasis: a phase III, multicentre, double-blind trial. Lancet 2005;366(9494):1367–74.

93. Kavanaugh A, van der Heijde D, McInnes IB, et al. Golimumab in psoriatic arthritis: one-year clinical efficacy, radiographic, and safety results from a phase III, randomized, placebo-controlled trial. Arthritis Rheum 2012;64(8):2504–17.

94. Kavanaugh A, McInnes IB, Mease P, et al. Clinical efficacy, radiographic and safety findings through 5 years of subcutaneous golimumab treatment in patients with active psoriatic arthritis: results from a long-term extension of a randomised, placebo-controlled trial (the GO-REVEAL study). Ann Rheum Dis 2014;73(9):1689–94.

95. Reich K, Ortonne JP, Gottlieb AB, et al. Successful treatment of moderate to severe plaque psoriasis with the PEGylated Fab' certolizumab pegol: results of a phase II randomized, placebo-controlled trial with a re-treatment extension. Br J Dermatol 2012; 167(1):180–90.

96. Griffiths CE, Strober BE, van de Kerkhof P, et al. Comparison of ustekinumab and etanercept for moderate-to-severe psoriasis. N Engl J Med 2010;362(2):118–28.

97. Papp KA, Kaufmann R, Thaci D, et al. Efficacy and safety of apremilast in subjects with moderate to severe plaque psoriasis: results from a phase II, multicenter, randomized, double-blind, placebo-controlled, parallel-group, dose-comparison study. J Eur Acad Dermatol Venereol 2013;27(3): e376–83.

98. Lovell DJ, Reiff A, Ilowite NT, et al. Safety and efficacy of up to eight years of continuous etanercept therapy in patients with juvenile rheumatoid arthritis. Arthritis Rheum 2008;58(5):1496–504.

99. Lovell DJ, Reiff A, Jones OY, et al. Long-term safety and efficacy of etanercept in children with polyarticular-course juvenile rheumatoid arthritis. Arthritis Rheum 2006;54(6):1987–94.

100. Ruperto N, Lovell DJ, Cuttica R, et al. Long-term efficacy and safety of infliximab plus methotrexate for the treatment of polyarticular-course juvenile rheumatoid arthritis: findings from an open-label treatment extension. Ann Rheum Dis 2010;69(4): 718–22.

101. Visvanathan S, Wagner C, Marini JC, et al. The effect of infliximab plus methotrexate on the modulation of inflammatory disease markers in juvenile idiopathic arthritis: analyses from a randomized, placebo-controlled trial. Pediatr Rheumatol Online J 2010; 8:24.

102. Biester S, Deuter C, Michels H, et al. Adalimumab in the therapy of uveitis in childhood. Br J Ophthalmol 2007;91(3):319–24.

103. Tynjala P, Kotaniemi K, Lindahl P, et al. Adalimumab in juvenile idiopathic arthritis-associated chronic anterior uveitis. Rheumatology (Oxford) 2008;47(3):339–44.

104. Gladman D, Fleischmann R, Coteur G, et al. Effect of certolizumab pegol on multiple facets of psoriatic arthritis as reported by patients: 24-week patient-reported outcome results of the RAPID-PsA study. Arthritis Care Res 2014;66:1085–92.

105. Chang CA, Gottlieb AB, Lizzul PF. Management of psoriatic arthritis from the view of the dermatologist. Nat Rev Rheumatol 2011;7(10):588–98.

106. Yeaw J, Watson C, Fox KM, et al. Treatment patterns following discontinuation of adalimumab, etanercept, and infliximab in a us managed care sample. Adv Ther 2014;31(4):410–25.

107. Thorlund K, Druyts E, Avina-Zubieta JA, et al. Anti-tumor necrosis factor (TNF) drugs for the treatment of psoriatic arthritis: an indirect comparison meta-analysis. Biologics 2012;6:417–27.

108. Lubrano E, Spadaro A. Pharmacoeconomic burden in the treatment of psoriatic arthritis: from systematic reviews to real clinical practice studies. BMC Musculoskelet Disord 2014;15:25.

109. Ruperto N, Lovell DJ, Cuttica R, et al. A randomized, placebo-controlled trial of infliximab plus methotrexate for the treatment of polyarticular-course juvenile rheumatoid arthritis. Arthritis Rheum 2007;56(9):3096–106.

110. Filer C, Ho P, Smith RL, et al. Investigation of association of the IL12B and IL23R genes with psoriatic arthritis. Arthritis Rheum 2008;58(12):3705–9.

111. Sato K, Suematsu A, Okamoto K, et al. Th17 functions as an osteoclastogenic helper T cell subset that links T cell activation and bone destruction. J Exp Med 2006;203(12):2673–82.

112. Malfait AM, Butler DM, Presky DH, et al. Blockade of IL-12 during the induction of collagen-induced arthritis (CIA) markedly attenuates the severity of the arthritis. Clin Exp Immunol 1998;111(2):377–83.

113. Gottlieb A, Menter A, Mendelsohn A, et al. Ustekinumab, a human interleukin 12/23 monoclonal antibody, for psoriatic arthritis: randomised, double-blind, placebo-controlled, crossover trial. Lancet 2009;373(9664):633–40.

114. van der Heijde D, Sharp J, Wassenberg S, et al. Psoriatic arthritis imaging: a review of scoring methods. Ann Rheum Dis 2005;64(Suppl 2):ii61–4.

115. Ritchlin C, Rahman P, Kavanaugh A, et al. Efficacy and safety of the anti-IL-12/23 p40 monoclonal antibody, ustekinumab, in patients with active psoriatic arthritis despite conventional non-biological and biological anti-tumour necrosis factor therapy: 6-month and 1-year results of the phase 3, multicentre, double-blind, placebo-controlled, randomised PSUMMIT 2 trial. Ann Rheum Dis 2014; 73(6):990–9.

116. Dommasch ED, Troxel AB, Gelfand JM. Major cardiovascular events associated with anti-IL 12/23 agents: a tale of two meta-analyses. J Am Acad Dermatol 2013;68(5):863–5.

117. Kimball AB, Papp KA, Wasfi Y, et al. Long-term efficacy of ustekinumab in patients with moderate-to-severe psoriasis treated for up to 5 years in the PHOENIX 1 study. J Eur Acad Dermatol Venereol 2013;27(12):1535–45.

118. Kimball AB, Leonardi C, Stahle M, et al. Demography, baseline disease characteristics, and treatment history of patients with psoriasis enrolled in a multicenter, prospective, disease-based registry (PSOLAR). Br J Dermatol 2014;171(1):137–47.

119. Varada S, Tintle SJ, Gottlieb AB. Apremilast for the treatment of psoriatic arthritis. Expert Rev Clin Pharmacol 2014;7(3):239–50.

120. Adamopoulos IE, Pflanz S. The emerging role of interleukin 27 in inflammatory arthritis and bone destruction. Cytokine Growth Factor Rev 2013; 24(2):115–21.

121. Genovese MC, Greenwald M, Cho CS, et al. Phase 2 randomized study of subcutaneous ixekizumab, an Anti-IL-17 monoclonal antibody, in biologic-naive or TNF-IR patients with rheumatoid arthritis. Arthritis Rheumatol 2014;66(7): 1693–704.

122. Papp KA, Leonardi C, Menter A, et al. Brodalumab, an anti-interleukin-17-receptor antibody for psoriasis. N Engl J Med 2012;366(13):1181–9.

123. Hueber W, Patel DD, Dryja T, et al. Effects of AIN457, a fully human antibody to interleukin-17A, on psoriasis, rheumatoid arthritis, and uveitis. Sci Transl Med 2010;2(52):52ra72.

124. Zhang L, Yang XQ, Cheng J, et al. Increased Th17 cells are accompanied by FoxP3(+) Treg cell accumulation and correlated with psoriasis disease severity. Clin Immunol 2010;135(1):108–17.

125. Chao CC, Chen SJ, Adamopoulos IE, et al. Anti-IL-17A therapy protects against bone erosion in experimental models of rheumatoid arthritis. Autoimmunity 2011;44(3):243–52.

126. McInnes IB, Sieper J, Braun J, et al. Efficacy and safety of secukinumab, a fully human anti-interleukin-17A monoclonal antibody, in patients with moderate-to-severe psoriatic arthritis: a 24-week, randomised, double-blind, placebo-controlled, phase II proof-of-concept trial. Ann Rheum Dis 2014;73(2):349–56.

127. Leonardi C, Matheson R, Zachariae C, et al. Anti-interleukin-17 monoclonal antibody ixekizumab in chronic plaque psoriasis. N Engl J Med 2012; 366(13):1190–9.

128. Mease P, Genovese MC, Gladstein G, et al. Abatacept in the treatment of patients with psoriatic arthritis: results of a six-month, multicenter, randomized, double-blind, placebo-controlled, phase II trial. Arthritis Rheum 2011;63(4):939–48.

129. Papp KA, Menter A, Strober B, et al. Efficacy and safety of tofacitinib, an oral Janus kinase inhibitor, in the treatment of psoriasis: a Phase 2b randomized placebo-controlled dose-ranging study. Br J Dermatol 2012;167(3):668–77.

130. Papp KA, Langley RG, Sigurgeirsson B, et al. Efficacy and safety of secukinumab in the treatment of moderate-to-severe plaque psoriasis: a randomized, double-blind, placebo-controlled phase II dose-ranging study. Br J Dermatol 2013;168(2): 412–21.

131. Available at: http://www.skinandallergynews.com/news/conference-news/american-academy-of-dermatology-annual-meeting-2013/single-article/psoriasis-drug-mk-3222-progresses-through-pipeline/eab1780ca1924cf44d735207b8823054.html. Accessed December 7, 2013. WSPdM-ptpSAN.

132. Jancin B. Secukinumab soars in phase III psoriasis studies. Rheumatology News Online 2013;2013.

133. SW. Psoriasis drug MK-3222 progresses through pipeline. Skin Allergy News 2013.

134. Sofen H, Smith S, Matheson RT, et al. Guselkumab (an IL-23-specific mAb) demonstrates clinical and molecular response in patients with moderate-to-severe psoriasis. J Allergy Clin Immunol 2014; 133(4):1032–40.

135. Ruperto N, Lovell DJ, Quartier P, et al. Abatacept in children with juvenile idiopathic arthritis: a randomised, double-blind, placebo-controlled withdrawal trial. Lancet 2008;372(9636):383–91.

136. Meyer SC, Levine RL. Molecular pathways: molecular basis for sensitivity and resistance to jak kinase inhibitors. Clin Cancer Res 2014;20(8):2051–9.

137. Zerbini CA, Lomonte AB. Tofacitinib for the treatment of rheumatoid arthritis. Expert Rev Clin Immunol 2012;8(4):319–31.

138. van der Heijde D, Tanaka Y, Fleischmann R, et al. Tofacitinib (CP-690,550) in patients with rheumatoid arthritis receiving methotrexate: twelve-month data from a twenty-four-month phase III randomized radiographic study. Arthritis Rheum 2013; 65(3):559–70.

139. Heinecke GM, Luber AJ, Levitt JO, et al. Combination use of ustekinumab with other systemic therapies: a retrospective study in a tertiary referral center. J Drugs Dermatol 2013;12(10):1098–102.

140. Ryan C, Korman NJ, Gelfand JM, et al. Research gaps in psoriasis: opportunities for future studies. J Am Acad Dermatol 2014;70(1):146–67.

141. Scarpa R, Cuocolo A, Peluso R, et al. Early psoriatic arthritis: the clinical spectrum. J Rheumatol 2008;35(1):137–41.

142. Fraser AD, van Kuijk AW, Westhovens R, et al. A randomised, double blind, placebo controlled, multicentre trial of combination therapy with methotrexate plus ciclosporin in patients with active psoriatic arthritis. Ann Rheum Dis 2005;64(6): 859–64.

143. Baranauskaite A, Raffayova H, Kungurov NV, et al. Infliximab plus methotrexate is superior to methotrexate alone in the treatment of psoriatic arthritis in methotrexate-naive patients: the RESPOND study. Ann Rheum Dis 2012;71(4):541–8.

144. Gottlieb AB, Langley RG, Strober BE, et al. A randomized, double-blind, placebo-controlled study to evaluate the addition of methotrexate to etanercept in patients with moderate to severe plaque psoriasis. Br J Dermatol 2012;167(3):649–57.

145. Fagerli KM, Lie E, van der Heijde D, et al. The role of methotrexate co-medication in TNF-inhibitor treatment in patients with psoriatic arthritis: results from 440 patients included in the NOR-DMARD study. Ann Rheum Dis 2014;73(1):132–7.

146. Kristensen LE, Geborek P, Saxne T. Dose escalation of infliximab therapy in arthritis patients is related to diagnosis and concomitant methotrexate treatment: observational results from the South Swedish Arthritis Treatment Group register. Rheumatology (Oxford) 2009;48(3):243–5.

147. Atzeni F, Boccassini L, Antivalle M, et al. Etanercept plus ciclosporin versus etanercept plus methotrexate for maintaining clinical control over psoriatic arthritis: a randomised pilot study. Ann Rheum Dis 2011;70(4):712–4.

148. Zangger P, Gladman DD, Bogoch ER. Musculoskeletal surgery in psoriatic arthritis. J Rheumatol 1998;25(4):725–9.

149. Shbeeb M, Uramoto KM, Gibson LE, et al. The epidemiology of psoriatic arthritis in Olmsted County, Minnesota, USA, 1982-1991. J Rheumatol 2000;27(5):1247–50.

150. Zangger P, Gladman DD, Urowitz MB, et al. Outcome of total hip replacement for avascular necrosis in systemic lupus erythematosus. J Rheumatol 2000;27(4): 919–23.

151. Glintborg B, Ostergaard M, Krogh NS, et al. Clinical response, drug survival, and predictors thereof among 548 patients with psoriatic arthritis who switched tumor necrosis factor alpha inhibitor

therapy: results from the Danish Nationwide DAN-BIO Registry. Arthritis Rheum 2013;65(5):1213–23.

152. Menter A, Feldman SR, Weinstein GD, et al. A randomized comparison of continuous vs. intermittent infliximab maintenance regimens over 1 year in the treatment of moderate-to-severe plaque psoriasis. J Am Acad Dermatol 2007;56(1): 31.e1–15.

153. Ramirez-Fort MK, Levin AA, Au SC, et al. Continuous versus intermittent therapy for moderate-to-severe psoriasis. Clin Exp Rheumatol 2013;31(4 Suppl 78):S63–70.

154. Jani M, Macphie E, Rao C, et al. Effectiveness of switching between biologics in psoriatic arthritis-results of a large regional survey. Clin Med 2014; 14(1):95–6.

155. de Vlam K, Gottlieb AB, Mease PJ. Current concepts in psoriatic arthritis: pathogenesis and management. Acta Derm Venereol 2014. [Epub ahead of print].

156. Friedewald VE, Cather JC, Gelfand JM, et al. AJC editor's consensus: psoriasis and coronary artery disease. Am J Cardiol 2008;102(12):1631–43.

157. Kimball AB, Gladman D, Gelfand JM, et al. National psoriasis foundation clinical consensus on psoriasis comorbidities and recommendations for screening. J Am Acad Dermatol 2008;58(6): 1031–42.

158. Costa L, Caso F, Atteno M, et al. Impact of 24-month treatment with etanercept, adalimumab, or methotrexate on metabolic syndrome components in a cohort of 210 psoriatic arthritis patients. Clin Rheumatol 2014;33(6):833–9.

159. Kilic B, Dogan U, Parlak AH, et al. Ocular findings in patients with psoriasis. Int J Dermatol 2013; 52(5):554–9.

160. van der Horst-Bruinsma IE, Nurmohamed MT, Landewe RB. Comorbidities in patients with spondyloarthritis. Rheum Dis Clin North Am 2012; 38(3):523–38.

Pharmacogenomics and the Resulting Impact on Psoriasis Therapies

Amy C. Foulkes, MD, Richard B. Warren, MD, PhD*

KEYWORDS

- Psoriasis • Pharmacogenomics • Pharmacogenetics • Next generation sequencing
- Metabolomics • Bioinformatics • Personalised medicine

KEY POINTS

- Pharmacogenomics is the study of the relationship between drug response and a genomic test, broadly to include changes in the genome, epigenome, transcriptome, proteome, or metabolome.
- Stratified medicine refers to the potential to make clinical decisions based on a pharmacogenomic test by adjusting dosage or choosing a different drug.
- Psoriasis is a model disease for the development of pharmacogenomic markers of treatment response, with ready access to diseased tissue and objective validated outcome measures.
- With the application of state-of-the-art technologies and investment in careful experimental design, the goal of stratified medicine in psoriasis may be possible.

INTRODUCTION

Pharmacogenomics

The way in which an individual responds to a drug is affected by many factors, including those related to the drug, the disease, and the individual. *Pharmacogenetics*, a term suggested by Vogel in 1959, is the study of relationships between genetic polymorphisms and drug response.[1]

A gene can be defined as exhibiting a polymorphism if the variant allele exists in the normal population at a frequency of at least 1% (Meyer 2000). The most frequent type of polymorphism is a single nucleotide polymorphism (SNP); however, they can take on several forms, including nucleotide repeat sequences. Polymorphisms may result in altered efficacy or toxicity of a given drug through mechanisms such as alteration of its absorption, distribution, metabolism, and elimination.

The presence of a genetic polymorphism is not the only way in which drug response may vary; the potential for posttranslational changes, including gene–environmental interactions, also is critical. Although the terms *pharmacogenetics* and *pharmacogenomics* are often used interchangeably, pharmacogenomics encompasses changes in not just the DNA code but also the transcriptome, metabolome, and epigenome and their interrelationships to identify their influence on response to treatment.

Disclosure: A.C. Foulkes has received educational support to attend conferences from or acted as a consultant for Pfizer, AbbVie, Leo Pharma, Novartis and Janssen, all of which manufacture therapies used in the treatment of psoriasis. R.B. Warren has acted as a consultant and/or speaker for Abbvie, Amgen, Janssen Cilag, Leo Pharma, Pfizer, Novartis and Schering-Plough (now MSD), all of which manufacture therapies used in the treatment of psoriasis.

The Dermatology Centre, Manchester Academic Health Science Centre, Salford Royal NHS Foundation Trust, The University of Manchester, Salford, Manchester M6 8HD, UK

* Corresponding author. The Dermatology Centre, Salford Royal Foundation Hospital, The University of Manchester, Salford, Manchester, M6 8HD, UK.

E-mail address: Richard.Warren@manchester.ac.uk

Dermatol Clin 33 (2015) 149–160
http://dx.doi.org/10.1016/j.det.2014.09.011

derm.theclinics.com

Personalized Therapies

When a pharmacogenomic investigation finds a marker or markers predictive of response to treatment, there is potential for making clinical decisions based on a pharmacogenomic test by adjusting the dosage or choosing a different drug. Drug treatment may be referred to as targeted, as each patient may have treatment selected based on their own rather than population characteristics. This process is referred to as *personalized* or *stratified* medicine. Advantages of the application of pharmacogenomics are far reaching, allowing minimization of treatment cost and the improvement of treatment safety through the reduction in adverse events. Furthermore, individualization of therapy may allow drug repositioning, as an existing therapy may be newly applied to a selected cohort of another disease. To achieve the goals of personalized medicine, testing in the field must be accurate in predicting drug response and be cost effective. The potential properties of an ideal pharmacogenomic test are shown in **Fig. 1.**

The Successes of Personalized Medicine in Other Fields

Translation of pharmacogenomic studies has resulted in major successes in personalized medicine, exemplified by progress in oncology.

A key example is that of the epidermal growth factor receptor (EGFR) pathway with activation being necessary before the development of non-–small cell lung cancer. As a result, EGFR has become a key focus for the development of targeted therapy[2,3] with certain chemotherapeutic agents only being suitable in individuals expressing specific mutation in the EGFR gene.[4] Diseased tissue, in the form of cancer biopsy specimens, allows ready testing of individual genetic/genomic markers but is often challenging to obtain because of anatomy or access. In the case of EGFR inhibitor therapies, a focus on the development of genomic markers extracted from blood rather than tissue may soon be possible.[5]

Inflammatory Conditions

Numerous studies have sought genetic determinants to therapies in the treatment of inflammatory conditions such as rheumatoid arthritis, asthma, and inflammatory bowel disease.

In the treatment of rheumatoid arthritis, the common tumor necrosis factor (*TNF*) −308G>A promoter-region polymorphism was found to be modestly predictive of poor responses to TNFI therapy, irrespective of the agent used.[6] Variation in the *CD84* gene, which encodes SLAM family member 5 (also known as leukocyte-differentiation antigen CD84), has been shown to be predictive of responsiveness to the soluble TNF receptor 2 fusion protein, etanercept ($P = 8 \times 10^{-8}$), and the *PDE3A–SLCO1C1* locus, which harbor the genes encoding cGMP-inhibited 3′,5′-cyclic phosphodiesterase A and solute carrier organic anion transporter family member 1C1, has been associated with response to the TNF inhibitors etanercept, infliximab, and adalimumab.

In the study of asthma, genes have been identified as important in the response to both inhaled corticosteroids and inhaled short-acting β-agonists.[7,8] Transcriptome profiling is now being used to offer a novel and comprehensive assessment of glucocorticoid response.[9] For those with severe disease, the drug pipeline of biologic therapies holds great promise, with TNF inhibitors forming only part of the number of agents, with others targets including interleukin (IL)-4, the IL-4 receptor, and IL-13. The hope is that these therapies may be personalized, and interaction has been shown between anti–IL-4 receptor-α therapy and IL4RA gene variation.[10]

However, none of the described associations have yet proven sufficiently predictive to inform clinical decisions regarding selection of the most appropriate therapy for individual patients.

Pharmacogenomics and Dermatology

Melanoma treatment

Improved survival in melanoma has been reported in those treated with the *BRAF* kinase inhibitor,

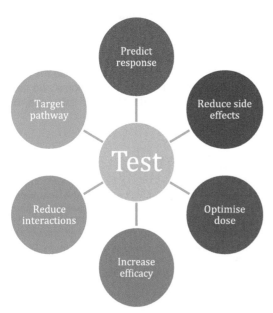

Fig. 1. Properties of an ideal pharmacogenomic test.

vemurafenib, with a V600E mutation in the *BRAF* gene. In a phase III clinical trial, treatment with vemurafenib was compared with the melanoma chemotherapy agent, dacarbazine.[11] At the time of study, dacarbazine was the only agent approved by the US Food and Drug Administration for the treatment of metastatic melanoma. Mutations in the proto-oncogene *BRAF* gene led to downstream activation of MAPK pathway and occur in 40% to 60% of melanomas with 90% of these mutations resulting in the substitution of glutamic acid for valine at codon 600 (*BRAF V600E*). Although these targeted therapies have shown some clinical promise, their use has been limited by partial response and high relapse rates.[12] The overall survival benefit is modest, with various mechanisms of drug resistance described, and future efforts may rely on the development of successful combination therapies aimed at simultaneously targeting tumor mechanisms and circumventing resistance strategies.[12,13]

Azathioprine dosing

Azathioprine dosing based on thiopurine methyltransferase (TPMT) measurement provides an example of the application of pharmacogenetics in dermatology. Common polymorphisms in TPMT, a key enzyme in thiopurine metabolism, can lead to variable levels of myelosuppression in individuals treated with azathioprine. A randomized, placebo-controlled, double-blind trial of azathioprine use in moderate-to-severe atopic eczema determined that with use of a TPMT-based azathioprine dose regimen, drug efficacy could be maintained while avoiding drug toxicity.[14]

Dapsone

Dapsone is a sulfonamide the licensed indications of which include use in dermatology for the treatment of dermatitis herpetiformis. Patients with glucose-6-phosphate dehydrogenase (G6PD) deficiency are susceptible to hemolysis when treated with oxidative drugs such as dapsone. G6PD exhibits high genetic diversity, and when dapsone treatment is planned, determination of G6PD status should be considered in at-risk populations.

With the assessment of TPMP and G6PD, enzyme activity is measured by the pretreatment test and not directly the patient genotype.

Pharmacogenomic Investigational Design for Psoriasis

To facilitate the advent of stratified medicine, pharmacogenomic studies must be designed with translation to the improvement of clinical care in mind. In the case of psoriasis, high-quality study design with use of adequately powered, well-phenotyped cohorts is necessary and may require application of one of the newer omics technologies. Because this field is rapidly evolving, these new technologies are briefly reviewed.

Technologies

Over recent years, the use of nucleic acid sequencing has increased exponentially as the ability to sequence has become accessible to research and clinical laboratories worldwide.[15] Next-generation sequencing refers to any technology that uses a high-throughput parallel approach to sequencing large numbers of different sequences (a library) in a single reaction. RNA profiling exploits recent advances in next-generation sequencing to provide a comprehensive measurement of the genes being expressed in a sample. RNA sequencing (RNA-Seq) can complement traditional histopathologic, immunologic, cytogenetic, and proteomic means of pharmacogenomic analysis.[16] The open platform offered by RNA-Seq also enables direct comparison with other open access research data. Although the association in genomic studies tends to be of one or more SNPs with either response to (or toxicity of) a therapy, in transcriptomic studies this may be in the form of a gene expression profile or signature of treatment response. Gene expression profiling from lesional versus nonlesional skin in a patient with psoriasis may play a key role in establishing biomarkers of treatment response in psoriasis.

Epigenetics is the study of mitotically heritable changes in gene expression that do not involve any alterations in the underlying DNA sequence. Compared with the largely static DNA sequence, the epigenetic status of the genome varies dynamically in different tissues. Identifying epigenetic abnormalities involved in the onset and progression of disease is of great relevance to the development of new therapeutic approaches because, unlike genetic mutations, epigenetic aberrations are potentially reversible with the use of pharmacologic agents. The 3 main epigenetic mechanisms are DNA methylation, histone modifications, and RNA-associated gene silencing.

Untargeted, global metabolite profiling, referred to as *metabolomics* (or *metabonomics*), can offer insight into disease processes, drug toxicity, and response to therapies.[17,18] Obtaining metabolic profiles from complex samples, such as biological fluids, requires powerful, high-resolution and information-rich analytical methods, for which spectroscopic technologies are generally used,[18] (eg, mass spectrometry). Metabolite separation techniques, including liquid chromatography, can reduce complexity and provide additional information on metabolite properties to aid metabolite identification.[17]

Pharmacogenomics of Psoriasis

Pharmacogenomic studies to date in psoriasis, as in many other areas of medicine, have been underpowered and have lacked robust, prospectively acquired data with clear delineation of disease response and adverse events, such that major advances in this important area have not been made. Studies have varied as to their application of available technologies, with some studies not designed as pharmacogenomic association studies but as investigations of genomic or transcriptomic changes with therapy that may lead to advances in understanding of psoriasis pathogenesis. These studies were, therefore, not designed primarily with power to detect association with treatment response. This finding has been exemplified by the lack of replication in studies to date.

Topical Therapies

Several early pharmacogenetic studies have evaluated a possible association between polymorphisms in the vitamin D receptor (VDR) with the clinical response to topical vitamin D analogue preparations.[19–21] Studies to date have varied in design, including the choice of topical agent and how it was administered to the patient, cohort size, time point of assessment of response, and how response has been measured (eg, patient self-reported data vs physician assessment). Studies varied in the technology applied and whether an association between the polymorphism evaluated and response to treatment was reported. When an association has been found with a polymorphism in the VDR,[22–25] the findings have not been replicated nor has the associated polymorphism been found to be functionally active. To date, no convincing biomarker of response has been found for any topical therapy used in the treatment of psoriasis.

Pharmacogenomics of Phototherapy

Pharmacogenomic studies in psoriasis patients treated with ultraviolet (UV) radiation are limited. One group investigated if interindividual differences in the cutaneous expression of a variety of drug-metabolizing and cytoprotective genes, including cytochrome P450s and drug transporters, occurred in those exposed to ultraviolet radiation.[26,27] The group found marked interindividual differences in the constitutive expression

of many drug-metabolizing enzymes. However, this study correlated the UV radiation treatment with change in gene expression rather than improvement of psoriasis. Thus, further research is required to determine the potential role of these genes as biomarkers of treatment response.

Genetic polymorphisms in the p53 gene and in the VDR gene have been evaluated in relationship to clearance of psoriasis with narrow-band UVB phototherapy in 2 studies.[28,29] The Arg/Arg homozygote state of the p53 gene was reported as significantly increased in the response group, but from patient-reported data the Taq1 VDR polymorphism was found to be predictive of remission duration.

In a study of 32 patients receiving either narrow-band UVB or bath psoralen ultraviolet A (PUVA) phototherapy, IL-6 levels were measured before and after courses of treatment, and IL-6 levels correlated with percentage reduction in the objective validated psoriasis outcome measure, Psoriasis Area and Severity Index (PASI).[30] Limitations of this approach include lack of description of participant phenotype, lack of control for additional therapies, and correlation of the investigated marker with a nonvalidated method of assessment of response.

Several studies have investigated the gene expression profile from lesional skin from patients with psoriasis treated with phototherapy,[31–33] which, although not originally intended to find a single pharmacogenomic marker of treatment response, are of interest to inform future pharmacogenomic work. An example of this work would be the identification of significant reduction in inflammatory cytokines including IL-20 and IL-23 in responding and not nonresponding plaques of psoriasis during treatment with narrow-band UVB phototherapy.[32] These findings can be taken forward for validation through adequately powered pharmacogenomic investigations.

Methotrexate

One of the largest and most comprehensive pharmacogenetic studies in psoriasis has been the evaluation of SNPs on treatment response to methotrexate.[34] Adults with chronic plaque psoriasis treated with methotrexate were recruited retrospectively, and 84 SNPs from 5 genes involved in pharmacodynamics factors related to methotrexate were analyzed. Three SNPs in the gene ABCC1 (from the efflux transporter ATP-binding cassette subfamily C) and 2 of the SNPs (introns 2 and 9) in the gene ABCG2 (ATP-binding cassette, subfamily G, member 2) were associated with response to methotrexate. No significant association was detected between clinical outcomes in patients with psoriasis treated with methotrexate and SNPs in 4 genes coding for enzymes involved in methotrexate intracellular metabolism.[35] An earlier study, which used some of the same patients studied by Warren and colleagues,[36] found that the reduced folate carrier 80A allele was associated with methotrexate toxicity and the thymidylate synthase 3′-UTR 6 base-pair deletion was associated with poor clinical response to methotrexate. Although of some promise, these studies have not been repeated and no clinical translation has yet ensued. Furthermore, characterization of treatment response retrospectively is a significant weakness of all these studies.

Acitretin

Acitretin is a synthetic retinoid that is a well-established second-line agent in the treatment of severe psoriasis. Although acitretin has relatively low efficacy and is poorly tolerated because of numerous side effects, including mucocutaneous dryness (the extent of which frequently limits dosing), hyperlipidemia, and teratogenicity,[37] it has a place as either monotherapy or in combination with phototherapy, in the treatment of a subset of patients with severe disease. There is limited pharmacogenomic work for this therapeutic agent, but polymorphisms of the apolipoprotein E gene (APOE) and the vascular endothelial growth factor gene (VEGF) have been evaluated as predictors of response to psoriasis patients treated with acitretin. Although the frequency of the APOE e4 allele (+3937C/+4075C) was higher in patients with chronic plaque and guttate psoriasis than in controls, there was no significant difference in the frequency of alleles in acitretin responders and nonresponders.[38] There was a significant increase in the frequency of the -460 TT genotype of the VEGF gene in patients who were nonresponsive to acitretin therapy compared with those who cleared with treatment, but the numbers of patients in these studies was small.[39]

Ciclosporin

Several studies have evaluated gene expression profiling during ciclosporin therapy.[40–42] All reported significant changes in disease-related genes in patients responding to ciclosporin.

All studies were limited by small cohort size. In 2 cases, the primary agent under investigation was a multifunctional cytokine, recombinant human IL-11, with ciclosporin-treated patients acting as a comparison cohort.[41,42]

Biologic therapies for psoriasis

Several pharmacogenomic studies have been carried out investigating potential predictors of biologic treatment response. Investigational approaches have varied in terms of agent(s) being studied the use of hypothesis free versus a candidate gene approach and therefore the technologies used. As in studies of biologic response in other inflammatory disorders, candidate genes for investigation include those known as markers of disease associations. Further candidates have been genes from relevant pathways of drug action including polymorphisms of receptor activity.

At least 44 SNPs in the tumor necrosis factor (TNF) gene have been identified, and 2 SNPs in the promoter region (G-to-A transitions at the -238 and -308 sites) seem to be functionally relevant, affecting TNF expression.[43] Tejasvi and colleagues[44] reported their study of 683 patients who received anti-TNF therapy or systemic agents for the treatment of psoriasis. SNPs in the promoter region of TNF were examined and compared with drug response (however, response was self-evaluated). An association was seen among adalimumab responders with the TNF-1031T/C polymorphism (overall risk, 4.43, $P = .04$).

The HLA-Cw*0602 allele of the human leukocyte antigen (HLA) class I HLA-Cw6 is the main genetic determinant of psoriasis, designated "psoriasis susceptibility" 1 (PSORS1).[45] Pharmacogenetic studies of the HLA-Cw*0602 allele have not shown an association with response to anti-TNF therapy. In a retrospective study of 98 patients with chronic plaque psoriasis treated with etanercept (n = 78) or adalimumab (n = 50), the presence of the HLA-Cw*0602 allele did not predict response to etanercept, and there was a nonsignificant trend suggesting that the HLA-Cw*0602–positive patients were more likely to respond to adalimumab.[46]

Gene expression profiling from lesional versus nonlesional skin in a patient with psoriasis may play a key role in establishing biomarkers of treatment response in psoriasis. Krueger and colleagues[47] evaluated gene expression profile from 15 patients treated with etanercept (50 mg twice weekly) at baseline and after 12 weeks of therapy. The primary outcome measure was to evaluate how "closely the transcriptome returned to the non-lesional state in responders." However, limitations of this approach include that response was determined histologically as described in the group's previous report[48] through epidermal thickness and keratin 16 immunohistochemistry from samples taken at 12 weeks of etanercept therapy (50 mg twice weekly.) The mean percentage clearance of the 16 responders from the original cohort of 20 patients was 74.5%. Improvements in objective validated outcome measures for psoriasis were not indicated.

Table 1
Checklist of requirements for pharmacogenomic study in psoriasis

Checklist Item	Subgroup	Details of Minimum Requirements	Ideal Requirements
Study design	Study protocol	Applied to all participants, especially where study conducted at multiple sites	Protocol or details published
	Power calculation	Description of determination of sample size	Power calculation declared Declare sample size where cannot reach the required and discuss
	Outcomes	Outcomes fully defined Where response to treatment, use of objective validated outcome measure, such as PASI at each visit Where numerous outcome measures recorded, clarify which score used as assessment of response in advance and which correlated with genomics	PASI 75 and 90 as measures of response to treatment, less than PASI 50 as nonresponse
	Proposed laboratory studies	Defined in advance	For genetic tests, biological plausibility discussed
Participant characteristics	Selection of participants	Description of selection process	
	Accurate phenotyping of psoriasis participants	Consultant diagnosis of psoriasis vulgaris Exclusion of other forms of psoriasis such as erythrodermic psoriasis and associated conditions, such as palmoplantar pustulosis	Designation type I or type II psoriasis ± HLA-C type
	Participant demographics	Participant details including presence or absence of PsA, washout from prior treatments and concurrent medication	
	Ethnicity	Ethnicity and ancestry of participants recorded	Ethnicity and ancestry of participants recorded and accounted for in analysis

Methodology	Publish full repeatable methodology	DNA studies to refer to checklist of requirements for pharmacogenetic study,[56] to include genotyping procedures and testing for Hardy-Weinberg equilibrium RNA studies to include reference to minimum standard of used technology, where exists[57,58] RNA studies to include details of technology used, eg, microarray chip or RNA-Seq platform, validation of microarray results using low-throughput techniques, eg, RT-PCR, assessment of RNA integrity and quality control of individual hybridizations
Results and analysis	Results reporting	Consistency of reporting of genes, gene products, and SNPs, with gene ontology listed as compliant with the HUGO Gene Nomenclature Committee and SNPs listed by accession number or reference SNP ID (rs) number
	Access to raw data	Open access to all raw data (for DNA and RNA studies) For microarray studies, MIAME-compliant microarray data deposited in a database GEO/ArrayExpress
	Statistical considerations	Genomic/transcriptomic considerations RNA studies to include listing of effect size criterion applied and derivation of P values
		Correction for multiple testing — Validated methodology

Abbreviations: PsA, psoriatic arthritis; RT-PCR, reverse transcriptase polymerase chain reaction.

The results indicated that 248 genes did not return to baseline expression after 3 months of treatment. Microarray work was conducted using a previously established psoriasis transcriptome and the current cohort assessed for resolution using the differently expressed genes from the group's previous works.[49] From these, genes with less than 75% improvement made up a residual disease genomic profile. In the group of upregulated genes, 76 probe sets (64 genes) did not improve beyond 75% with treatment and 206 probe sets (184 genes) from downregulated genes did not show 75% improvement. The microarray chips did not reliably detect several key cytokines, including interferon-γ, IL-17, and IL-22.

The team also hypothesize that altered expression of genes associated with structural cell types leaves a molecular scar in resolved plaques of psoriasis. Many of the genes that did not completely resolve with treatment involved structural cutaneous components, including markers of lymphatic endothelial cells. Biologic pathways were evaluated for gene changes. Only selected pathways are presented in the data, including the leptin pathway, in which the change was 56% improvement with treatment.

This group has further attempted to develop a genomic profile to predict histologic response to the anti-CD2 fusion protein, alefacept.[50] In a cohort of 22 patients treated with a total of 12 weekly intravenous 7.5-mg doses of alefacept, response was determined histologically as described in their earlier work.[51] Gene expression profiling was conducted on peripheral blood mononuclear cells from baseline samples, and 23 threshold genes were selected to form a classifier to predict response using the pretreatment blood measurements. The study used only a small cohort, and 2 of the nonresponding patients were misclassified as responders. Of interest, gene expression profiling was conducted in peripheral blood mononuclear cells at 24 hours of therapy. At this early time point, there was suppression of inflammatory genes, although data are not illustrated. The group previously published work on the agonistic mechanism of alefacept[52] from data from the same cohort. In this earlier work, gene expression profiling was conducted at baseline, 1, 6, and 24 hours and weeks 2, 4, and 13 (before alefacept administration). A significant increase was seen in the proinflammatory genes STAT1 and MIG within the first day of treatment, but gene expression normalized by week 13 of treatment. However, several immune-related genes were downregulated with treatment, and the group hypothesized that their results supported "negative regulation of genomic pathways in T

cells that could influence long-term activation or reactivation responses of T cells." Gene expression profiling was separated by histologic response to therapy, and Foxp3, a marker of regulatory T cells, was induced in responders preferentially to nonresponders 6 hours after treatment.

The relationship between the presence of the HLA-Cw*0602 genotype in patients with psoriasis has also been evaluated in relationship to response to the biologic agents, efalizumab and ustekinumab. A 2009 abstract publication reported that the presence of HLA-Cw6 predicted response to efalizumab therapy.[53] No participant details, including phenotype details, details of drug administration including duration, or how response to treatment was assessed were provided.

An Italian cohort of 51 patients with moderate-to-severe chronic plaque psoriasis treated with at least one ustekinumab injection underwent HLA genotyping and evaluation of response to treatment at or after 3 months from initial injection.[54] An association between the presence of HLA-Cw*0602 and ustekinumab response was reported, with higher rates of response in terms of PASI 75 at 4, 12, and 28 weeks of therapy (at week 28, 96.3% patients with a positive response reached PASI 75 vs 72.7% of patients with a negative response $P<.008$). There was no listing of inclusion or exclusion criteria, specifically, no mention of psoriasis phenotype for included participants or an inclusion of only participants with a certain qualifying psoriasis severity index. Although the presence of HLA-Cw*0602 is known to be more strongly associated with type I psoriasis, age of onset of psoriasis for the cohort was listed with standard deviation and range (22.5 $\pm$ 11.3; 1–59). Participants had a washout period from other biologic agents of at least 3 months, but no mention was made of preceding or concurrent systemic medication. Statistical analysis for the categorical data was performed with a simple χ^2 test, with the only report of multivariate logistical regression analysis that age of onset of psoriasis was not related to response to ustekinumab. There is no discussion of the high rates of ustekinumab response in HLA-Cw*0602–negative patients nor a comparison of investigation data with published ustekinumab clinical trial response data. In a cohort of Chinese patients with psoriasis treated with ustekinumab (n = 66), significantly more HLA-Cw*0602–positive patients achieved a PASI 50, 75, or 90 response[55] than HLA-Cw*0602–negative patients. However, the study was at risk of significant bias, with participants selected retrospectively.

Translation of Pharmacogenomic Studies in Psoriasis

There is no convincing predictive biomarker for any drug used to treat psoriasis. Problems with methodologic quality may in part be responsible for the lack of replication present in the field of pharmacogenomics.[56] There are several methodologic areas that may be more thoroughly considered in the planning and conducting of future pharmacogenomic studies to improve the quality of results of any one study. Furthermore, the generation of huge datasets from newer technologies and the open access of such data for effective meta-analysis are crucial to future translation of potential biomarkers.

Standardization of Approach to Pharmacogenomic Studies

Future pharmacogenomic studies in psoriasis should adhere to a standardized approach, using a checklist, which includes reference to several previously published standards (**Table 1**). Examples already exist of the implementation of criteria to standardize studies, such as in drug-induced skin injury, in which efforts have been made to standardize phenotypes of participants.[59,60] In psoriasis research, this approach is feasible by using simple clinical criteria, for example, a diagnosis of psoriasis vulgaris confirmed by a dermatologist and designation of age of onset of psoriasis vulgaris and exclusion of erythrodermic psoriasis, pustular psoriasis, and palmo-plantar pustulosis.

This checklist ensures adequate details are provided about key aspects of study design, including participant phenotype and participant characteristics, methodology, and the presentation of results and analysis.

Adherence

Given the significant contribution of adherence to drug response, the validity of results cannot be assessed without ensuring that adherence to therapy has been adequately taken into account. For those studies in the clinical trial setting, there are recognized problems with existing tools for the self-reporting of adherence and a need to determine whether the existing self-report tools are suitable for measuring medication-taking behaviors in patients with psoriasis.[61] This issue has been highlighted for pharmacogenomic studies of warfarin dosing and the recommendation made that consideration is given to assessing adherence when designing future pharmacogenomic studies of warfarin and other drugs.[62]

Recommendations to Researchers and Journals

Journals and journal editors may contribute to future translation of pharmacogenomic studies in psoriasis by ensuring that minimum standards are truly adhered to in published pharmacogenomic studies. These professionals can also contribute through ensuring sufficient expertise in the peer review of submitted studies, with additional support from bioinformaticians or statisticians when the data pipeline is not entirely familiar to the dermatologist reviewer.

Open access publication of all results remains vital. In this way, study quality may be subjected to rigorous assessment and studies compared one to another. Ultimately, with uniformity in the generation of genomic data, bioinformaticians will be in a position to overlay DNA, RNA, proteome, and metabolome data for a complete pharmacogenomic assessment. Future work may include meta-analysis of appropriate genomic studies in which their results are comparable. Meta-analysis methods that integrate the results of separate genomic assessments are now being used to allow the identification of cellular components, biological processes, molecular functions, pathways, networks, and individual genes in diseases such as epilepsy.[63] This strategy could be used in psoriasis, in which sufficient comparable genomic data exist.

SUMMARY

Psoriasis is a model disease for the development of pharmacogenomic markers of treatment response, with ready access to diseased tissue and objective validated outcome measures. With the application of state-of-the-art technologies and investment in careful experimental design, the goal of stratified medicine in psoriasis may be possible. Current pharmacogenomic studies in psoriasis show excellence in many areas, including the investigation of a broad range of psoriasis therapies. To facilitate the advent of stratified medicine in psoriasis, uniformity of study design is required, with high quality, consistent phenotyping strategies for participants; definitions of outcome; and the publication of reproducible methodologies. Improvements in these areas would facilitate future meta-analyses and may ultimately allow us to treat patients who have psoriasis with more effective and safe drugs at the outset of their disease onset.

REFERENCES

1. Vogel F. Modern problem der humangenetik. Ergeb Inn Med Kinderheilkd 1959;12:52–125.

2. Rosell R, Carcereny E, Gervais R, et al. Erlotinib versus standard chemotherapy as first-line treatment for European patients with advanced EGFR mutation-positive non-small-cell lung cancer (EURTAC): a multicentre, open-label, randomised phase 3 trial. Lancet Oncol 2012;13(3):239–46.

3. Mitsudomi T, Morita S, Yatabe Y, et al. Gefitinib versus cisplatin plus docetaxel in patients with non-small-cell lung cancer harbouring mutations of the epidermal growth factor receptor (WJTOG3405): an open label, randomised phase 3 trial. Lancet Oncol 2010;11(2):121–8.

4. Weng L, Zhang L, Peng Y, et al. Pharmacogenetics and pharmacogenomics: a bridge to individualized cancer therapy. Pharmacogenomics 2013;14(3):315–24.

5. Weber B, Meldgaard P, Hager H, et al. Detection of EGFR mutations in plasma and biopsies from non-small cell lung cancer patients by allele-specific PCR assays. BMC Cancer 2014;14(1):294.

6. Maxwell JR, Potter C, Hyrich KL, et al. Association of the tumour necrosis factor-308 variant with differential response to anti-TNF agents in the treatment of rheumatoid arthritis. Hum Mol Genet 2008;17(22): 3532–8.

7. Wechsler ME, Kunselman SJ, Chinchilli VM, et al. Effect of beta2-adrenergic receptor polymorphism on response to longacting beta2 agonist in asthma (LARGE trial): a genotype-stratified, randomised, placebo-controlled, crossover trial. Lancet 2009; 374(9703):1754–64.

8. McGeachie MJ, Wu AC, Chang HH, et al. Predicting inhaled corticosteroid response in asthma with two associated SNPs. Pharmacogenomics J 2013;13(4): 306–11.

9. Himes BE, Jiang X, Wagner P, et al. RNA-Seq transcriptome profiling identifies CRISPLD2 as a glucocorticoid responsive gene that modulates cytokine function in airway smooth muscle cells. PLoS One 2014;9(6):e99625.

10. Slager RE, Otulana BA, Hawkins GA, et al. IL-4 receptor polymorphisms predict reduction in asthma exacerbations during response to an anti-IL-4 receptor alpha antagonist. J Allergy Clin Immunol 2012;130(2):516–22.e4.

11. Chapman PB, Hauschild A, Robert C, et al. Improved survival with vemurafenib in melanoma with BRAF V600E mutation. N Engl J Med 2011; 364(26):2507–16.

12. Bombelli FB, Webster CA, Moncrieff M, et al. The scope of nanoparticle therapies for future metastatic melanoma treatment. Lancet Oncol 2014;15(1): e22–32.

13. Eggermont AM, Spatz A, Robert C. Cutaneous melanoma. Lancet 2014;383(9919):816–27.

14. Meggitt SJ, Gray JC, Reynolds NJ. Azathioprine dosed by thiopurine methyltransferase activity for moderate-to-severe atopic eczema: a double-blind, randomised controlled trial. Lancet 2006;367(9513): 839–46.

15. Grada A, Weinbrecht K. Next-generation sequencing: methodology and application. J Invest Dermatol 2013;133(8):e11.

16. Tang W, Hu Z, Muallem H, et al. Clinical implementations of RNA signatures for pharmacogenomic decision-making. Pharmgenomics Pers Med 2011;4:95–107.

17. Want EJ, Wilson ID, Gika H, et al. Global metabolic profiling procedures for urine using UPLC-MS. Nat Protoc 2010;5(6):1005–18.

18. Theodoridis GA, Gika HG, Want EJ, et al. Liquid chromatography-mass spectrometry based global metabolite profiling: a review. Anal Chim Acta 2012;711:7–16.

19. Kontula K, Valimaki S, Kainulainen K, et al. Vitamin D receptor polymorphism and treatment of psoriasis with calcipotriol. Br J Dermatol 1997;136(6):977–8.

20. Mee JB, Cork MJ. Vitamin D receptor polymorphism and calcipotriol response in patients with psoriasis. J Invest Dermatol 1998;110(3):301–2.

21. Chen ML, Perez A, Sanan DK, et al. Induction of vitamin D receptor mRNA expression in psoriatic plaques correlates with clinical response to 1,25-dihydroxyvitamin D3. J Invest Dermatol 1996; 106(4):637–41.

22. Saeki H, Asano N, Tsunemi Y, et al. Polymorphisms of vitamin D receptor gene in Japanese patients with psoriasis vulgaris. J Dermatol Sci 2002;30(2):167–71.

23. Giomi B, Ruggiero M, Fabbri P, et al. Does the determination of the Bb vitamin D receptor genotype identify psoriasis vulgaris patients responsive to topical tacalcitol? J Dermatol Sci 2005;37(3):180–1.

24. Halsall JA, Osborne JE, Pringle JH, et al. Vitamin D receptor gene polymorphisms, particularly the novel A-1012G promoter polymorphism, are associated with vitamin D3 responsiveness and non-familial susceptibility in psoriasis. Pharmacogenet Genomics 2005;15(5):349–55.

25. Dayangac-Erden D, Karaduman A, Erdem-Yurter H. Polymorphisms of vitamin D receptor gene in Turkish familial psoriasis patients. Arch Dermatol Res 2007; 299(10):487–91.

26. Smith G, Dawe RS, Clark C, et al. Quantitative real-time reverse transcription-polymerase chain reaction analysis of drug metabolizing and cytoprotective genes in psoriasis and regulation by ultraviolet radiation. J Invest Dermatol 2003;121(2):390–8.

27. Smith G, Wolf CR, Deeni YY, et al. Cutaneous expression of cytochrome P450 CYP2S1: individuality in regulation by therapeutic agents for psoriasis and other skin diseases. Lancet 2003;361(9366):1336–43.

28. Hairutdinov VR, Moshkalov AV, Samtsov AV, et al. Apoptosis-deficient Pro allele of p53 gene is associated with the resistance of psoriasis to the UV-based therapy. J Dermatol Sci 2005;37(3):185–7.

29. Ryan C, Renfro L, Collins P, et al. Clinical and genetic predictors of response to narrowband ultraviolet B for the treatment of chronic plaque psoriasis. Br J Dermatol 2010;163(5):1056–63.

30. Lo YH, Torii K, Saito C, et al. Serum IL-22 correlates with psoriatic severity and serum IL-6 correlates with susceptibility to phototherapy. J Dermatol Sci 2010; 58(3):225–7.

31. Hochberg M, Zeligson S, Amariglio N, et al. Genomic-scale analysis of psoriatic skin reveals differentially expressed insulin-like growth factor-binding protein-7 after phototherapy. Br J Dermatol 2007;156(2):289–300.

32. Johnson-Huang LM, Suárez-Fariñas M, Sullivan-Whalen M, et al. Effective narrow-band UVB radiation therapy suppresses the IL-23/IL-17 axis in normalized psoriasis plaques. J Invest Dermatol 2010;130(11):2654–63.

33. Gu X, Nylander E, Coates PJ, et al. Effect of narrowband ultraviolet B phototherapy on p63 and microRNA (miR-21 and miR-125b) expression in psoriatic epidermis. Acta Derm Venereol 2011;91(4):392–7.

34. Warren RB, Smith RL, Campalani E, et al. Genetic variation in efflux transporters influences outcome to methotrexate therapy in patients with psoriasis. J Invest Dermatol 2008;128(8):1925–9.

35. Warren RB, Smith RL, Campalani E, et al. Outcomes of methotrexate therapy for psoriasis and relationship to genetic polymorphisms. Br J Dermatol 2009;160(2):438–41.

36. Campalani E, Arenas M, Marinaki AM, et al. Polymorphisms in folate, pyrimidine, and purine metabolism are associated with efficacy and toxicity of methotrexate in psoriasis. J Invest Dermatol 2007;127(8): 1860–7 [Erratum appears in J Invest Dermatol 2008;128(10):2545–6].

37. Ormerod AD, Campalani E, Goodfield MJ. British Association of Dermatologists guidelines on the efficacy and use of acitretin in dermatology. Br J Dermatol 2010;162(5):952–63.

38. Campalani E, Allen MH, Fairhurst D, et al. Apolipoprotein E gene polymorphisms are associated with psoriasis but do not determine disease response to acitretin. Br J Dermatol 2006;154(2):345–52.

39. Young HS, Summers AM, Read IR, et al. Interaction between genetic control of vascular endothelial growth factor production and retinoid responsiveness in psoriasis. J Invest Dermatol 2006;126(2):453–9.

40. Haider AS, Lowes MA, Suárez-Fariñas M, et al. Identification of cellular pathways of "type 1," Th17 T cells, and TNF- and inducible nitric oxide synthase-producing dendritic cells in autoimmune inflammation through pharmacogenomic study of cyclosporine A in psoriasis. J Immunol 2008; 180(3):1913–20.

41. Oestreicher JL, Walters IB, Kikuchi T, et al. Molecular classification of psoriasis disease-associated genes through pharmacogenomic expression profiling. Pharmacogenomics J 2001;1(4):272–87.

42. Trepicchio WL, Ozawa M, Walters IB, et al. Interleukin-11 therapy selectively downregulates type I cytokine proinflammatory pathways in psoriasis lesions. J Clin Invest 1999;104(11):1527–37.

43. Li C, Wang G, Gao Y, et al. TNF-alpha gene promoter -238G>A and -308G>A polymorphisms alter risk of psoriasis vulgaris: a meta-analysis. J Invest Dermatol 2007;127(8):1886–92.

44. Tejasvi T, Stuart PE, Nair RP, et al. Preliminary pharmacogenetic assessment of tumour necrosis factor (TNF) polymorphisms in psoriasis: response to anti-TNF and systemic therapies. Br J Dermatol 2008;159(6):1391.

45. Russell TJ, Schultes LM, Kuban DJ. Histocompatibility (HL-A) antigens associated with psoriasis. N Engl J Med 1972;287(15):738–40.

46. Ryan C, Kelleher J, Collins P, et al. A study to examine if the HLA Cw*0602 allele is a predictor or response to TNF-a inhibitors in the treatment of psoriasis. Br J Dermatol 2009;161(Suppl):21–69.

47. Suárez-Fariñas M, Fuentes-Duculan J, Lowes MA, et al. Resolved psoriasis lesions retain expression of a subset of disease-related genes. J Invest Dermatol 2011;131(2):391–400.

48. Zaba LC, Cardinale I, Gilleaudeau P, et al. Amelioration of epidermal hyperplasia by TNF inhibition is associated with reduced Th17 responses. J Exp Med 2007;204(13):3183–94.

49. Zaba LC, Suárez-Fariñas M, Fuentes-Duculan J, et al. Effective treatment of psoriasis with etanercept is linked to suppression of IL-17 signaling, not immediate response TNF genes. J Allergy Clin Immunol 2009;124(5):1022-10.e1–395.

50. Suárez-Fariñas M, Shah KR, Haider AS, et al. Personalized medicine in psoriasis: developing a genomic classifier to predict histological response to Alefacept. BMC Dermatol 2010;10:1.

51. Chamian F, Lowes MA, Lin SL, et al. Alefacept reduces infiltrating T cells, activated dendritic cells, and inflammatory genes in psoriasis vulgaris. Proc Natl Acad Sci U S A 2005;102(6):2075–80.

52. Haider AS, Lowes MA, Gardner H, et al. Novel insight into the agonistic mechanism of alefacept in vivo: differentially expressed genes may serve as biomarkers of response in psoriasis patients. J Immunol 2007;178(11):7442–9.

53. Gulliver W. HLA-Cw6 polymorphism predict response to the biologic therapy efalizumab in patients with chronic plaque psoriasis. J Am Acad Dermatol 2009;60(3 Suppl 1):AB162.

54. Talamonti M, Botti E, Galluzzo M, et al. Pharmacogenetics of psoriasis: HLA-Cw6 but not LCE3B/3C deletion nor TNFAIP3 polymorphism predisposes to clinical response to interleukin 12/23 blocker ustekinumab. Br J Dermatol 2013;169(2):458–63.

55. Chiu HY, Wang TS, Chan CC, et al. HLA-Cw06 as a predictor for the clinical response to ustekinumab, an interleukin -12/23 blocker, in Chinese patients with psoriasis: a retrospective analysis. Br J Dermatol 2014. [Epub ahead of print].

56. Jorgensen A, Williamson P. Methodological quality of pharmacogenetic studies: issues of concern. Stat Med 2008;27(30):6547–69.

57. Brazma A, Hingamp P, Quackenbush J, Sherlock G, Spellman P, Stoeckert C, et al. Minimum information about a microarray experiment (MIAME)-toward standards for microarray data. Nature Genetics 2001;29(4):365–71.

58. Bustin SA, Benes V, Garson JA, Hellemans J, Huggett J, Kubista M, et al. The MIQE guidelines: minimum information for publication of quantitative real-time PCR experiments. Clinical Chemistry 2009;55(4):611–22.

59. Pirmohamed M, Friedmann PS, Molokhia M, et al. Phenotype standardization for immune-mediated drug-induced skin injury. Clin Pharmacol Ther 2011;89(6):896–901.

60. Pirmohamed M, Aithal GP, Behr E, et al. The phenotype standardization project: improving pharmacogenetic studies of serious adverse drug reactions. Clin Pharmacol Ther 2011;89(6):784–5.

61. Thorneloe RJ, Bundy C, Griffiths CE, et al. Adherence to medication in patients with psoriasis: a systematic literature review. Br J Dermatol 2013; 168(1):20–31.

62. Jorgensen AL, Hughes DA, Hanson A, et al. Adherence and variability in warfarin dose requirements: assessment in a prospective cohort. Pharmacogenomics 2013;14(2):151–63.

63. Mirza N, Vasieva O, Marson AG, et al. Exploring the genomic basis of pharmacoresistance in epilepsy: an integrative analysis of large-scale gene expression profiling studies on brain tissue from epilepsy surgery. Hum Mol Genet 2011;20(22): 4381–94.

Psoriasis: The Future

M. Alan Menter, MD[a],*, Christopher E.M. Griffiths, MD, FMedSci[b]

KEYWORDS

- Drug safety • Phenotypical variants • Personalized medicine • Psoriatic arthritis • Systemic disease
- Biosimilars

KEY POINTS

- Personalized or stratified medicine will become increasingly important.
- The cost-effectiveness of treatments will be ever more germane to health care providers.
- Psychological comorbidities and their management will be an integral part of psoriasis management.
- The identification of, and management plans for, subpopulations of patients with psoriasis will become important aspects of clinical practice.

INTRODUCTION

The articles that constitute this detailed review of psoriasis have each focused on specific areas of interest in this fascinating disease which affects 120 million people globally. The authors have assimilated specific areas of interest discussed in prior articles with their personal views into a coherent "The Future" review of interest to clinicians and researchers alike. The scope and interest of this final article is what is anticipated to change the landscape of both our understanding of psoriasis and implications for therapy by 2020.

We are fortunate to have a full range of therapeutic options available for our patients with psoriasis, ranging from topicals to phototherapy to systemic and biological agents. Scientific research, in which our International Psoriasis Council (IPC) members are committed to maintaining their leading role, will, we believe, drive the optimal use, cost-effectiveness, and safe utilization of this spectrum of therapies allied to new agents in the pipeline.

MANUSCRIPT

The preceding articles in this issue of *Dermatologic Clinics* devoted to psoriasis have detailed the full extent of this complex, immune-mediated, genetic disorder and included measurements of outcome used in clinical trials and clinical practice. In addition, the life cycle stages of this lifelong disease from childhood to old age are reviewed, as are the significant comorbidities associated with psoriasis.

Will it be possible in the future to assess each patient with psoriasis *ab initio* from a genetic perspective, building on a new molecular taxonomy for the disease so that appropriate therapy can be tailored to the individual thereby affording them a normal lifestyle? The IPC's proposal toward completing the genetic map of psoriasis is, we believe, one of the most important current research projects likely to change our understanding of the disease. The intricacies of protein variants may enable targeting of specific therapies to the wide spectrum of psoriasis phenotypes (**Figs. 1–8**) with a significantly higher likelihood of clinical success.

Disclosures: See last page of article.
[a] Division of Dermatology, Baylor University Medical Center at Dallas, Dallas, TX, USA; [b] Dermatology Centre, Salford Royal Hospital, The University of Manchester, Manchester Academic Health Science Centre, Manchester M6 8HD, UK
* Corresponding author.
E-mail address: amderm@gmail.com

Dermatol Clin 33 (2015) 161–166
http://dx.doi.org/10.1016/j.det.2014.09.012

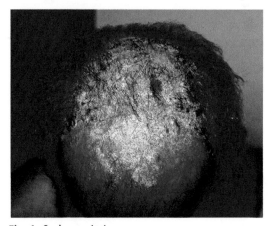

Fig. 1. Scalp psoriasis.

This task is not easy; witness the 18-year gap following the discovery of the first locus for psoriasis (PSORS2) outside MHC by modern genetic technology in 1994[1] before CARD 14, an epidermal regulator of nuclear factor–kappa B, was shown to be the specific protein involved.[2]

THE CLINICAL SPECTRUM OF PSORIASIS (PHENOTYPICAL VARIANTS)

Understanding the diverse clinical phenotypes of psoriasis,[3] the complex genetic architecture that determines them, and their mutual relationship to the pathogenesis of the disease is a daunting task and one that has significant implications for future patient care. Although most new therapeutic agents introduced over the past decade have been biological agents for moderate to severe psoriasis,[4] the need for new topical and small molecule oral agents for milder disease is paramount. This latter category of patients comprises at a minimum 75% of the total number of patients worldwide (ie, 90 million). Our most potent topical agent for treating this large group of patients, clobetasol propionate, was introduced more than 4

decades ago[5] and the newest, calcipotriol, 25 years ago. Thus, in the future, our ability to develop new classes of topical agents that are effective, cosmetically acceptable, and of low-frequency application are mandated. In addition, the use of specific topicals for defined areas of involvement (eg, flexures, including genitalia [frequently involved but seldom evaluated or discussed by clinicians and patients alike] and scalp) is currently very much a stochastic process that will necessitate new clinical and investigative approaches. Fortunately, there are a host of new topical agents in various stages of development with the likelihood of at least one or two of them emerging as important new classes for our patient population (**Box 1**).

When considering the future of systemic therapies, it is interesting to note that methotrexate, like clobetasol propionate, was also introduced more than 4 decades ago and is still the first-line systemic agent used for psoriasis worldwide despite only showing effectiveness in 40% to 45% of patients.[6] Cost obviously plays a very significant role in methotrexate retaining its leadership position. However, targeting methotrexate to specific patients with the potential of an optimized response and with lower toxicities is a definitive future need. Likewise, the introduction of new methotrexate-based molecules is emerging with a recent phase 1 study of an aminopterin (the original precursor of methotrexate) enantiomer showing superior absorption and tolerability with less accumulation in cerebral spinal fluid.[7] Phase 2 studies are in the late stages of development.

Future oral as well as biological therapies have been well covered in prior articles with a great deal of excitement surrounding the oral, small molecule technologies, such as apremilast and tofacitinib, and the three interleukin (IL)-17 inhibitors brodalumab, ixekizumab, and secukinumab.

Appropriate comparator studies with the IL-17 inhibitors against the three tumor necrosis factor

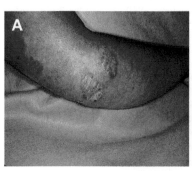
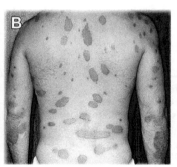
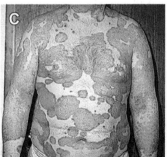

Fig. 2. Plaque psoriasis. (*A*) Mild. (*B*) Moderate. (*C*) Severe.

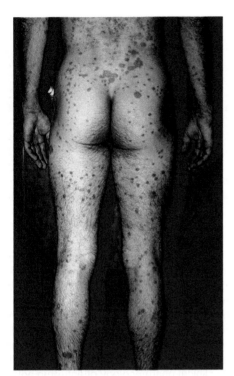

Fig. 3. Guttate psoriasis.

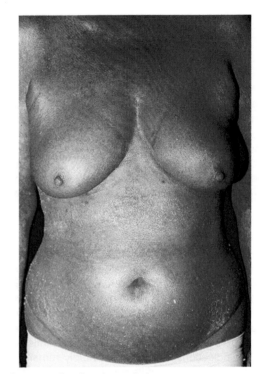

Fig. 5. Erythrodermic psoriasis.

(TNF) inhibitors in use for psoriasis and ustekinumab inhibitors have yet to be completed. We believe these will provide important information not only for short-term efficacy up to one year but also for safety purposes. This idea is because more than 3 million patients across all indications have been treated with the TNF inhibitors since first marketed more than 15 years ago and more than 70,000 patients have received ustekinumab since its introduction more than 5 years ago. Thus, despite the IL-17 inhibitors' seeming superior efficacy in current clinical trials, their adoption as first-line agents once they come to market (2015) will have to be monitored carefully from a

safety perspective. Most clinical trials performed on all biological agents for chronic plaque psoriasis over the past 15 years have been as monotherapy. It is hoped that future studies will include other phenotypic variants, such as palmar plantar disease, which is notoriously recalcitrant to all therapeutic modalities.

An important difference between clinical trials of therapies for psoriasis, versus those for psoriatic arthritis and rheumatoid arthritis, is that psoriasis studies always use monotherapy as compared with arthritis whereby methotrexate and even low stable dosages of prednisolone are allowable and used in up to 50% of clinical trial patients. Thus, we believe future studies should facilitate appropriate combination therapies thereby mirroring clinical practice. Safety considerations with these combinations (eg, methotrexate plus a biologic) are obviously important. However, psoriasis registries around the world, including the British Association of Dermatologists Biologic Interventions Register and European registries including the PsoNET conglomerate and the US Psoriasis Longitudinal Assessment and Registry,[8] are finally allowing us the benefit of real-life pharmacovigilance data on large numbers of patients akin to information on other immune-mediated inflammatory disease (IMIDs) treated with systemic therapies (eg, rheumatoid arthritis). These data will allow for the detection of rare but potentially fatal

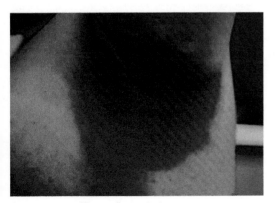

Fig. 4. Inverse (flexural) psoriasis.

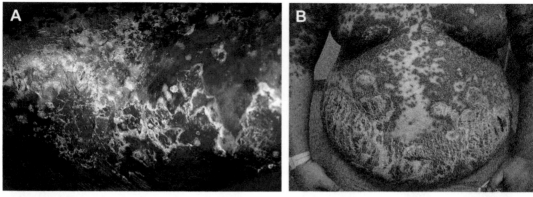

Fig. 6. Pustular psoriasis. (*A*) Localized. (*B*) Generalized.

side effects, such as the 3 cases of progressive multifocal leukoencephalopathy (PML), which led to the withdrawal of efalizumab after more than 40,000 patients had received the drug. Of interest is the significantly higher incidence of PML in other current agents used for chronic immune-mediated disorders (eg, rituximab in rheumatoid arthritis and other indications, which will inevitably remain on the market because of its essential and important therapeutic profiles).[9]

It is highly likely that within the next decade stratified medicine will start to influence the prescribing of systemic therapies for psoriasis. Knowledge gained from the study of disease and drug response endotypes and the development of companion diagnostics, based on algorithms, will dictate which is the best biological therapy for an individual patient. Furthermore, knowledge of the clinical pharmacology of anti-drug antibody production and determinants of non-adherence to

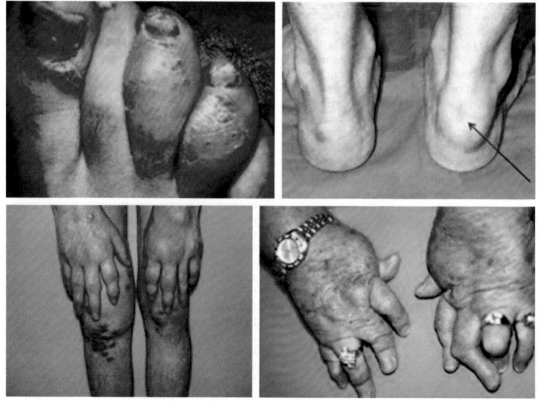

Fig. 7. Psoriatic arthritis.

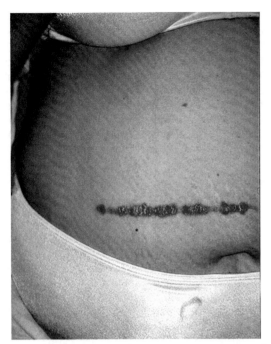

Fig. 8. The Koebner phenomenon-appearance of psoriasis in an appendectomy scar.

therapy will enable minimum dosing and cost-effective prescribing.

It is likely that in the future, patients' views of what are important consequences of treatment, beyond physical measures, such as psoriasis area severity index (PASI), will start to be used as important end points known as patient-reported outcomes; these will be aligned to holistic measures of response to therapy.

A recent publication by Ryan and colleagues,[10] on behalf of the American Academy of Dermatology's Guidelines of Care psoriasis 12-person group, has focused on this issue. Five important future study groups were recommended for future consideration:

1. Studies to address patient, physician, treatment, and economic factors that result in patients with psoriasis not remaining under long-term control
2. Studies based on patients' view points as to what they consider is the optimal response individually
3. Studies based on therapeutic needs of patients relating to all aspects of their disease
4. Individualized therapy as discussed previously
5. Studies to assess better outcome measures that will be used more frequently in clinical practice and not just in clinical trials

The cost considerations of management in our psoriasis population who are, as compared with their counterparts in rheumatology and gastroenterology, significantly undertreated, are significant. With the psychosocial detriment faced by patients with severe psoriasis at least on a par with, and often higher than, patients with rheumatoid arthritis or inflammatory bowel disease, why is it that so many of this psoriasis subgroup (approximately 24 million worldwide) remain undertreated? In the United States, with a population of 1.4 million patients with moderate to severe psoriasis, less than 300,000 (21%) are currently receiving any form of systemic or biological treatment. Given that topical therapies are irrelevant to rheumatologists and gastroenterologists, would they and their patient organizations accept this figure and lack of appropriate therapy despite the higher cost of their biological and systemic agents?

Over the next 2 to 5 years, biosimilar agents will be introduced into the psoriasis market as our current TNF inhibitors lose patent protection worldwide. It is important to recognize that despite having biological agents for psoriasis available for more than 10 years, different batches, despite being manufactured in the same plant with complex production and purification procedures, may differ slightly from year to year in their chemical composition mainly because of the heterogeneity of glycosylation.[11] Thus, unlike methotrexate, for instance, which is manufactured by multiple pharmaceutical companies in different plants across the world, follow-up biological agents will be very slightly different to the parent compound, hence the term *biosimilar*.

Already two biosimilar agents for infliximab have received approval from the European Medicines Agency (EMA), with other countries, including Canada, recently giving approval for this biosimilar agent for various disease indications. There is a strong need for dermatologists, as well as patients, to understand all aspects of biosimilar agents, their manufacturing processes, and their equivalence to the parent biological

---

Box 1
Emerging psoriasis treatments: topical agents

1. Janus kinase inhibitors (JAK)
2. Phosphodiesterase inhibitors (PDE-4)
3. New vitamin D analogues and combinations
4. Cysteine protease inhibitors
5. Lymphocyte migration inhibitors
6. High mobility group box antagonist (HMGB 1)

drug to enable an appropriate "comfort factor." In the future, prescribing of biosimilar agents, likely to be 25% to 30% cheaper than the parent compound, will be of inestimable benefit to health care costs globally. Approval of these biosimilar products is already strongly regulated across medical agencies in Europe and North America.

The advent of biosimilars will have a major impact on prescribing habits. It is hoped, this will allow the millions of psoriasis patients not being adequately treated presently to enjoy the benefits of biologics, and thus improve their quality of life.

SUMMARY

The future of psoriasis management from the perspective of investigation and therapeutic development has reached an exciting stage. For a disease, known since biblical times, to have lagged behind other IMIDs in therapies, but not basic science interrogation, is unacceptable, especially as our psoriasis population has quality-of-life detriment in excess of most other IMIDs. Fortunately, with the endeavors of leading IPC scientists and clinicians as presented in articles in this psoriasis review, appropriate advances in the clinical and nonclinical sciences across the full spectrum of the disease will maintain momentum. The consequent health and lifestyle gains will be of benefit not only to psoriasis patients but also to society worldwide.

DISCLOSURES

Dr A.M. Menter has served on advisory boards for AbbVie, Allergan, Amgen, Boehringer ingelheim, Genentech, Janssen Biotech Inc, LEO Pharma, and Pfizer. Dr A.M. Menter has been consultant for AbbVie, Allergan, Amgen, Convoy Therapeutics Inc, Eli-Lilly, Janssen Biotech Inc, LEO Pharma, Novartis, Pfizer, Syntrix, Wyeth, XenoPort. Dr A.M. Menter has been an investigator for AbbVie, Allergan, Amgen, ApoPharma, Boehringer Ingelheim, Celgene, Convoy Therapeutics Inc, Eli-Lilly, Genentech, Janssen Biotech Inc, LEO Pharma, Merck, Novartis, Pfizer, Symbio/Maruho, Syntrix, and Wyeth. Dr A.M. Menter has been a speaker for AbbVie, Amgen, Janssen Biotech Inc, LEO Pharma, and Wyeth. Dr A.M. Menter has received grants from AbbVie, Allergan, Amgen, ApoPharma, Boehringer Ingelheim, Celgene, Convoy Therapeutics Inc, Genentech, Janssen Biotech Inc, LEO Pharma, Merck, Pfizer, Symbio/Maruho, and Syntrix. Dr A.M. Menter has received honoraria from AbbVie, Allergan, Amgen, Boehringer Ingelheim, Convoy Therapeutics Inc, Eli-Lilly, Genentech, Janssen Biotech Inc, LEO Pharma, Novartis, Pfizer, Syntrix, Wyeth, and Xenoport. A.M. Menter has no personal financial stake in any pharmaceutical company. Dr C. Griffiths has received honoraria and/or research grants from AbbVie, Actelion, Amgen, Celgene, Eli Lilly, Galderma, GSK-Stiefel, Janssen, LEO, MSD, Novartis, Pfizer, Sandoz, Trident, and UCB.

REFERENCES

1. Tomfohrde J, Silverman A, Barnes R. Gene for familial psoriasis susceptibility mapped to the distal end of human chromosome 17q. Science 1994;264: 1141–5.
2. Jordan CT, Cao L, Roberson ED, et al. PSORS2 is due to mutations in CARD14. Am J Hum Genet 2012;90:784–95.
3. Griffiths CEM, Christophers E, Barker JN, et al. A classification of psoriasis vulgaris according to phenotype. Br J Dermatol 2007;156:258–62.
4. Mansouri B, Patel M, Menter A. Biological therapies for psoriasis. Expert Opin Biol Ther 2013;13:1715–30.
5. Allenby CF, Main RA, Marsden RA, et al. Effect on adrenal function of topically applied clobetasol propionate (Dermovate). Br Med J 1975;4:619–21.
6. Heydendael VM, Spuls PI, Opmeer BC, et al. Methotrexate vs cyclosporine in moderate-to-severe chronic plaque psoriasis. N Engl J Med 2003;349: 658–65.
7. Menter A, Thrash B, Cherian C, et al. Intestinal transport of aminopterin enantiomers in dogs and humans with psoriasis is stereoselective: evidence for a mechanism involving the proton-coupled folate transporter. J Pharmacol Exp Ther 2012; 342:696–708.
8. Naldi L, Addis A, Chimenti S, et al. Impact of body mass index and obesity on clinical response to systemic treatment for psoriasis. Evidence from the Psocare project. Dermatology 2008;217:365–73.
9. Clifford DB, Ances B, Costello C, et al. Rituximab-associated progressive multifocal leukoencephalopathy in rheumatoid arthritis. Arch Neurol 2011;68: 1156–64.
10. Ryan C, Korman NJ, Gelfand JM, et al. Research gaps in psoriasis: opportunities for future studies. J Am Acad Dermatol 2014;70:146–67.
11. Strober BE, Armour K, Romiti R, et al. Biopharmaceuticals and biosimilars in psoriasis: what the dermatologist needs to know. J Am Acad Dermatol 2012;66:317–22.

Index

Note: Page numbers of article titles are in **boldface** type.

Dermatol Clin 33 (2015) 167–173
http://dx.doi.org/10.1016/S0733-8635(14)00128-4
0733-8635/15/$ – see front matter © 2015 Elsevier Inc. All rights reserved.

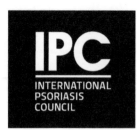

IPC
INTERNATIONAL PSORIASIS COUNCIL

CELEBRATING
10 YEARS
2004 - 2014

ABOUT THIS ISSUE OF DERMATOLOGIC CLINICS

This collection of Dermatologic Clinic articles on psoriasis, written by board members and councilors of the International Psoriasis Council covers cutting edge topics on our current understanding of the pathogenesis and treatm of the disease and how these may inform futur research and patient management. The treatise provides a comprehensive, yet manageable, prir of advances in psoriasis.

ABOUT THE INTERNATIONAL PSORIASIS COUNCIL

Founded in 2004, the International Psoriasis Council (IPC) is a dermatology-led, voluntary, global nonprofit organization dedicated to innovation across the full spectrum of psoriasis through research, education and patient care.

IPC GLOBAL PSORIASIS LEADERSHIP

With over one hundred board members and councilors from twenty-four countries, IPC embodies the global expertise of multi-specialty psoriasis key opinion leaders. These leaders include representatives from basic science, translational research, genetics, epidemiology, cardiology, international clinical trials, and direct patient care.

IPC MISSION

IPC'S mission is to empower this network of global key opinion leaders to advance the knowledge of psoriasis and its associated comorbidities, thereby enhancing the care of patients worldwide.

IPC BOARD OF DIRECTORS

Executive Board Officers

Christopher EM Griffiths ▪ President
United Kingdom
Peter van de Kerkhof ▪ Immediate Past President
The Netherlands
Alexa B. Kimball ▪ Vice President and President Elect
United States
Craig L. Leonardi ▪ Treasurer
United States
Hervé Bachelez ▪ Secretary
France
Steve O'Dell ▪ CEO
United States

Board Members

Jonathan Barker, *United Kingdom*
Robert Holland III, *United States*
Bruce Strober, *United States*
Wolfram Sterry, *Germany*

Alan Menter ▪ Founding President
United States

VISIT THE IPC WEBSITE TO ACCESS:
- Semi-annual Review of Top 5 Papers in Psoriasis Research
- Continuing Medical Education Programs
- Psoriasis Image Library
- International Calendar of Psoriasis Programs and Events

www.psoriasiscouncil.org